Matt Cartmill

Lachman's
Case Studies in Anatomy

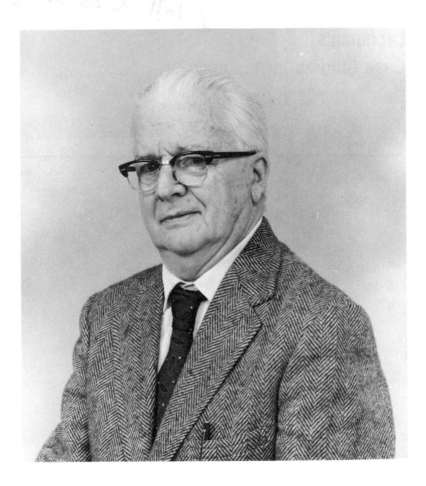

ERNEST LACHMAN, 1901–1979

LACHMAN'S CASE STUDIES IN ANATOMY

FOURTH EDITION

Revised by
DONALD R. CAHILL

New York   Oxford
OXFORD UNIVERSITY PRESS
1997

Oxford University Press

Oxford New York
Athens Auckland Bangkok Bogota
Bombay Buenos Aires Calcutta Cape Town
Dar es Salaam Delhi Florence Hong Kong Istanbul
Karachi Kuala Lumpur Madras Madrid
Melbourne Mexico City Nairobi Paris
Singapore Taipei Tokyo Toronto

and associated companies in
Berlin Ibadan

Library of Congress Cataloging-in-Publication Data
Cahill, Donald R.
Lachman's case studies in anatomy.—4th ed. /
rev. by Donald R. Cahill.
p. cm.
Rev. ed. of: Case studies in anatomy /
Ernest Lachman, in collaboration with
Kenneth F. Faulkner. 3rd ed. 1981.
Includes bibliographical references.
ISBN 0–19–510297–5
1. Anatomy, Pathological—Case studies.
I. Lachman, Ernest, 1901–1979
Case studies in anatomy. II. Title.
[DNLM: 1. Anatomy, Regional—case studies.
2. Pathology—case studies.
QZ 4 C132L 1997] RB31.L3 1997 616'.09—dc20
DNLM/DLC   for Library of Congress   96–2397

9 8 7 6 5 4 3 2 1

Printed in the United States of America
on acid-free paper

Preface

I am very pleased to revise this distinguished book by Ernest Lachman. Almost from the beginning of my anatomical studies, his cases in anatomy guided my learning and subsequently my teaching toward an emphasis on clinical anatomy because they are so solidly based on anatomy as applied to patient care. I have endeavored to maintain Lachman's chatty and humanistic manner of writing, which I always found compelling. His style eagerly invites reader involvement with the anatomical and clinical details needed to solve the clinical problems, and his artfully subtle way of engaging the reader with well-placed and instructive questions and then supplying timely answers quickly when interest is at its highest is Lachman's literary and educational hallmark.

In keeping with the original version, each chapter begins with a short history, followed by physical findings, diagnosis, therapy, discussion, and further course. The chapter entitled "Central Venous Catheterization" has been added to the text, and the remaining chapters have been updated with current therapies and diagnostic methods; many have been supplied with new figures including CT's and MRI's. The chapters on cholecystectomy, prolapse of the uterus, and knee injury have undergone extensive revision; the other chapters required less amendment.

Case Studies in Anatomy is intended primarily for students. It is designed to reinforce and enhance their anatomic knowledge and to expand their logical and critical thinking abilities for use in clinical practice. It should also be of value to teachers. I frequently use the case studies as lecture themes in gross anatomy to stimulate student interest in anatomy through its treatment of practical applications. I also use the text for constructing clinically relevant examination questions because the cases so thoroughly weave the anatomic details related to diagnosis and the principles of patient care.

I am most indebted to Robert J. Leonard, Ph.D., for his outstanding scholarship that entailed the reading and sage critiquing of all parts of the manuscript. I also take great pleasure in thanking the following colleagues in clinical medicine and anatomy who contributed generously to this text by commenting on the chapters that dealt with their particular areas of skill and wisdom: Peter C. Amadio, M.D.; Oliver H. Beahrs, M.D.; William A. Cliby, M.D.; Bradford L. Currier, M.D.; Arthur F. Dalley II, Ph.D.; Francis Helminski, J. D.; Bruce R. Krueger, M.D.; Sandy C. Marks, Jr., Ph.D., D.D.S.; Richard A. McLeod, M.D.; Matthew J. Orland, M.D.; David W. Page, M.D.; Steve G. Peters, M.D.; Carl C. Reading, M.D.; Glenn Roberts, Ph.D.; Michael E. Torchia, M.D.; Burton A. Sandok, M.D.; and Franklin H. Sim, M.D. Especially warm thanks are rendered to Ruth Pedersen, my secretary.

It is a pleasure to thank Jeffrey House, Vice President, Oxford University Press, for asking me to revise this book and for all his help and expertise in bringing this book to fruition.

I hope those who study this book will find it worthwhile.

Rochester, Minnesota   D. C.
January 1996

Preface to the First Edition

In the teaching program in Gross Anatomy we face the well-known dilemma that at the time the student has to master a large body of anatomical information he is not aware of its application to clinical medicine. On the otehr hand when he is ready to utilize his knowledge at the bedside, he has forgotten a substantial part of this material. Yet the importance of anatomical reasoning and the application of anatomical principles in the explanation of clinical signs and events and in the design of therapeutic procedures can be exemplified almost from the first week of the basic course. This will strengthen the student's motivation for learning and satisfy his thirst for information relating to clinical medicine. We cannot afford to stifle this basic interest which has brought a large proportion of our students to medicine. The student can be made to realize from the beginning that his day-by-day learning is meaningful in terms of his future work as a physician.

Thus, the case studies presented in this book are directed specifically to the first and second year medical student for collateral reading either in the basic anatomy course or in advanced courses in the field. Elective courses in the clinical years can readily be based on the exercises presented here, particularly if they are supplemented by pertinent and specialized dissections, executed by the student himself. Residents may find these case reports useful in their review studies, particularly for board examinations.

In each case a short history, physical findings, diagnosis, therapy, and further course are given. This is followed by a discussion of the material from the anatomical viewpoint, generally in the form of questions posed and answers given. The underlying anatomy is illustrated by drawings. This presentation lends itself to self-study since all questions formulated are answered in detail and in a comprehensive discussion of the subject matter.

The individual exercises are based on case histories chosen from the literature and from the author's experience and present a composite picture that exemplifies the characteristic anatomical features of the problem under discussion. In a few instances the history is taken from one of the classical collections of masterfully composed case studies available in the literature, such as the works of Hertzler, Cabot, or Kanavel. This type of presentation should call the student's attention to a stimulating form of medical instruction. In this connection it may be worth noting that in law classes in American universities the case method has been utilized for many years, even in the freshman year, whereby principles of law are illustrated by actual cases and real-life legal problems.

All case histories contained in this book have appeared previously in *The New Physician,* but in many instances their format has been changed, a large number have been revised and amplified.

Grateful acknowledgement is made to *The New Physician* and its editorial staff for permission to utilize these case histories.

Permission was also granted by the C. V. Mosby Company to use part of two case histories from Hertzler's *Clinical Surgery by Case Histories;* by the W. B. Saunders Company to utilize a portion of one case history published in Volume I of Cabot's *Differential Diagnosis;* by Lea and Febiger to use a case history from Kanavel's *Infections of the Hands;* by Doctors R. D. Duncan and M. E. Myers, Dr. L. B. Rose, and Dr. D. H. O'Donoghue to utilize material from individual case histories published by them. To these publishers and authors I express my grateful appreciation.

Thanks are due to the artists Mr. E. F. Hiser and Dr. J. E. Allison for their fine co-operation in executing the drawings, and to Frank Romano.

I am greatly indebted to Doctors G. H. Daron and K. K. Faulkner for many thoughtful suggestions.

Especially warm thanks are rendered to Mrs. Pat Friedel, our department secretary, whose tireless efforts were so helpful in bringing the work to speedy completion.

Oklahoma City   E. L.
October 1964

Contents

V   PELVIS AND PERINEUM

VI   UPPER LIMB

VII   LOWER LIMB

APPENDIX

I   HEAD AND NECK

1   Facial Paralysis
(Bell's Palsy)

A 36-year-old woman librarian slept close to an open window with a cold draft one night. She woke up the next morning with some aching pain in and around her right ear; the right side of her face felt numb and swollen. On arising she noticed that her face was distorted and deformed, and she could not close her right eye. She had some difficulty in speaking, eating, and drinking. Food seemed to collect between her teeth and right cheek. Saliva and liquids that she tried to drink ran out of the right corner of her mouth, although she had no difficulty swallowing. She became apprehensive that she had suffered a stroke and consulted a physician two days later.

EXAMINATION

On examination the right side of the patient's face appears immobile and without expression. All wrinkles have disappeared from her right forehead; the right nasolabial fold is less distinct than the left. The right eyebrow droops, and the right lower eyelid sags. She is emotional and although both eyes exhibit tearing, tears run down only the right side of her face. Her mouth and nose seem deviated toward the unaffected side, and the right corner of her mouth is sagging.

On further examination, the following facial movements prove to be affected. The patient cannot frown on the right side when asked to do so. When she attempts to shut her eyes, the right eye does not close completely. She cannot purse her lips tightly, whistle, or puff out her cheeks. Asked to show her teeth, she uncovers them only on the unaffected left side, and her lips seem to be drawn to the left side. When she attempts to laugh, the distortion of her face becomes considerably more noticeable and disfiguring. Corneal reflex is absent on the right. She is embarrassed by her appearance and does not want anyone to see her in this condition.

DIAGNOSIS

All signs and symptoms point to a disease known as facial paralysis, or Bell's palsy, the latter term perpetuating the name and memory of Charles Bell, the British anatomist and surgeon who first described the disease in 1821.

THERAPY AND FURTHER COURSE

The patient is advised to avoid cold weather and wind and to protect her eye with a patch as necessary. Massage and electrical stimulation are used to prevent muscle atrophy. After five weeks the patient has almost completely recovered, and only traces of the previous paralysis, particularly around the mouth, can be demonstrated.

DISCUSSION

The exact cause of the condition is not known, but paralysis of the facial nerve is commonly presumed to be due to an inflammation of the facial nerve in the facial canal (Fig. 1-1). In some cases it seems to be triggered by exposure to cold. Remember the course of the facial nerve in the facial canal of the petrous portion of the temporal bone, where even slight swelling of the nerve within its tight-fitting bony surroundings would subject the nerve to destructive pressure. What is the name of the foramen at the lower end of the canal, through which the nerve emerges from the skull? Is this also the site of entrance of an artery that supplies the facial nerve within the canal? Of what artery is it most commonly a branch? The facial nerve emerges from the skull through the stylomastoid foramen, which is the site of entrance of the stylomastoid artery, a branch of the posterior auricular artery of the external carotid artery.

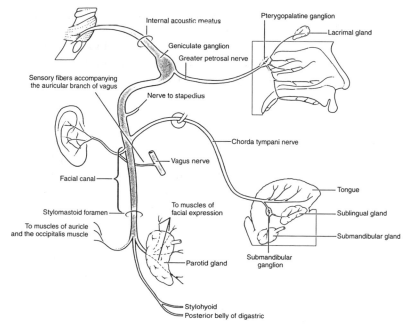

Figure 1-1. Schematic of the facial nerve.

Effects of paralysis on facial muscles

The motor deficiencies in this case exemplify the actions of the muscles of facial expression innervated by the seventh cranial nerve. These muscles are responsible for voluntary movements of the face and for emotional expression. Why do the wrinkles of the forehead and certain facial folds disappear in facial paralysis? It must be realized that some folds of the skin are brought about by muscular activity, as on the forehead in frowning and around the eyes in squinting. With paralysis of the facial muscles, such as the frontalis, which is normally responsible for transverse folds on the forehead, or the orbicularis oculi, which causes "crow's feet," the tonus of these muscles, which attach in part to the skin, is lost and the folds disappear.

Paralysis of which muscle explains the inability to close the right eye and causes the sagging of the lower eyelid? Paralysis of the orbicularis oculi prevents the patient from closing her eye as in squinting, but more importantly it prevents blinking. Blinking distributes tears over the cornea, which is necessary to keep it moist and to prevent its drying and consequent ulceration, the most serious complication of facial paralysis. The sagging of the lower lid, due to loss of muscle tone, results in its eversion and the spilling of tears, as in this case.

What muscle opens the eye? Is it affected in facial palsy? The muscle responsible for opening the eye is the levator palpebrae superioris, which in its larger skeletal portion is supplied by the unaffected oculomotor nerve; its smooth-muscle component is innervated by unaffected sympathetic fibers from the superior cervical ganglion. Unfortunately, the eye in patients with facial paralysis remains partially open because of the unopposed pull of the levator palpebrae superioris against the paralyzed orbicularis oculi. Education of patients involves teaching them to use droplets of artificial tears during the day and ointment and taping the eyes shut at night to prevent desiccation of the cornea.

Where do tears normally drain? Tears normally drain through the lacrimal puncta and canaliculi into the lacrimal sac and from there via the nasolacrimal duct into the nose, where they are sniffed or blown away.

Why is the patient's face distorted (asymmetrical) in appearance, particularly when she is smiling? The distortion is partially due to a shift of her face toward the side that remains innervated due to the unopposed pull of the innervated muscles.

Why is the corneal reflex absent? How is this reflex tested and what are its pathways? The physician stimulates the reflex by lightly stroking the cornea with a wisp of cotton, which should evoke a responsive blink. The pathways for this reflex include a sensory limb that is carried by the ophthalmic division of the trigeminal nerve, central connections located in the pons and midbrain, and a motor pathway carried by the facial nerve. Paralysis of the facial nerve in this patient interrupted the motor limb of the corneal reflex.

Paralysis of which important muscle causes food to collect between the cheek and teeth and is responsible for the inability to whistle? The buccinator has the essential function of maintaining the tension of the cheek and keeping food from passing between the cheek and teeth. It also prevents the mucous membrane of the cheek from being caught between the teeth in the act of mastication.

The inability to purse the lips and show the teeth of the affected side is due to paralysis of the orbicularis oris, which through its action as a whole or in parts can either protrude the lips as in pouting or draw them against the teeth.

The absence of the expressions of smiling and laughter is the result of the dysfunction of numerous small facial muscles, such as the zygomaticus, the risorius, the nasalis, and the levator labii superioris, all of which have in common a superficial subcutaneous location, the absence of a muscle fascia, and insertion into the skin. Their paralysis is responsible for the previously mentioned characteristic feature of Bell's palsy: loss, on the paralyzed side, of expression of emotion, such as surprise and attention, joy and sorrow.

Movements of the scalp muscles (frontalis and occipitalis) and the extrinsic muscles of the ear as well as of the stylohyoid and posterior belly of the digastric muscle are difficult to demonstrate.

How do you account for the aching pain in and around the ear and the sensation of numbness in the face? Does the facial nerve contain any pain fibers? In which ganglion are their cell bodies located? The geniculate ganglion contains the cell bodies of these somatic sensory fibers. The peripheral course of the fibers mediating pain from the ear in facial palsy is somewhat uncertain. Two pathways are possible: one by way of a communication from the facial nerve in the lowest part of the facial canal to the auricular branch of the vagus and with it to the external ear, the other by way of sensory fibers accompanying the motor fibers of the posterior auricular branch of the facial nerve. Whether the facial nerve contains fibers mediating deep sensibility of the face, including deep-seated pain, is disputed.

The absence of clinically demonstrable signs of involvement of the chorda tympani may not help in locating the site of the lesion because the mouth may still contain sufficient saliva to keep it moist, even though the parasympathetic impulses to the sublingual and submandibular glands have been lost on the affected side. Alternate pathways provided by connections of the trigeminal nerve with the facial nerve often make it impossible to demonstrate taste deficiencies in case of damage to the chorda tympani. It should be recalled, however, that taste in the anterior two thirds of the tongue is carried predominantly by the chorda tympani.

Localization of the lesion

Occasionally, the stapedius muscle also is paralyzed. Would that give a clue as to the site of paralysis along the facial nerve? It may if every branch central to the nerve to the stapedius is intact. In that case, paralysis of the stapedius would occur if the facial nerve is affected in the facial canal at the origin of its branch to the stapedius muscle. Because it is the function of the stapedius muscle to dampen the vibrations of the ossicles, what is the result of paralysis of this muscle? It increases the acuity of the sense of loud noises (hyperacusis), which may be quite annoying to patients. Our patient, however, does not describe any hearing disturbance.

Because the patient produced tears during the examination in apparently similar amounts from both eyes, we can conclude that the nervous pathways for lacrimation, including the greater petrosal branch of the facial nerve, are functioning normally. The greater petrosal nerve carries parasympathetic fibers to the pterygopalatine ganglia, which reach the lacrimal gland after joining the lacrimal branch of the maxillary nerve.

Where is the lesion to the right facial nerve located? Because all branches located proximal to the stylomastoid foramen are functioning normally, and those distal to the foramen are not, the lesion must be located at or near the level of the foramen.

2   Trigeminal Neuralgia

A 60-year-old woman has suffered attacks of sharp, stabbing pain on the right side of her nose and cheek and the right upper lip for more than one year. These paroxysms (sudden attacks) of pain last only a few seconds but seem to the patient so unbearable that she requests immediate help. She reports that when the pain started it was less intense, occurred less often, and was felt only at the side of the nose rather than in the larger area where it is now located. She also states that the pain ceased for a period of four months but returned in greater intensity and frequency. She had several teeth extracted in the upper jaw and underwent drainage of the maxillary sinus, without relief. Chewing, drinking, washing, drying her face, or blowing her nose will bring on these attacks. A light touch to the side of the nose often likewise precipitates a paroxysm of pain. The patient protects her face against touch and cold drafts with a scarf. On questioning, she states that the pain is always confined to her right side and never crosses the midline.

EXAMINATION

During the examination an attack is observed during which the patient winces and contorts her face in a ticlike fashion. Because of difficulties in eating and drinking, she has lost fifteen pounds and appears dehydrated. On neurological examination no motor defects or interference with any modality of sensation conducted by the trigeminal nerve can be discovered. Examination of the function of other cranial nerves is also negative. Except for the patient appearing anxious and tense, the physical examination is noncontributory.

DIAGNOSIS

The diagnosis is neuralgia (tic douloureux) of the maxillary division of the trigeminal nerve.

THERAPY AND FURTHER COURSE

The patient is given tranquilizers and analgesics, and several medications are tried, including carbamazepine and phenytoin. The patient is seen regularly, but treatment gives only temporary relief. When the pain returns, she requests surgical measures. With the patient under local anesthesia, 1 ml of 95 percent alcohol is injected into the maxillary division of the trigeminal nerve within the pterygopalatine fossa just beyond the exit of the nerve from the foramen rotundum.

For the next nine months, the patient has complete relief from the attacks of pain. She gains weight and is quite comfortable but complains of annoying numbness and paresthesia (tingling and burning) in the areas supplied by the maxillary division (Fig. 2-1 and Fig. 2-2).

A year and a half after the alcohol injection, she again begins to suffer recurrence of excruciating pain. The maxillary division is blocked for the second time with an alcohol injection in the pterygopalatine fossa. This time the pain-free period lasts only about eight months. Consequently, a more radical approach is selected: cutting the sensory root of the trigeminal nerve posterior to the trigeminal ganglion (rhizotomy).

A temporal extradural approach to the sensory root of the trigeminal nerve is chosen. The patient is put in a sitting position in a chair, akin to a dental chair, with the head held upright. General anesthesia is applied. A vertical incision is made in front of the external auditory meatus and extended upward from the zygoma. The temporal fascia and the underlying temporalis muscle are split and retracted.

With a burr, an opening is drilled through the squama of the temporal bone and enlarged to 4 cm in diameter. By blunt dissec-

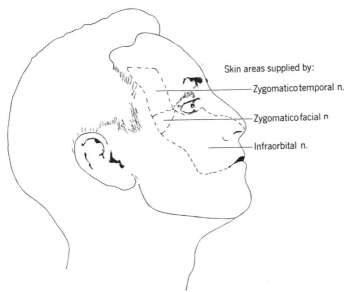

Skin areas supplied by:

Zygomaticotemporal n.

Zygomaticofacial n

Infraorbital n.

Figure 2-1. Skin areas supplied by the maxillary division of the trigeminal nerve.

tion, the dura is stripped from the anterior slope of the petrous part of the temporal bone and the floor of the middle cranial fossa. The middle meningeal artery is located at the foramen spinosum, cut, coagulated, and ligated. Further stripping of the dura uncovers the mandibular division of the trigeminal nerve at the site where it enters the foramen ovale, medial to and in front of the foramen spinosum. Following the posterior border of the mandibular division (V_3), the surgeon is led to the trigeminal (Gasserian) ganglion and from there in a posteromedial and upward direction to its sensory root. This root is uncovered by incision into the trigeminal cave (Meckel's cave), a dural/arachnoidal sleeve of the ganglion and sensory root. Thus, the subarachnoid space around these structures is opened, a procedure that resulted in a flow of cerebrospinal fluid, which is aspirated until the field is dry. It is the intent of the surgeon to sever only the sensory root fibers from the maxillary and mandibular divisions of the trigeminal nerve, but not the ophthalmic. As these occupy a fairly well-defined position within the lateral part of the root, a subtotal section of the root is possible. This section is

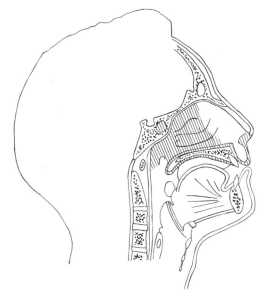

Figure 2-2. Mucosal areas supplied by the maxillary division of the trigeminal nerve. Keep in mind that areas of anesthesia after injection or surgical
intervention are somewhat smaller because of overlap by other divisions of
the trigeminal and other cranial and cervical nerves.

undertaken about 0.5 cm posterior to the ganglion and does not
include the sensory fibers of the ophthalmic division or the motor
root of the mandibular division (Fig. 2-3). The sensory fibers of the
ophthalmic division occupy a superomedial location within the sensory root of the trigeminal nerve. Occasionally, they are separated
from the fibers of the other two divisions by a cleft, which of course
makes selective sectioning easier. The motor root of the trigeminal
nerve can be identified by its somewhat more opaque appearance,
by its direction, and especially by its position deep to the sensory
root. The motor root runs obliquely downward and forward to join
the sensory part of the mandibular division at the foramen ovale.
After all bleeding points are controlled, the incision is closed by
approximating and suturing the cut ends of the temporal muscle,
temporal fascia, and skin. The patient recovers speedily from the
operation and is free of pain. Her only complaint is numbness of the

right side of her face. From previous alcohol injections, the patient is familiar with these side effects and tolerates them well.

DISCUSSION

General definition of trigeminal neuralgia

This patient suffered from trigeminal neuralgia involving the maxillary division (second division, V_2, also called the maxillary nerve) of the trigeminal nerve. It was temporarily relieved by alcohol injection into the nerve but required further treatment by subtotal retroganglionic neurotomy (rhizotomy). The patient was typical in terms of age, sex, and the involved division of the trigeminal nerve. The disease is most common in elderly women, but it also occurs in men. Although not fatal, trigeminal neuralgia represents one of the most catastrophic afflictions of humans; the pain can be so intense as to drive the sufferer to suicide.

The neuralgia consists of paroxysmal attacks of pain that involve

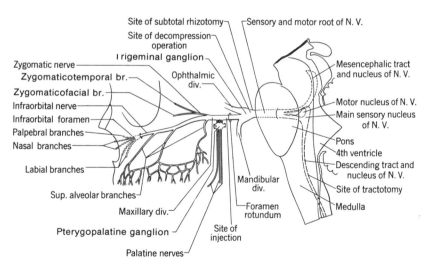

Figure 2-3. Trigeminal nuclei and tracts, root, ganglion, and divisions of the trigeminal nerve and distribution area of maxillary division. Notice the sites of surgical intervention: tractotomy, rhizotomy, decompression, and alcohol injection.

the area of the sensory distribution of one or more divisions of the trigeminal nerve. The attacks are characterized by their short duration, by intervals of relief from pain, by their unilaterality, by the absence of objective neurological findings (either on clinical examination or at autopsy), and by the frequent presence of trigger zones in the face or the mucosa. These zones, when lightly touched, may induce an attack. In a limited number of cases, infections and neoplasms as well as toxic, vascular, or nutritive factors play a role in bringing about this condition, but, in most instances no cause can be found. As in our patient, there is no involvement of the paranasal sinuses, and extraction of teeth brings no relief.

Tic douloureux (painful twitch) is a somewhat misleading term in that it might be deduced that a muscular spasm is the cause of the pain. Actually, the sequence is reversed. It is the excruciating pain that causes the patient to wince and grimace by contorting the facial muscles.

Course and distribution of the maxillary nerve and the applied anatomy of maxillary nerve block

The only division involved in our case is the maxillary division of the trigeminal nerve. What is its course to its peripheral area of distribution, and what regions of skin and mucosa does it supply? The maxillary nerve, as this division also is frequently called, runs from the middle portion of the trigeminal ganglion along the lateral wall of the cavernous sinus. It leaves the middle cranial fossa through the foramen rotundum to enter the pterygopalatine fossa. Here it can be reached by alcohol injection, as done in our case (Fig. 2-3). Inspection of a skull demonstrates that the injection needle must be inserted into the infratemporal fossa below the zygomatic arch and in front of the neck of the mandible. It passes through the pterygomaxillary fissure into the pterygopalatine fossa, where it reaches the maxillary nerve just after the latter leaves the foramen rotundum and before it has divided into its branches of distribution.

What regions of skin and mucosa are supplied by branches of the maxillary division? The skin over the anterior part of the temple and part of the cheek are innervated by the zygomatic nerve, one of the smaller terminal branches. The main branch, the infraorbital, enters the orbit through the inferior orbital fissure, passes along the infraorbital groove and canal, and emerges on the face through the infraorbital foramen to supply the skin of the lower eyelid, the lateral side of the nose, and the skin and mucous membrane of the upper lip. Other branches supply the mucous membrane of the paranasal sinuses, the nasopharynx, the palatine tonsil, the soft palate, the teeth and gingiva of the upper jaw, the inside of the nasal cavity, and the conjunctiva of the lower eyelid (Figs. 2-1, 2-2, and 2-3).

The sites mentioned define the location of the excruciating pain in neuralgia of this division, although the pain may be confined to smaller areas of skin or mucosa, such as the infraorbital region or parts of the palate. We also understand why, in neuralgia of this division, the upper teeth are so often extracted and the paranasal sinuses drained, as in our patient, unfortunately with negative results.

The area of anesthesia after alcohol injection into the maxillary division roughly coincides with the anatomical distribution of its branches. Allowance must be made, however, for some overlap in the sensory supply of skin and mucosa from other divisions of the trigeminal nerve and from other cranial and cervical nerves. As a result of the anesthesia, after blocking the maxillary division or sectioning its root, the patient often complains of disturbing numbness in the denervated area.

What is the explanation for the frequent recurrence of neuralgic pain after alcohol injection into the nerve, as in our patient? The alcohol injection leads to disintegration of the sensory nerve fibers and therefore to interruption of pain transmission. The relief is generally only temporary, as nerve fibers regenerate from their proximal ends above the site of injection. Recurring injections become less and less successful because the scarring and fibrosis in the nerve prevent the alcohol from reaching all the fibers.

Applied anatomy of trigeminal ganglion injection

Attempts to avoid the pitfall of regeneration of the sensory fibers and recurrence of neuralgia have been made by alcohol injection into the ganglion itself. Here the injection destroys the cell bodies of the sensory fibers, which then cannot regenerate; however, this procedure has fallen into disfavor because of the dangers and complications connected with it.

The possible harmful effects of trigeminal ganglion destruction by injection can be understood through familiarity with its anatomy.

The trigeminal (semilunar or Gasserian) ganglion is homologous to a dorsal root ganglion of a spinal nerve and contains pseudounipolar cell bodies. These cell bodies send out T-shaped processes that divide into a central fiber that runs in the sensory root of the trigeminal nerve to the brain stem, and a peripheral fiber hat conducts sensory impulses from the periphery to the ganglion cell. The trigeminal ganglion lies in a slight depression in the apex of the petrous portion of the temporal bone within the middle cranial fossa. The ganglion is surrounded by a diverticulum of the subarachnoid space filled with cerebrospinal fluid, termed the trigeminal (Meckel's) cave, which extends over the posterior portion of the ganglion. The danger of injection of the ganglion lies in its close relation to the subarachnoid space. Customarily, the ganglion is injected through the foramen ovale. If the needle enters the subarachnoid space and not the ganglion, the alcohol may be injected directly into the cerebrospinal fluid and may cause severe, even permanent central nervous system complications. Other dangers are based on the close relationship of the ganglion to the cavernous sinus, wherein the injecting needle may perforate the sinus and enter the internal carotid artery. The danger to the motor portion of the trigeminal nerve is another complication.

Subtotal retroganglionic neurotomy

As stated, after failure of alcohol injections into the involved division, the treatment of choice is subtotal retroganglionic neurotomy by way of a temporal approach (Fig. 2-3). The operation has been described. The mortality rate is around 1 percent, lower in the hands of experienced neurosurgeons. Subtotal, in contrast to complete, section of the sensory root is possible by virtue of the fact that the fibers in the sensory root posterior to the ganglion are still arranged according to the three divisions of the nerve. Fibers from the ophthalmic division are more medial and superior, whereas those of the maxillary and mandibular divisions are located more lateral and inferior. Why did the surgeon in our case not just sever the fibers coming from the maxillary division, as these were the only ones involved, rather than include the mandibular fibers? The maxillary and mandibular components are not as easily separated from each other as they are from the ophthalmic division. A second important reason is the frequent spread of trigeminal neuralgia from the second to the third division and vice versa, with the ophthalmic division being only rarely involved. Such spread would necessitate a second intracranial operation, which is thus avoided. It is most important to preserve the fibers of the ophthalmic division, if at all possible, because destruction of the sensory fibers from the cornea leads to abolishment of the protective corneal reflex. The absence of this reflex makes the cornea susceptible to inflammation and ulceration as a result of desiccation and trauma. Serious keratitis and possible loss of eyesight on this side may follow denervation of the ophthalmic division.

The other portion of the trigeminal nerve to be spared is the motor root, which is not too difficult to separate from the sensory root. The minor portion of the trigeminal nerve, as the motor root is frequently called, runs along the undersurface of the major portion from medial to lateral, to join the mandibular nerve (division) with which it passes through the foramen ovale. The mandibular nerve is a mixed nerve containing both motor and sensory fibers, whereas the maxillary and ophthalmic divisions are sensory only. Can you name the eight muscles supplied by the mandibular nerve? From which branchial arch do they derive? It is convenient to separate these eight muscles into two groups: four that are primary muscles of mastication and four that are not. The primary muscles of mastication are the temporalis, masseter, medial pterygoid, and lateral pterygoid. The four others are the tensor tympani, tensor veli palatini, mylohyoid, and anterior belly of the digastric. All muscles supplied by the mandibular nerve are derivatives of the first branchial arch.

Interruption of the middle meningeal artery

In the description of the surgical procedure used in our patient, it was mentioned that after stripping the dura from the middle cranial fossa, the meningeal artery was cut and coagulated. Coagulation at the site of sectioning protects against the risk of future extradural hemorrhage. Where does the middle meningeal artery come from, and how does it enter the skull? What does the artery supply, and how well is its interruption tolerated? The middle meningeal artery is a branch of the first part of the maxillary artery and enters the skull through the foramen spinosum. It is a major source of blood supply to the adjacent skull bones in addition to providing for the dura mater. After ligation of the middle meningeal artery, meningeal branches from other sources assume the distribution of arterial blood to the areas previously supplied by it. Which other arteries supply the dura mater and provide collateral circulation to the dura? The anterior meningeal artery branches from the anterior ethmoidal artery and supplies the floor of the anterior cranial fossa. An anastomotic branch from the ophthalmic artery joins the middle meningeal artery and may replace it. The posterior meningeal artery, which is frequently a direct branch from the external carotid, supplies the posterior cranial fossa.

Physiology of paresthesias

The main complication of trigeminal root section, however, is numbness, which is unavoidable and well tolerated by the great majority of patients, and paresthesias, such as creeping sensations, burning, and itching. About 10 percent of patients who undergo this operation are severely disturbed by this effect, which is not paroxysmal as the original neuralgia, but is continuous and unremitting (anesthesia dolorosa). Some patients have declared that they are unhappier after the surgery than before. The cause of these paresthesias is difficult to establish. One might postulate that the absence of sensory input from other nerves might disturb the balance of perception.

Decompression operation

New approaches are still under investigation. One is based on the assumption that trigeminal neuralgia may be due to compression of the nerve before the ganglion by an abnormal artery looping over it or by a bony anomaly pressing on it. The operation consequently consists of direct visualization of the trigeminal nerve in the pontine cistern between the pons and the petrous apex and removal of the abnormal arterial loop or bony anomaly that may be compressing the nerve.

Gangliolysis and the surgery of intentional trauma to the ganglion

Gangliolysis is obtained by the introduction under anesthesia of an insulated needle through the skin of the cheek into the foramen ovale and the application of a controlled radio-frequency current to damage the trigeminal ganglion thermally. Because the operation is rather short and not too traumatic, it is particularly indicated in elderly or debilitated patients. It can be repeated if relapse occurs. Deliberate traumatization of the ganglion by mechanical compression has also been tried with apparent success. Thus, trigeminal neuralgia, although its cause is still obscure, is being attacked medically and surgically with good results.

3   Septic Thrombosis of the Cavernous Sinus

A 32-year-old business executive returns from a hunting trip, where living conditions had been rather primitive, with high fever and severe headaches and in a generally bad state of health. He relates that about six days earlier he developed a boil on the right upper lip, which resulted from a cut while shaving. He concedes that he had squeezed the boil. He is seen by his family physician, who gives him penicillin injections and keeps him under close observation. The patient does not improve but becomes extremely restless and rather delirious and is transferred the same day to the hospital.

On admission the patient is found to be acutely ill with high temperature and frequent chills. He vomits at intervals, and from time to time becomes delirious. In his clearer moments he complains of nausea and severe headache, particularly on the right side.

EXAMINATION

On examination of this vigorous and athletic patient, the physician observes marked rigidity of his neck muscles and various other clinical signs of meningeal irritation. His upper lip is hard and markedly swollen to about twice its normal size and is dusky red. Some dark crusts cover the right side of the upper lip, and some pus oozes from several points. The right cheek and right side of his nose are swollen and hard. The right upper and lower eyelids are swollen, as are the palpebral and bulbar conjunctivae. The right eyeball protrudes farther than the left (exophthalmos).

Examination of the right eye is made difficult by the temporarily delirious state of the patient and the swelling of the eyelids. The fundus of the right eye shows dilation and engorgement of the retinal veins and some edema of the optic nerve at the papilla. All voluntary movements of the right ocular muscles, including the superior oblique and lateral rectus muscles, are abolished. In his more lucid moments, the patient complains of severe pain in his right eye, in which vision is severely impaired. He also notices tingling and burning (paresthesia) of the right forehead, the right side of his nose, and the upper portion of his face. There seems to be some hardening along the course of the right facial vein.

On later examination he also shows some swelling of the left eyelid with protrusion of the left eyeball and inability to abduct the left eye completely. Repeated blood cultures are positive for *Staphylococcus aureus*. The patient has marked leukocytosis (increase of leukocytes in the bloodstream). His differential blood count also indicates the presence of an acute infection.

DIAGNOSIS

The patient is diagnosed as having deep-seated staphylococcic infection of the subcutaneous tissue of the upper lip (carbuncle), infectious cavernous sinus thrombosis on the right, and beginning cavernous sinus thrombosis on the left, with right-sided paralysis of all ocular muscles (ophthalmoplegia), abducens paralysis on the left, and staphylococcic septicemia.

THERAPY AND FURTHER COURSE

The patient is immediately put on intravenous antibiotics, which include large doses of nascillin for the staphylococci septicemia. Local warm, moist dressings are applied to both eyes and the right side of his face, and narcotics are given to stop the pain.

The patient responds only slowly to the antibiotic treatment. His septic temperatures and severe illness persist for several days and only gradually subside. There is some sloughing of the subcutaneous tissue of the upper lip. Ocular function improves gradually but finally returns to normal. Antibiotic treatment is continued for about two weeks. The patient is discharged after three weeks, having made a complete recovery.

DISCUSSION

We are dealing here with infectious cavernous sinus thrombosis, a condition that is almost invariably fatal if not diagnosed and treated properly. Where did the infection start? The infection began as an innocuous-appearing boil in the hair follicles of the upper lip, a rather common occurrence. How did it spread to the cavernous sinus? There is a rich venous plexus of labial veins superficial to the main muscle mass of the lips, the orbicularis oris. Squeezing the boil by the patient and the never-ceasing motion of the labial muscles, which are traversed by numerous veins, led to propagation of infected material. It passed first through the finer venules, then through the smaller and larger veins draining the lips, with resulting infectious thrombosis of these veins (thrombophlebitis).

Facial vein, its tributaries and communications

Into what vein do the labial veins drain? The labial veins are tributaries of the facial vein, which usually terminates in the internal jugular vein. Was the facial vein involved in our case? What is its course in the face? The facial vein was thrombosed and could be felt as a hardened cord. It runs posterolateral to the facial artery in front of the masseter muscle, where it passes across the lower border of the mandible. More important for the spread of the disease is the communication of the beginning of the facial vein, the angular vein, with the superior ophthalmic vein, and through it with the cavernous sinus (Fig. 3-1). The infection spreads discontinuously by means of an embolus (detached clot) from the face via the facial and angular veins and through the superior ophthalmic vein into the cavernous sinus, or there is an infectious thrombosis extending by continuity through the same vascular channels. The end result is a septic thrombosis of the cavernous sinus.

Is there an anatomical feature that facilitates the spread of infection to the cavernous sinus? The absence of valves in the veins of the face makes it possible for the venous blood to flow in either direction, toward the neck and the internal jugular vein or in the opposite direction toward the beginning of the facial vein at the inner angle of

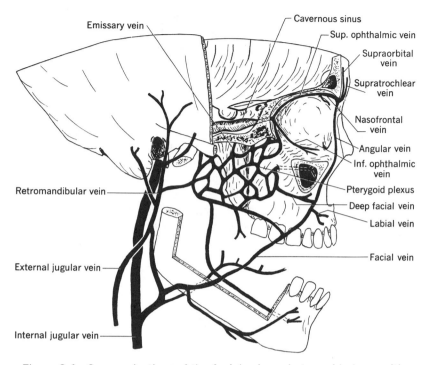

Figure 3-1. Communications of the facial vein and pterygoid plexus with the cavernous sinus.

the eye. How is the angular vein at this site formed? The supratrochlear and supraorbital veins descend from the forehead to unite at the upper medial corner of the orbit to form the angular vein, which then continues across the face as the facial vein, receiving tributaries from the eyelids, the side of the nose, and the lips. It is the important communication of the angular vein with the superior ophthalmic vein that is responsible for the serious prognosis when there is infection in the area drained by the facial vein (Fig. 3-1).

Are there fascial layers surrounding the facial muscles that might limit the spread of infection? The muscles of facial expression are located in the subcutaneous tissue and are intimately connected with the skin. Because they lack fascial septa, no barrier prevents propagation of infection. On the contrary, as has been mentioned, the contraction of these muscles, as in speaking or eating, tends to milk infectious material along the venous channels.

Are there other venous channels to the cavernous sinus that could bypass the ligated vein? There is a large communication from the facial vein via the deep facial vein to the pterygoid plexus. The latter anastomoses with the cavernous sinus by means of emissary veins that pass through foramina in the base of the skull. Is opening of the carbuncle on the upper lip indicated? No, cutting through infected tissues may spread the infection and generally results in worsening of the condition.

Are there other areas in the face besides the upper lip from which the infection could be propagated to the cavernous sinus? Any portion of the skin of the face that is drained by the facial vein can serve as the site of a primary focus. Boils of the nasal cavity and cellulitis of the cheeks, eyelids, eyebrows, forehead, and lower lip have at times been the source of this dangerous complication.

Emissary veins

Could a deeper region of the head be the primary site of the infection that is transmitted via venous channels to the cavernous sinus? Anatomically formulated, the question is: What veins besides the facial vein establish communications with the cavernous sinus and can serve as a pathway for the spread of infectious material to the sinus? The pharyngeal and pterygoid plexuses communicate with the cavernous sinus by way of emissary veins that pass through the foramen ovale and adjacent foramina. The pterygoid plexus also anastomoses with the inferior ophthalmic vein by a vein traversing the inferior orbital fissure. The inferior ophthalmic vein is a direct or indirect tributary of the cavernous sinus (Fig. 3-1). All the aforementioned veins, as well as the previously discussed superior ophthalmic vein, drain important regions of the head that frequently harbor infection. Thus, we understand that tonsillar and paratonsillar abscesses, dental infections (particularly after extractions), infections of the paranasal sinuses and the orbit, and posttraumatic infections of the face, the maxilla, and the frontal bone all may lead to infectious cavernous sinus thrombosis.

What is the definition of an emissary vein? What is the direction of blood flow in emissary veins? Emissary veins are communications between intracranial venous sinuses and extracranial veins. They are thin-walled, valveless vessels that pass through cranial openings generally termed emissary foramina. Blood in them may flow in either direction. Their presence represents a safety mechanism that comes into play when there is an increase in intracranial venous pressure that might otherwise endanger the brain. On the other hand, the blood flow may be reversed, passing from the outside to the sinuses, if there is an obstruction in the extracranial veins as in our case of thrombosis of the facial vein. Ophthalmic veins establish a communication between the facial veins and the cavernous sinus, and, in a sense, can be regarded as emissary veins. Again, the blood flow can be in either direction, toward the cavernous sinus or toward the facial veins, depending on the ever-changing venous pressure conditions.

Cavernous sinus

The superior ophthalmic vein is the main tributary of the cavernous sinus. It enters the sinus at the superior orbital fissure. How does the cavernous sinus drain? It is continuous posteriorly at the apex of the petrous bone with, and drains its blood into, the superior and inferior petrosal sinuses and through them into the transverse sinus and the internal jugular vein. Retrograde spread of infection from the ear via the petrosal sinuses represents an additional and important route leading to cavernous sinus thrombosis. If one keeps in mind that cerebral and meningeal veins also drain into the cavernous sinus, other serious complications, such as brain abscess and spreading meningitis, can be understood on the basis of retrograde spread. Signs of meningeal irritation, such as rigidity of the neck and headache, were also present in our case.

What anatomical features does the cavernous sinus share with other sinuses, and in what respect does it differ? Like other intracranial venous sinuses, it is located between two layers of dura, is lined by endothelium, but lacks a muscular coat. It differs from other dural sinuses, however, in that it is traversed by numerous trabeculae, which give it a spongelike appearance. This arrangement also makes it more susceptible to stasis and thrombosis. Embedded in its lateral wall are the oculomotor, trochlear, and first and second divisions of the trigeminal nerve; the internal carotid artery, with its sympathetic plexus and the abducens nerve, course through its lumen (Fig. 3-2).

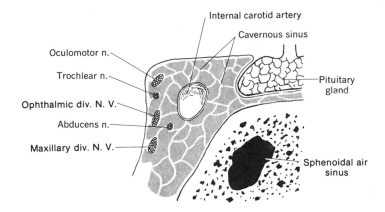

Figure 3-2. Cross section of the right cavernous sinus showing its important nerve and arterial contents.

Eye signs in cavernous sinus thrombosis

How do you explain the swelling of the eyelids and conjunctiva, the exophthalmos, the congestion of the retinal vessels, and edema of the optic nerve in this patient? All these signs are caused by interference with the blood flow in the sinus and connecting veins as a result of the thrombosis. The latter causes retrograde congestion of the ocular veins and edema (swelling) of the orbital structures. What signs do we have in our case that the right third, fourth, and sixth cranial nerves are affected by the sinus thrombosis? How would you test for specific involvement of the abducens and trochlear nerves? Detailed examination pertaining to function of individual eye muscles was difficult in our patient because of swelling of the right eye and his poor and irrational condition, but it was found that all voluntary movements of the eyeball were abolished. The oculomotor nerve supplies all muscles moving the eyeball with the exception of the superior oblique and lateral rectus muscles, which are innervated by the trochlear and abducens nerves, respectively. How would you test the functions of these two muscles? If the superior oblique is functionless as a result of involvement of the fourth cranial nerve, there is loss of downward movement of the eyeball if it is adducted. In case of paralysis of the lateral rectus, there is loss of full abduction of the eyeball. Both of these motions were abolished in our case. The impairment of vision in the right eye can be explained on the basis of edema of the optic nerve with congestion of the central vein of the retina, which drains into the superior ophthalmic vein.

Can permanent blindness develop? We have already mentioned that retinal congestion was observed. Blindness is a definite possibility and would occur if the thrombosis completely blocked flow in the superior ophthalmic vein, because the central vein of the retina does not anastomose with other veins. Are there clinical indications that the upper two divisions of the trigeminal nerve, which lie in the wall of the sinus, were also involved? Yes, there were sensory disturbances (paresthesias) in the face along the distribution of these two divisions.

Later protrusion and swelling of the left eye with abducens paralysis indicate involvement of the left cavernous sinus also. Are there anatomical pathways for the spread of the thrombosis from the right to the left sinus? The two cavernous sinuses are connected by anterior and posterior intercavernous sinuses, which may readily spread the infection from one sinus to the other. The abducens nerve, being in a more exposed position within the sinus, is often the first of the nerves supplying the eye muscles to be involved in sinus thrombosis. Occasional reports of cases that have come to autopsy note infectious thrombosis of the internal carotid artery within the sinus. This path, of course, could be the route of the spread of infection to the brain by means of anterior and middle cerebral arteries.

The presence of positive blood cultures in this case indicates that the infection had spread beyond the confines of the cranium. The final happy outcome of the case is gratifying and can be ascribed to the vigorous constitution of the patient. Such a positive result is not as common as one might expect in this era of intensive antibiotic treatment. Indeed, one author reports 80 percent mortality and that 75 percent of survivors have some aftereffects, mainly involving eye muscles and changes in visual acuity. Disappearance of local signs in our patient can be explained on the basis of subsidence of the infection and recanalization of the thrombosed sinus as well as by development of a collateral circulation bypassing the sinus.

4 Cancer of the Lip with Radical Neck Dissection

A 58-year-old farmer who had been chewing tobacco for forty years comes to the outpatient department with an ulcerated swelling involving parts of the red portion of the lower lip on the left. He states that the lesion started as a scab about six years earlier and that it generally enlarged. From time to time it heals over, but then it breaks open again and occasionally bleeds.

EXAMINATION

On examination the left portion of the lower lip shows an area of induration that is centrally ulcerated. The ulcer is about 2 cm in its largest diameter and is located at the vermilion border of the lower lip close to the left angle of the mouth. The borders of the ulcer are elevated and hard. When slightly scraped, the ulcer bleeds readily. There are several hard, nontender, enlarged nodes palpable in the left submandibular and carotid triangles. Otherwise, examination is negative. There is no sign of involvement of other nodes besides the cervical nodes.

DIAGNOSIS

The patient has cancer of the lip with probable metastasis to the cervical nodes. Biopsies of the primary lesion of the lip and needle biopsy of one of the enlarged submandibular nodes confirm the diagnosis of squamous cell cancer.

THERAPY AND FURTHER COURSE

The patient is admitted to the hospital for surgery. With the patient under general anesthesia, the primary ulcerated tumor is removed by a V-shaped excision, which includes a 5-mm-wide margin of normal-appearing tissue around the tumor. The defect is closed by a flap of approximately the same shape from the surface of the left upper lip, which is rotated around to form a new corner of the mouth.

The next step in the operation is a radical neck dissection, which aims at removal of all deep cervical lymph nodes on the diseased side from the lower margin of the mandible to the clavicle, and from the anterior midline of the neck to the anterior border of the trapezius. From superficial to deep, it includes the lymphatics between the deep surface of the platysma and the prevertebral fascia.

The operation consists of removal in one block of the deep cervical lymphatics, particularly those in the submandibular and submental triangles, around the internal jugular vein and surrounding the accessory nerve and the transverse cervical vessels. The procedure includes sacrifice of the submandibular salivary gland, the sternocleidomastoid muscle, the accessory nerve, the internal jugular vein, the cutaneous branches of the cervical plexus, and the ansa cervicalis.

Skin flaps are widely reflected to expose the anterior and posterior triangles of the neck. The skin flaps include the platysma muscle. Attention is given to preserving the marginal mandibular branch of the facial nerve where it courses along the lower margin of the mandible superficial to the facial artery and vein. These vessels are ligated and cut. The first structure met is the external jugular vein, which is ligated and resected to allow later removal of the sternocleidomastoid muscle, which this vein crosses superficially. The sternocleidomastoid muscle at the site of its distal attachment to the sternum and clavicle and the posterior belly of the omohyoid are divided. The internal jugular vein is doubly ligated and severed just above the clavicle. Attention is given to preservation of vagus and phrenic nerves and the roots of the brachial plexus. The phrenic nerve and the roots of the brachial plexus lie deep to the prevertebral fascia, which may or may not be removed in this operation. Likewise, the common, external, and internal carotid arteries and the thoracic duct on the left are kept intact. The accessory nerve is cut close to its entrance into the trapezius muscle.

Next the surgeon removes all areolar and lymphatic tissue, starting in the posteroinferior region of the posterior triangle and working forward and upward. Here the transverse cervical vessels, and usually the suprascapular vessels, are ligated and severed and the supraclavicular nerves cut. The other cutaneous branches of the cervical plexus are also sacrificed at this time. The bulk of tissues consisting of the sternocleidomastoid and omohyoid muscles, the internal jugular vein, and the areolar and fatty tissue with the lymphatics is reflected upward. The common carotid artery and its two divisions with the lower branches of the external carotid artery are exposed. The ansa cervicalis has been sacrificed previously to allow opening of the carotid sheath and removal of the internal jugular vein and adjacent lymph nodes. The important tributaries of the internal jugular vein are ligated and cut. The upper end of the internal jugular vein is clamped, ligated, and sectioned as high as possible. Again, special care is taken to avoid injury to the vagus nerve. The attachment of the sternocleidomastoid muscle to the mastoid process is cut as is the attachment of the omohyoid to the hyoid bone. The proximal end of the accessory nerve is likewise severed.

These steps are followed by removal of all fat and lymph nodes from the carotid, submental, and submandibular triangles. In the latter, the submandibular salivary gland is removed and its duct ligated, but care is taken not to injure the lingual and hypoglossal nerves. Removal of the submental nodes from the opposite side, in this case, entails crossing the midline and requires exposing the anterior belly of the opposite digastric muscle. The mass of tissue dissected out is removed in one block with the aim of eliminating all possibly cancerous lymphatics without cutting into them, thus avoiding dispersal of cancer cells.

After the dissection is completed, all bleeding is controlled by sutures and the wound is closed. A drain is left inside along the course of the common carotid artery and brought out through the surgical wound.

The postoperative course in this patient is uneventful. He is up and about on the second day and is discharged from the hospital ten days later. Examination six months, one, two, and three years after surgery shows no signs of recurrence.

DISCUSSION

In the design of this operation, it is noted that cancer of the lip spreads by way of the deep cervical lymphatics but generally remains confined to the head and neck. Death from unchecked cancer occurs when large masses of cancerous cervical nodes interfere with swallowing, leading to gradual starvation, and slowly compress the air passages, thus strangling the patient, or erode the great vessels, resulting in an acute and profuse fatal hemorrhage. Hence, the goal of radical neck dissection is removal of all deep cervical lymph nodes that may harbor metastatic cancer cells having arrived there by way of lymphatic vessels.

The classic radical neck dissection, described by Crile in 1905, was performed in this case. It sacrifices the sternocleidomastoid and omohyoid muscles, the spinal accessory nerve, the internal and external jugular veins, and adjacent lymph nodes and vessels. This procedure is indicated for most squamous cell carcinomas of the head and neck. For selected lesions, however, the neck dissection can be modified to preserve one or all of these structures except for those lymphatic tissues into which primary lesions have spread.

There is no standard definition of a modified neck dissection. The term means that if one or more structures normally sacrificed in a radical neck dissection are preserved, the procedure becomes a modified neck dissection. How the radical neck dissection is modified becomes descriptive in each operation.

Lymphatic drainage of lower lip

What is lymphatic drainage of the lower lip? The lymph vessels from the lateral portion of the lip pass downward to the submandibular nodes of the same side in the submandibular triangle, whereas the more medial portions of the lip drain in part also to submental nodes in the submental triangle to both sides of the midline. Lymph vessels, even from the lateral portions of the lower lip, may cross the midline to submental nodes of the other side, but the danger of contralateral spread increases the closer the lesion is to the midline

(Fig. 4-1). The possibility of this spread is the rationale for removing all lymph nodes in the submental triangle on both sides of the midline, as done in our case. The submandibular and submental nodes represent the first relay station of the lymphatics of the lower lip.

What are the other lymphatic channels along which cancer of the lower lip would spread after it invades the submandibular or submental nodes or with which an occasional lymph vessel from the lip, which bypasses these nodes, would connect? The chain of deep cervical nodes is the final pathway into which all lymph vessels from the head and neck drain. It consists of a large and variable number of lymph nodes that are related to the carotid sheath, particularly to the internal jugular vein. Many of these nodes lie directly under the sternocleidomastoid muscle (Fig. 4-2). This important vein and the sternocleidomastoid muscle must be resected in order not to leave any potentially cancerous lymph structures behind that are in close contact with them.

As mentioned, the omohyoid muscle is generally resected. It divides the deep cervical lymphatic chain into a superior group and an inferior group at the site where it crosses the internal jugular vein. If the surgeon is reasonably certain that cancerous invasion has not progressed beyond the superior deep cervical lymph nodes, a

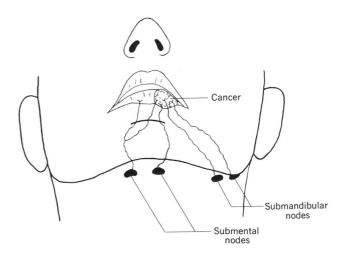

Figure 4-1. Cancer of the lower lip with first relay of potentially involved lymph nodes.

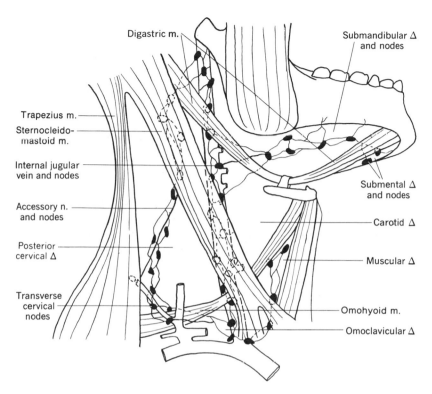

Figure 4-2. Cervical triangles and deep cervical lymph nodes.

supraomohyoid dissection is done, carrying the dissection only to the crossing point of the omohyoid muscle. The superior deep cervical nodes drain in part into the inferior nodes. Parts of their efferent vessels contribute to the formation of the jugular trunk that receives lymph from the inferior deep cervical group. A number of deep cervical nodes occupy a position away from the internal jugular chain around the accessory nerve and the transverse cervical and suprascapular vessels (Fig. 4-2). Removal of these nodes therefore entails sacrifice of this important motor nerve and these vessels.

Triangles of the neck and their lymph nodes

In the radical neck dissection, what six triangles of the neck are encompassed and from which all fatty areolar and lymphatic tissue is removed? All triangles of the neck are involved in this operation: the submandibular, submental, carotid, and muscular triangles, all of which are parts of the anterior triangle, and the occipital and subclavian subdivisions of the posterior triangle. Identify the boundaries of these triangles from Figure 4-2. Are lymph nodes present in all these triangles, and where are they most prevalent? The submental and submandibular nodes are present in the triangles of the same name. The nodes in the unpaired submental triangle lie on the mylohyoid muscle between the anterior bellies of the digastric muscles. Why must the submandibular salivary gland and its duct be sacrificed in removing the submandibular lymph nodes? These nodes lie within the fascial sheath of and in close relation to this salivary gland and cannot be removed properly without removing the gland. The close relationship of some of the smaller lymph nodes in this group to the facial vessels requires ligation and sacrifice of these vessels. Most of the superior deep cervical nodes lie in the carotid triangle and deep to the sternocleidomastoid muscle. A number of nodes of the cervical chain overflow into the muscular triangle and the two divisions of the posterior triangle. A number of important nodes are located in the posterior triangle around the accessory nerve and the transverse cervical and suprascapular vessels (Fig. 4-2). Again this entails removal of this nerve and ligation and sacrifice of these vessels.

What is the origin of the transverse cervical and suprascapular arteries, and where do their corresponding veins drain? The arteries are branches of the thyrocervical trunk of the subclavian artery, and the veins are generally tributaries of the external jugular vein, which is likewise ligated and removed. How does this latter vein drain? It is a tributary of the subclavian vein.

Loss of the internal jugular vein

The most important structure that must be sacrificed is the internal jugular vein, including its tributaries, particularly the lingual, pharyngeal, facial, the superior and middle thyroid, and occipital veins. If one realizes that the internal jugular vein is the largest vein of the head and neck draining blood from the brain, face, and neck and that the external jugular vein, which also drains part of the head and neck, is likewise removed, it is surprising that the loss of these veins is generally well tolerated. One might ask why total extirpation of the internal jugular vein from the site of its cranial exit to the level of the clavicle is necessary. All surgeons who have participated in the design of radical neck dissection agree on the need to remove this vein. It is surrounded by cervical lymph nodes that may readily be adherent to it and that cannot be completely eliminated without concomitant resection of the vein.

How is venous drainage from the head and neck effectuated after removal of the internal jugular vein? Because of ample communications across the midline, the contralateral internal jugular vein will easily adjust to the additional blood flow into it. The vertebral venous plexus also participates in the venous drainage from the brain and other parts of the head.

The cross-sectional area of the vertebral system of veins is greater than the entire system of jugular veins. Therefore, one or both jugular veins can be removed without causing mortality. There may be a transient, harmless increase in intracranial pressure after unilateral ligation of the internal jugular vein, but only in rare cases will there be a serious rise reflected in headache, slow pulse, and high blood pressure. Lumbar puncture with withdrawal of cerebrospinal fluid is the treatment of choice in these cases.

Motor and sensory nerves sacrificed in radical neck dissection

What muscles does the accessory nerve supply? The accessory nerve supplies two important muscles in the field of this operation, the sternocleidomastoid and the trapezius muscle, of which the former is resected during the operation. How does denervation of the trapezius affect the patient? Generally, loss of function of the trapezius is well tolerated although noticeable by a slight shoulder droop. It is possible that some motor function remains in this muscle as it receives additional motor fibers from the third and fourth cervical nerves that otherwise furnish proprioceptive fibers to the trapezius muscle. What muscles could replace the action of the trapezius in elevating and retracting the scapula? The levator scapulae and the rhomboid muscles are synergists of the trapezius in this action. What other motor nerves are resected in this operation, and what muscles do they supply? The ansa cervicalis lying on or in the anterior layer of the carotid sheath must be sacrificed. It supplies the infrahyoid muscles, whose denervation on one side is well tolerated. Attention is given to preservation of one small motor nerve, the marginal mandibular branch of the facial nerve, which runs along the lower edge of the mandible just superficial to the site where the facial vessels that are ligated cross the bone. If it must be resected, some disfigurement around the mouth results, particularly when smiling, and some difficulty closing the mouth.

What sensory nerves are sacrificed? Where are they located, and of what are they branches? The cutaneous branches of the cervical plexus are removed in the dissection of the posterior triangle, where they emerge along the posterior border of the sternocleidomastoid. They are the lesser occipital, great auricular, transverse cervical, and supraclavicular nerves, all derived from ventral rami of C2–C4. The resulting anesthesia and numbness is well tolerated and gradually decreases. What is the explanation for this phenomenon? It can be assumed that sensory nerves in the neighborhood gradually take over the function in the desensitized area by sending fibers into it. What nerves would be most likely to participate in this sensory resupply? The chief source would be the cutaneous branches of the dorsal rami of cervical nerves C2–C4. It is also conceivable that nerve fibers from the distal ends of the central stumps may gradually grow out and reach the skin to resume their sensory innervations.

Vagus, lingual, and hypoglossal nerves

Attention should of course be given to preservation of the vagus nerve. What is its relation to the internal jugular vein and the common and internal carotid arteries? It lies between the vein and arteries and on a somewhat deeper plane. Would section of the vagus nerve on one side be fatal? Injury of one vagus nerve is not followed by serious cardiac or pulmonary complications but will result in unilateral vocal cord paralysis with partial obstruction of the air passages. This complication would require watchful nursing care with particular attention to the air passages and tracheostomy in case of breathing difficulties.

In the rather difficult dissection of the submandibular triangle, attention is given to avoiding injury to the hypoglossal and lingual nerves. Removal of the submandibular salivary gland and duct, of all areolar tissue and lymph nodes, as well as ligation of the facial vessels facilitate display of these important nerves. Quite frequently, the lower pole of the parotid gland is also amputated, and some surgeons recommend separation of the posterior belly of the di-

gastric and stylohyoid muscles from the hyoid bone and their resection. What muscles form the floor of the submandibular triangle that
must be defined in this operation? Portions of the mylohyoid and the
hyoglossus muscles constitute the deep boundary of the submandibular triangle, with the mylohyoid overlapping the hyoglossus
superficially. In the area where the two muscles overlap, do the
lingual and hypoglossal nerves run superficial to the mylohyoid,
deep to it (that is, between it and the hyoglossus muscle), or deep to
the hyoglossus? They run between the mylohyoid and hyoglossus
muscles, with the lingual nerve superior to the hypoglossal nerve
and with the duct of the submandibular gland between them. The
hypoglossal nerve is exposed to injury, where it hooks around the
occipital artery to enter the carotid triangle inferior to the posterior
belly of the digastric muscle. It returns to the submandibular triangle by traveling deep to the digastric muscle.

5   Bilateral Dislocation of the Temporomandibular Joint (TMJ)

About forty-five minutes before being referred to the clinic, a 22-year-old college student took a large bite of an apple. She immediately experienced sharp, severe pain on both sides of her face just in front of the ear. Since that moment she has been unable to close her mouth completely and cannot speak clearly. She also complains of pain in both temporomandibular joints when she tries to open or close her mouth. The pain radiates to the ear and the skin above it.

EXAMINATION

On examination, the patient appears to have a severe malocclusion with her lower jaw protruding beyond her upper jaw (prognathism). She is unable to bring her upper and lower teeth together when she tries to close her mouth. On both sides there is an obvious dimpling of the skin and a depression in the preauricular area that corresponds to the mandibular fossa.

DIAGNOSIS

The diagnosis is bilateral anterior dislocation of the mandible.

THERAPY AND FURTHER COURSE

The patient is admitted to the hospital and given a general anesthetic preceding surgery. After complete relaxation of the facial musculature by an injection of muscle relaxant, it is possible to reduce the dislocation of first one side and then the other by downward bimanual pressure on the lower molar teeth, followed by a backward push of the mandible. To obviate the possibility of recurrence of the dislocation after recovery from the anesthesia and the muscle relaxant, the jaw is immobilized by intermaxillary wiring. After three weeks the wires are removed and movement of the mandible allowed. One year later the patient reports that no further incidence of dislocation had occurred.

DISCUSSION

The TMJ (temporomandibular joint) is the only synovial joint in the skull with the exception of those between the ear ossicles. It is also the only joint in the body where a dislocation can occur spontaneously by exaggerated, but otherwise normal, movements in articulation. Most often this happens during yawning, but it can also occur while laughing, singing, or biting into an apple. It can also take place in a dentist's chair when the mouth is opened too widely. Traumatic dislocation is not as common as the spontaneous variety.

The TMJ

Bones, cartilage, and capsule.   To understand the readiness with which dislocations occur, we must look at the anatomy of this somewhat complex joint. The uninitiated observer may assume that the TMJ is a simple hinge joint, with the upward and downward movements of the jaw taking place around a horizontal axis laid through the joint. Actually, the joint has two compartments, an upper and a lower, completely separated by an articular disk composed of dense fibrous connective tissue and areas of fibrocartilage (Fig. 5-1). Superiorly, the bony articular surface consists of the anterior portion of the mandibular fossa and the downward protruding articular tubercle (eminence); both are parts of the temporal bone. Below, the bony articular surface is formed by the condylar head of the mandible. In contrast to other freely movable joints, in which the articulating surfaces are covered by hyaline cartilage, avascular fibrous tissue covers all parts of the articular bony portions.
    Superiorly, the disk is convex over the mandibular fossa and

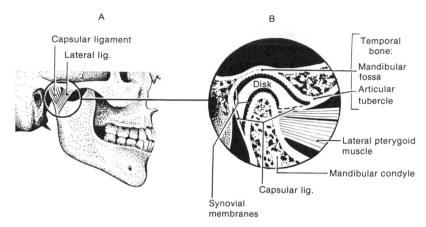

Figure 5-1. A. Lateral view of the articular capsule of of the temporomandibular joint. B. Sagittal section through the temporomandibular joint. Note the fibrocartilaginous disk and attachments of the internal pterygoid muscle.

concave over the articular tubercle. Inferiorly, it is concave for the convex head of the mandible, thus harmonizing the two bony surfaces. The disk also acts as a shock absorber. It is thicker at the periphery, where it attaches to the joint capsule. The capsule, lined by synovial membrane, is rather loose and attaches above and below to the margins of the bony parts of the joint.

Many times the articular disk may be displaced, which becomes evident in two ways: Opening the mouth, the patient may hear a "snap" in the ear, followed by a "click" every time the patient opens the mouth. The patient may also suffer occasional attacks of locking and salivation. The disk must be either reduced by a dentist or physician, or it may reduce itself. When this occurs, the discomfort and pain cease.

Ligaments. The tonus of the muscles responsible for joint movement is of major importance in stabilizing the joint. The ligaments play only an ancillary role in maintaining the position of the mandible, but they aid in limiting exaggerated movements (Fig. 5-2). The most important of these ligaments is the lateral (temporomandibular) ligament, which extends from the zygoma (zygomatic process of the temporal bone) to the lateral and posterior parts of the neck of the mandible and restrains mainly the backward movement of the jaw. The two ligaments on the medial side of the mandible, the sphenomandibular and the stylomandibular, are not very significant for the function of the joint.

Movements of the joint. The expected hinge action takes place in the lower compartment between the inferior surface of the disk and the condyle of the mandible, but opening the mouth is always accompanied by the forward gliding motion of the disk and condyle of the mandible onto the articular tubercle. Because the summit of the articular tubercle reaches more inferiorly than the inferior surface of the mandibular fossa, the forward movement of the mandible in itself results in a separation of the teeth. Thus, the motion of opening the mouth actually takes place in both compartments, with the axis of the combined motion running transversely through the mandibular foramina located on the medial sides of the two mandibular rami, approximately at their center. This location prevents the unnecessary stretching of the alveolar nerves and blood vessels at their points of entrance into the mandible when the mouth is opened. A reverse series of motions takes place in all parts of the joint when the mouth is closed. Other movements of the joint, such as protrusion

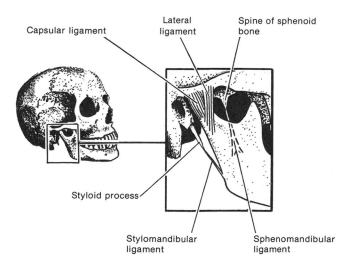

Figure 5-2. Lateral view of the ligaments of the temporomandibular joint.

(protraction) and retraction and grinding (side-to-side) motion, ar-
ediscussed along with the muscles executing them.

Muscles controlling the movements.   Which muscles control the
movements of the mandible in the joint? All motions of the jaw are
the result of highly integrated and closely coordinated performances
of the muscles listed below, but it should not be forgotten that the
finer and more complex movements are individually attuned to the
shape and position of the teeth and differ from one person to
another.

The muscles of the two sides act either in unison (as in depression, elevation, protrusion, and retrusion of the mandible) or alter-
nately on the two sides (as in the side-to-side gliding motion in
grinding the teeth or chewing).

As we have seen, movement of the mandible in opening the
mouth consists of a simultaneous forward gliding of the mandible
with its disk onto the articular tubercle and depression of the mandible as a result of the hinge action within the lower compartment of
the joint. The forward motion is effectuated by the lateral pterygoid
muscle, which runs horizontally backward from its origin in the
infratemporal fossa to its attachment to the disk of the TMJ and the
neck of the mandible (Fig. 5-1). The mandible is depressed by contraction of the digastric and mylohoid muscles and the infrahyoid
muscles (thyrohyoid, sternothyoid, and sternohoid). Thus, the digastric and mylohyoid muscles are linked inferiorly to the sternum
through the infrahyoid muscles by their common attachments to the
hyoid bone.

The opposite action of elevation of the jaw in closing the mouth
is brought about by the powerful contraction of the masseter, temporalis, and medial pterygoid muscles. These muscles arise from the
bones of the lateral side of the skull. Where do they insert? The
temporalis inserts onto the coronoid process and the anterior border
of the ramus of the mandible, and the medial pterygoid inserts on
the medial surface of the mandible near its angle, whereas the masseter is inserted into the lateral surface of the mandible near its
angle. (See the case study dealing with fracture of the mandible in
Chapter 7). The strength of the closing motion can be seen in circus
athletes who can dangle themselves, and even a companion, by
biting onto a bar suspended in the air by the force of the three
contracted muscles. Protrusion of the chin is brought about by mus-

cles that arise anterior to the joint and course backward, such as the lateral, and, to a lesser extent, the medial pterygoid muscles. The opposite motion of retraction takes place mainly when the posteroinferior portion of the temporalis muscle contracts. In grinding and chewing (side-by-side motions), the movements of the two sides are coordinated, but the right and left lateral pterygoid muscles generally act in alternating contraction.

Causes, clinical signs, and symptoms of dislocation

How are traumatic or spontaneous, but generally bilateral, dislocations brought about? Practically all dislocations consist of an abnormal anterior displacement of the mandible, which takes place when a blow to the chin or an exaggerated opening of the mouth causes the articular disk and condyles of the mandible to be pulled over the summits of the articular tubercles (Fig. 5-3). This movement is due mainly to forcible involuntary contraction of the lateral pterygoid muscles while spasm of the superioinferiorly directed muscles (such as the temporalis, medial pterygoid, and the deep part of the masseter) keep the jaw arrested in the infratemporal fossa with the mouth half open.

In some disease states, such as tetanus, the patient cannot open the mouth because of muscular spasm of these masticatory muscles. This muscular spasm is called trismus and is often very painful. It may be relieved by muscle relaxants or general anesthesia.

In examining the patient, it was mentioned that the heads of the mandible could not be palpated from within the external acoustic

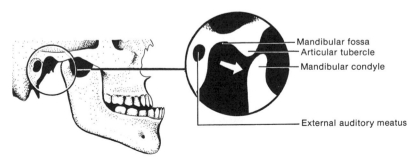

Figure 5-3. Lateral view of the dislocation of the temporomandibular joint. Note the overriding of the articular tubercle by the mandibular condyle.

meatuses. This is a common diagnostic procedure in examination of the TMJ, as the joint lies directly in front of the external meatus. The examiner lets the tip of a finger slide over the tragus of the external ear into the meatus. The examiner then can analyze by palpation the movements of the mandibular heads on opening and closing the mouth, in protrusion and retraction of the chin, and on grinding motions. In this case the absence of the heads from the articular fossae was easily diagnosed and confirmed by the depression and dimpling of the skin that could be felt and seen in front of the ears.

The patient also rather typically complained of pain in the joint that radiated into the external ear and the temporal region. The nerve, which is mainly responsible for the sensory supply of the joint, including its capsule, is the auriculotemporal from the mandibular division of the trigeminal nerve (V_3). It courses right behind the joint and in front of the ear and then ascends over the temple posterior to the superficial temporal artery. During this course it supplies, in addition to the joint, the external acoustic meatus, the outer surface of the tympanic membrane, and the lower lateral region of the scalp. This explains the radiation of the pain to the ear and temporal region. It also confirms Hilton's law, that "a joint is supplied by the same nerve trunk that supplies the skin over the joint and also the muscles crossing the joint." In the latter connection, it is interesting to note that the nerves to the masseter and temporalis muscles from the mandibular division of the trigeminal also provide sensory branches to the temporomandibular joint.

Clinically, it must be realized that once bilateral dislocation has occurred, it can easily happen again, and people afflicted with this condition are known as chronic dislocators. Some are asymptomatic, but others suffer a great deal of pain in the area of the TMJ. For relief of the latter group, the height of the articular tubercle may be surgically reduced to allow unrestricted anterior movement of the mandibular condyles and to eliminate the pain associated with dislocation. This surgery may cause dislocation to occur more frequently, however.

One final comment in regard to terminology seems of interest. In describing the therapy applied to this patient, the common surgical term intermaxillary wiring was used. Intermaxillary fixation, also often found in surgical textbooks, refers to immobilization of the jaw by wires extending between maxilla and mandible. The term intermaxillary originated at a time when maxilla, following its Latin usage, designated both upper and lower jaws (superior and inferior maxillae), which also explains the frequent and now obsolete term submaxillary salivary gland, which is more correctly called the submandibular salivary gland. On the other hand, the term mandible was used for centuries for either the upper or lower jaw in insects.

6 Rheumatoid Arthritis of the Temporomandibular Joint (TMJ)

The patient is a 39-year old female lawyer with a 12-year history of rheumatoid arthritis (RA). For the past nine months, she has noticed pain in the right TMJ. The pain is aggravated by opening and closing her mouth and in chewing, movements that have become more difficult during the last year. At present she can open her mouth only enough to admit liquid and semiliquid nourishment and occasionally some soft foods. Pain and stiffness in the TMJ are particularly severe on rising but diminish as the day progresses. The patient states that she has lost 10 pounds during the last few months.

EXAMINATION

On physical examination the previously mentioned restriction of motion is noted. The patient can open her mouth wide enough to admit the tip of the little finger, a distance of about 5 mm, compared with the normal average maximum opening of about 40 mm, as measured between the incisal edges of the incisor teeth. There is some swelling in the tissue around the right TMJ, and with a stethoscope placed over the right joint, crepitation (crackling sounds) can be heard during attempted jaw movement. There is no discernible anterior movement of the head (condyle) of the mandible. Accompanying pain is poorly localized but frequently radiates to the right ear and temple.

Radiographic examination of the left TMJ is within normal

limits, but the right joint is grossly abnormal, with narrowing of the joint space and osteosclerotic and osteolytic changes in the temporal bone and the head of the mandibular condyle. The head of the condyle is flattened and irregular in contour with alteration of the normal cortical bone. Overall inspection of the patient reveals typical deformities of the small articulations of the fingers and muscular wasting in the hands.

DIAGNOSIS

Rheumatoid arthritis of the right TMJ is diagnosed.

THERAPY AND FURTHER COURSE

Medications in the past have included aspirin and cortisone to reduce pain and inflammation. These give temporary symptomatic relief and allow the patient to carry out normal daily activities. Physical therapy, such as heat applications and passive exercises, are initiated and symptomatic drug therapy is continued. Contact with the patient's family physician is established, and close observation of the changes in her TMJ joints is planned. Future surgical intervention is not excluded and would consist of either total or subtotal condylectomy and replacement of the disk by interposition of some inert material such as Teflon or a noncorrosive stainless steel. This implant is positioned over the stump of the totally or partially resected condyle with the idea that it will prevent further restriction of motion and food intake.

DISCUSSION

The patient is afflicted with rheumatoid arthritis, a chronic inflammatory disease that may occur anywhere in the body but quite often starts in the interphalangeal joints and may involve the TMJ in 25 to 50 percent of all cases. It belongs to a group of diseases that were once autoimmune-connective tissue diseases. The cause of these diseases is not known but has been attributed to an autoimmune reaction between an abnormal protein or antigen and an antibody, which has been produced perhaps in response to a bacterial or viral infection. Other diseases in this group are systemic lupus erythematosus, scleroderma, periarteritis nodosa, and rheumatic fever.

Historically, arthritis is an ancient disease dating back as far as 2750 B.C. It has been found in an Egyptian mummy that displayed involvement of hands and the TMJ, but this was apparently osteoarthritis, which is characterized by cartilage degradation, joint-space narrowing, and an absence in blood tests for rheumatoid factors.

Rheumatoid arthritis appears to be a more recent disease with a skeletal record of less than 500 years. It is most common in adults aged 20 to 50 (80%) and is said to occur two to three times more frequently in women. The patient in this case falls into both categories. It also affects children. Initial involvement, which is often symmetrical, takes place in the small joints of the fingers, followed by the knees, elbows, shoulders, wrists, and ankles. In the early stages of the disease the symptoms in the TMJ are often only subjective, consisting of transient pain and muscle spasms with negative radiographic findings. One of the striking features of the disease is the pronounced tendency for exacerbations and remissions.

The opening distance of the mouth is the result of a small hinge movement and a large translational movement of the mandibular condyle anteriorly along the articular eminence of the temporal bone. The hinge movement accounts for only a few millimeters of the 40-mm opening distance. The absence of any translational movement in RA accounts for the limited opening.

Anatomy

The anatomy and physiology of the TMJ was described in the case study dealing with bilateral dislocation of the mandible. Here it may be added that in structure and function it is one of the most complicated joints in the body. It is subject to continued use in speech and eating. Important nerves and blood vessels are in its immediate neighborhood. Its articular fossa, the mandibular fossa, is considerably larger than its movable counterpart, the head of the mandible, but its most characteristic feature is the presence of the articular disk, a fibrocartilaginous plate, thinner in the center and thicker in the periphery. This disk divides the joint into upper and lower compartments. As stated, the bony articulating surfaces are covered by avascular fibrocartilaginous tissue. The joint capsule surrounds the articulating parts rather loosely and is lined by synovial membrane (synovium) in the portions of the joint not exposed to pressure. Consequently, synovial membrane is absent over the articular parts of the condyle, the mandibular fossa, the disk, and the articular tubercle. The synovium may send folds (plicae) into the joint, thus diminishing friction. The same function is exercised by the synovial fluid (synovia), which lubricates the joint and perhaps contributes to the nourishment of the fibrous tissue within the joint.

Pathology

The characteristic feature of RA of the TMJ is a progressive inflammation of all joint structures. The disease starts in the synovium, which becomes edematous and hyperemic. The synovial fluid is less viscous than normal. If the RA progresses, it forms an inflammatory granulation tissue that grows over the articular surfaces and gradually erodes the cartilaginous portions of the joint, including the disk. The fibrous capsule and finally the articulating parts of the bones become involved. The end result may be fibrous or bony fixation and immobility of the joint (ankylosis). Thus, it may reach a terminal stage in which the disease has burned itself out with reparative fibrous or osseous bridging and complete absence of motion.

Pain

The pain of which the patient complains is due to the inflammation and swelling of all structures in the joint and also to the accompanying muscle spasms (see the case study dealing with fracture of the mandible). These spasms (trismus) are quite painful and affect the muscles that are the prime movers of the joint. The joint itself receives its sensory supply mainly from the auriculotemporal nerve, which runs posterior to the joint; however, the nerves to the temporalis and masseter muscles also contain sensory fibers to the joint. The factor of spastic contractions of such a large number of muscles is probably responsible for the poor localization of the pain.

It can be difficult to diagnose TMJ pain because it may be perceived by the patient as coming from an ear, a tooth, or a paranasal sinus, all structures innervated, at least in part, by the trigeminal nerve. Conversely, pain caused by to disease in the teeth, paranasal sinuses, and ear may be perceived as TMJ pain because of the poorly explained phenomena of referred pain.

Radiography

In discussing the appearance of the disease in the TMJ, one should keep in mind the limitations inherent in the method. The radiographically visible "joint space" corresponds anatomically to the articular cartilage, the disk, and the synovial folds. Because the density of these structures approximates that of water and other soft tissues, the structures themselves cannot be visualized, and the inflammation, edema, and destruction of the previously mentioned structures cannot be detected by this method. Thus, clinical signs and symptoms may long precede radiographic changes. Rare widening of the joint space caused by abnormal fluid collection or, more commonly, narrowing of the space caused by destruction of the articular cartilage may be the first radiographic sign. In later stages we observe demineralization of the bone in and around the joint (osteoporosis), flattening of the mandibular condyle, and cortical sclerosis of the bony margins with the appearance of small subcortical cysts and irregularities in the contour of the articulating bones from erosion. Often there is no forward movement of the head of the condyle on attempting to open the mouth. Most of these radiographic signs are found in our patient. The final changes, which are not present in this case, are an expression of ankylosis with complete disappearance of the joint space and occasionally bony bridging between the mandibular fossa and the head of the mandible.

7   Fracture of the Mandible

A 23-year-old man was seen in the emergency department shortly after a car accident. His car was struck broadside by another car just after he entered an intersection near his home. His head impacted violently against the door frame. He regained consciousness in the ambulance, but he could not close his mouth or speak clearly. The pain in the left side of his jaw is intense and blood-stained saliva drools from his lips.

EXAMINATION

Oral examination in the emergency department reveals a malocclusion with a steplike deformity of the mandibular teeth in the left canine area. There is evidence of hemorrhage from a tear in the mucoperiosteum. A hematoma is beginning to form in the floor of the mouth, medial to the tear. Gentle bimanual examination reveals abnormal mobility of the left part of body of the mandible, which is quite painful even when slight pressure is applied. There is circumscribed tenderness in the left mandibular canine region. When the patient attempts to bring his teeth together, the left posterior portion of the mandible is displaced medially and superiorly. There is anesthesia and numbness over the left side of the chin and left lower lip near the midline.

Radiographic examination reveals a break in the continuity of the mandible between the left canine and second premolar teeth

posterior to the mental foramen. There is displacement of the fragments as described previously. The first left lower premolar is miss-
ing and presumably was avulsed by the blow.

DIAGNOSIS

Left-sided fracture of the body of the mandible with displacement of
the fragments is diagnosed.

THERAPY AND FURTHER COURSE

The patient receives a general anesthetic although regional anesthesia by means of an inferior alveolar nerve (mandibular) block
would have been effective as well. What is the site of this block, and
why would it be effective? The mandibular block is performed by
injecting an anesthetic near the mandibular foramen. This is the
method dentists commonly use to anesthetize the mandibular teeth
for dental procedures on the mandibular teeth because it blocks the
inferior alveolar nerve before this nerve enters the mandible.

After the anesthesia takes effect, the oral surgeon drills holes on
either side of the fracture line near the inferior border of the mandible. A stainless steel wire is placed across the fracture line through
the holes. This loop of wire is twisted and tightened, thus reducing
the displacement of the osseous fragments. The teeth are placed into
proper position of occlusion and held there by interdental wiring
between the mandibular teeth anterior and posterior to the fracture
and also between corresponding maxillary and mandibular teeth.
The jaw is immobilized for about six weeks to allow osseous callus to
develop and unite the fragments. Antibiotics are also prescribed to
avoid infection of the bone. Follow-up study shows healing of the
fracture in good position and alignment as well as normal function.

DISCUSSION

Site and typical displacement of fractures

With the exception of the nasal bone, fractures of the mandible
occur more frequently than any other bone in the skull. They make
up about two thirds of all facial fractures (common in fistfights as well

as automobile accidents). Seventy-three percent of these fractures occur in men. Fractures just posterior to the mental foramen, as in this case, are rather common. Other favorite sites that predispose to fractures are areas of structural weakness, such as the region of the incisive fossa near the symphysis, the angle of the mandible, and the neck of the mandible. A look at the structure of the mandible as it appears on cross section at various levels is indicated (Fig. 7-1). The mandible, the heaviest and strongest bone of the head, consists of spongy or cancellous bone surrounded by heavy compact bone on its outer (buccal) and inner (lingual) surfaces as well as on its lower border, where the compact bone is particularly well developed. The mandibular canal, which transmits the important inferior alveolar nerve and blood vessels of the lower jaw, passes through the spongy inner part with only a thin protective shell of dense bone around it.

As in most cases of fracture of the mandible, the fracture is compound, extending through an alveolus (tooth socket) and the mucosa of the oral cavity and, therefore, into a contaminated area, the oral cavity. This is the reason for the application of antibiotics in the patient. Oral surgeons generally regard the danger of osseous infection from the oral cavity as minimal unless there are teeth in the line of fracture. In these instances, traumatic disruption of the blood supply to the pulp results in an infarction of the pulpal tissue. The tooth may develop an apical abscess that is followed in many cases by osteomyelitis (inflammation of the bone marrow and adjacent bone).

What determines displacement of the fragments in fractures of the mandible and, therefore, the malocclusion? Important factors in all fractures are the direction of the initial force, the structure of the bone at the site of the fracture, and, most significantly, the traction of the muscles that attach to the fragments. Our case report states that the posterior fragment was displaced upward and medially. The muscles responsible for this misalignment are the masseter, medial pterygoid, and temporalis muscles, all three of which are elevators of the mandible, a function that can be deduced from their origins and insertions. The medial pterygoid, which is directed downward and laterally from its origin to insertion, accounts for the medial displacement. On the other hand, the anterior fragment of the mandible is displaced by the action of the digastric, geniohyoid, and, minimally, the mylohyoid muscles. All of these pull the anterior part of the body of the mandible downward toward the hyoid bone when the latter is in a fixed position (Fig. 7-2).

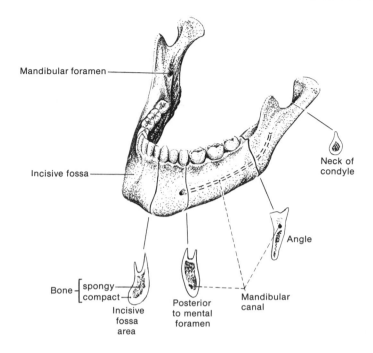

Mandibular foramen

Incisive fossa

Neck of
condyle

Angle

Bone $\left[\begin{array}{l}\text{spongy}\\\text{compact}\end{array}\right.$

Incisive
fossa
area

Posterior
to mental
foramen

Mandibular
canal

Figure 7-1. Mandible as it appears on cross section (1) at the incisive fossa, (2) posterior to the mental foramen, (3) at the angle, and (4) at the neck of the condyle.

Arterial supply of the mandible

Because the fracture intersected the mandibular canal, it interrupted the continuity of the inferior alveolar vessels. In our case this was borne out by a considerable hemorrhage at the site of the fracture and the developing hematoma in the floor of the mouth.

The inferior alveolar artery, a branch of the first part of the maxillary artery, enters the mandible through the mandibular foramen (Fig. 7-3). It traverses the mandibular canal to the mental foramen and divides into its two terminal branches, the larger mental and the smaller incisive arteries. In its course through the mandibular canal, it gives off dental branches to the roots of the lower teeth. These branches enter the pulp cavity as minute vessels through the apices of the roots. Other branches supply alveolar septa, adjacent bone, the periodontal ligaments, and then terminate in the gingiva. The incisive branch anastomoses with the incisive artery of the other side. The mental (L. mentum, chin) branch passes through the mental foramen to emerge under the skin and anastomoses with its partner on the other side and also with labial branches on the same side.

Fortunately, the anastomoses of the inferior alveolar artery with branches of the labial, buccal, and submental arteries and their counterparts on the opposite side are rich; so the ample blood supply not only discourages infection but also promotes healing of the fracture. For this reason, it is advisable to avoid extensive manipulation of the fragments, which might further traumatize the tissues and blood vessels.

Healing of the fracture by callus formation is dependent on a sufficient blood supply to the mandible, where the blood vessels have been torn. As the resulting hematoma organizes, blood vessels proliferate and are transformed into small arteries for the supply of

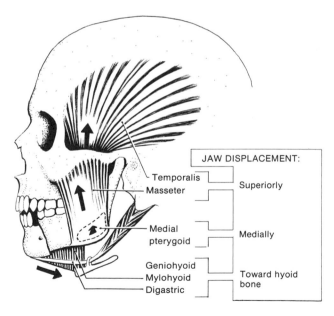

Figure 7-2. Displacement of the fractured manibular body caused by the contraction of attached muscles. The temporalis and masseter pull the mandible superiorly; the medial pterygoid pulls the mandible medially; and the geniohyoid, digastric, and mylohyoid pull it toward the hyoid bone.

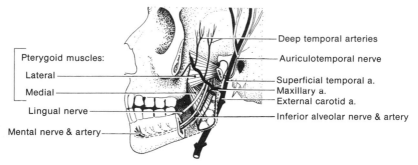

Figure 7-3. Lateral view of the arterial and nerve supply of the mandible.
Note the inferior alveolar artery and nerve in the mandibular canal.

the callus, periosteum, cortex, and spongy portion of bone. The
callus passes through various stages, from soft connective tissue into
spongy and finally dense bone, which is heavily calcified. The described healing process generally takes several months, which is the
reason for the total immobilization of the jaws in the stage of callus
formation.

Sensory nerve supply to the mandible

Interference with the sensory nerve supply has taken place in this
case, indicated by the anesthesia and numbness around the chin and
anterior portion of the lower lip. The inferior alveolar nerve from the
mandibular division of the trigeminal nerve (V_3) has been interrupted. More important than the anesthesia around the mouth is the
deficiency in the nerve supply to the anterior teeth (i.e., the incisors
and canine). Loss of sensory nerve supply may result in a devitalized
tooth. The inferior alveolar nerve follows the inferior alveolar artery
in its course through the mandibular canal (Fig. 7-3). It provides
dental branches that form plexuses in the bone like the corresponding arteries. These supply the molar and premolar teeth by fine
fibers that enter the pulp cavity through the apices of the root canals.
Interdental branches supply the adjacent alveolar bone, periodontal
ligament, and gingiva. As with the artery, the terminal incisive
nerve continues the direction of the inferior alveolar nerve and supplies the canine and incisor teeth, their alveolar septa, and the labial

aspect of the gingiva. The mental nerve continues through the mental foramen to supply the chin and anterior lower lip.

During the healing process, slow regeneration of the nerve within the mandibular canal takes place starting from the proximal stump of the interrupted nerve; this may take many months for complete regeneration. Other nerves, such as fibers from the gingival portions of the buccal and lingual nerves, contribute to recovery of the sensory innervation and, after some time, no sensory defect can be detected in the supply of teeth, skin, and mucosa.

8   Tracheostomy

Deeply troubled parents bring their 11-month-old infant daughter to the emergency department of the hospital with a history of cough of two days' duration and noisy respiratory efforts. The infant seems to struggle for air and appears quite frightened.

EXAMINATION

On examination, the patient's face, and particularly the lips, display bluish discoloration (cyanosis), the nostrils dilate with every breath, and the child struggles for air. In breathing, the accessory muscles of respiration are also used. The infant has a rapid pulse and a temperature of 101° F. From time to time, she has noisy coughing spells. The throat and larynx appear red and inflamed. On auscultation, coarse *rales* (abnormal respiratory sounds) are heard over the chest.

DIAGNOSIS

The patient has acute inflammation of the upper respiratory passages, including the trachea and bronchi, with swelling of the mucosa, resulting in partial obstruction of the air passages.

THERAPY AND FURTHER COURSE

The infant is placed in a steam tent to create a highly humid environment, and medication induces expectoration to expel the mucus blocking her airway. The infant becomes more restless and her cyanotic discoloration increases. She has an anxious expression and seems to become more exhausted and weaker. The infant is therefore sent to the operating room and prepared for tracheostomy.

Local anesthetic is applied to the site of the projected incision. The patient's head is fully extended by placing a sandbag under her shoulders. A nurse is stationed at the head of the table to ensure that rotation of the infant's head is avoided. A transverse incision is made one finger breadth above the jugular (suprasternal) notch and is about 3 cm long. This incision passes through the skin, superficial fascia, platysma, and investing layer of the deep cervical fascia. These structures are widely retracted to give ample access to the area. All superficial veins encountered in the field are ligated and divided. The fascia over the infrahyoid muscles is incised from the thyroid cartilage to the jugular notch of the sternum, and the infrahyoid muscles are retracted laterally. The isthmus of the thyroid gland is pulled superiorly. The pretracheal fascia is incised, and the second, third, and fourth tracheal cartilages are identified and divided in the midline together with the mucosal lining of the trachea (Fig. 8-1). The margins of the tracheal incision are spread apart by hooks, and the opening in the trachea (tracheostomy) is enlarged. A mucous plug is expelled spontaneously through the opening in the trachea. The infant takes a deep breath followed by a deep sigh. A tracheostomy tube is then inserted. The upper and lower ends of the subcutaneous incision are closed by sutures. The tracheostomy tube is held in place by a loose tape around the neck. The margins of the skin wound and the area around the tube are covered with moist gauze dressings.

The infant is placed in an oxygen tent, and the air is humidified to keep the mucous membrane of the trachea moist and to prevent secretions from drying. The inner tube of the tracheostomy tube is removed and cleaned frequently, and suction of the trachea is employed to aspirate mucus. Antibiotics are given. Within the next ten days, the respiratory infection subsides. Before removal of the tracheostomy tube, the lumen of the tube is obstructed in stages by being gradually plugged over a three-day period, using first a stopper obstructing only 50 percent of the lumen and then a full plug. The child is discharged as cured.

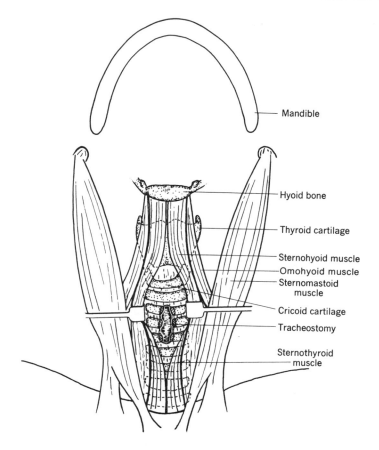

Figure 8-1. Site of the tracheostomy in the second, third, and fourth tracheal cartilages. Notice the structures in the midline above the tracheostomy site. Infrahyoid muscles are retracted.

DISCUSSION

We are dealing here with an infant in severe respiratory distress. What is the explanation for the cyanosis, particularly noticeable on the lips? The cyanosis is due to insufficient oxygenation of blood in the lungs and can be most easily detected by inspection of the lips, where a translucent epithelium covers a rich network of blood vessels.

What accessory muscles of respiration are used in case of respiratory difficulties? In dyspnea (shortness of breath), the auxiliary muscles of respiration are called into action to add their strength to the normal muscular and mechanical elements. These affect breathing by alternating changes in the superoinferior, transverse and anteroposterior diameters of the chest. In forced inspiration the scalene and sternocleidomastoid muscles stabilize and elevate the first rib and clavicle, respectively. The serratus anterior and pectoralis major and minor muscles increase the capacity of the thorax by elevating the ribs to which they attach, with the shoulder girdle and arms fixed by the action of other muscles. In doing so, the customary origins and insertions are reversed.

The inspiratory widening of the nasal opening in this case is an indication that all available muscles are called on to assist in breathing. In forced expiration maximal contraction of the abdominal muscles is called into play to enhance the action of the normal expulsive forces.

Tracheostomy is the surgical formation of an artificial opening in the trachea. Tracheostomy is indicated in this case to establish an open airway in the presence of inflammatory laryngeal obstruction and to evacuate tracheobronchial secretions that block the windpipe further down.

What is the purpose of fully extending the neck at the time of surgery? Will the normal curve of the cervical part of the vertebral column be enhanced or decreased by this maneuver? Why is close attention given to avoiding rotation of the head and neck?

The advantages of full extension of the neck include lengthening the trachea (which is pulled upward from the mediastinum), forward displacement of the trachea into the operative field by the increased anterior convexity of the cervical portion of the vertebral column, and tensing of the skin and fascia, which facilitates a clean-cut incision. Straightening the neck will line up the superior notch of the thyroid cartilage, trachea, and jugular notch of the sternum in a straight line for better identification of the trachea. On the other hand, rotation of the head and neck, particularly under emergency conditions, leads to displacement of the trachea and may induce the operator to miss the trachea entirely and insert the tracheostomy tube into the lax paratracheal connective tissue.

Cervical fascia encountered in tracheostomy

Besides the superficial fascia, which may contain fair amounts of subcutaneous fat, what fascial layers are encountered in this operation? With the exception of the superficial fascia (subcutaneous layer), all fascial layers present in the anterior triangle of the neck are derivatives of the deep fascia of the neck. The first fascial layer that is incised in approaching the trachea, after skin and superficial fascia have been retracted, is the investing layer of the deep cervical fascia. This layer bridges the anterior triangle as a sheet with offshoots that surround the infrahyoid muscles. The investing layer of the deep cervical fascia splits inferiorly to attach to both anterior and posterior aspects of the manubrium of the sternum, thus forming a suprasternal space that extends upward for a variable distance. It is therefore frequently opened in tracheostomy. What are the contents of this suprasternal space? Along with fat and possibly some lymph nodes, it contains an important anastomosis between the right and left anterior jugular veins, often called the jugular arch vein.

Identify the two pairs of infrahyoid muscles that are closest to the midline in the area of the operation and that must be retracted. Which of these muscle pairs almost reaches the midline just above the jugular notch of the sternum? The sternohyoid is the more superficial, and the sternothyroid is the deeper, but it is the sternothyroid muscles that converge from the thyroid cartilage to the midline at the site of their attachment to the posterior surface of the manubrium and thus make the operative field narrow if a low tracheostomy is undertaken (Fig. 8-1).

The next fascial layer that must be divided is the pretracheal fascia, another part of the deep cervical fascia. It covers the larynx and trachea and forms a sheath for the thyroid gland. It continues inferiorly behind the sternum into the mediastinum.

Landmarks in the midline

With the cutting of the pretracheal fascia, the level of the trachea has been reached, and it is now time to review the important landmarks in the infrahyoid part of the midline of the neck. Identify these on yourself by palpation, and with the help of a mirror point them out, passing from superior tő inferior.

The hyoid bone is a subcutaneous structure that can be easily felt below the mandible and above the larynx. It is somewhat moveable from side to side. Inferior to the hyoid bone and connected to it by the thyrohyoid membrane is the thyroid cartilage, which is characterized by the laryngeal prominence in the midline, the "Adam's apple," with the laminae of the thyroid cartilage on each side of the prominence. They form the superior thyroid notch just superior to the prominence. Inferior to the thyroid cartilage we palpate the arch of the cricoid cartilage. Connecting these two cartilages in the midline is the strong cricothyroid ligament. Below the cricoid cartilage are the tracheal rings, which give the trachea its corrugated surface. Partly masking the trachea in the midline is the isthmus of the thyroid, which usually overlaps the second and third and sometimes the fourth tracheal rings. The trachea recedes as it descends toward the mediastinum, and in the adult lies at about a depth of 4 cm from the surface at the superior border of the manubrium.

In infants the neck is, of course, very short so that the field of operation is quite small. The isthmus of the thyroid gland can be easily dislodged by retracting it upward or downward and snipping through the loose fibrous tissue that attaches it to the trachea. It can also be bisected and the parts retracted after ligation of bleeding vessels.

Larynx, trachea, and esophagus

If the site of tracheostomy is not properly identified by palpation, tracheostomy may be done too far superiorly. In that case, the cricoid and even the thyroid cartilages may be damaged, and laryngeal stenosis and severe interference with the voice may result.

Are the cartilaginous rings of the trachea complete, or are they deficient in some portion of their circumference? The approximately twenty rings of hyaline cartilage, which form the supporting framework of the trachea, occupy only two thirds of the tracheal circumference; they are U-shaped and open posteriorly. The membranous portion of the trachea, consisting of fibrous connective tissue and smooth muscle, closes this gap posteriorly.

Does the absence of firm cartilage from the posterior wall of the trachea have any bearing on the complications of tracheostomy? What organ lies in contact with the posterior aspect of the trachea, with only a small amount of areolar tissue intervening? The posterior membranous portion of the trachea may be perforated, particularly in emergency operations, and a tracheoesophageal communication may be established. This accident is frequently fatal, as milk and solid food may be aspirated into the lung through this fistula, causing an aspiration pneumonia. This complication is more apt to occur in infants because of their small tracheas, the diameter of which may be still further reduced by the protrusion of the anterior esophageal wall into the lumen of the trachea during swallowing and coughing spells. In small children, under emergency conditions, even the anterior surface of the vertebral column located just posterior to the esophagus has been injured by the knife of the surgeon.

Recent procedures concerned with disaster care of older children and adults encourage establishing an artificial airway through the cricothyroid membrane as a lifesaving operation under adverse and catastrophic conditions. The procedure is termed cricothyrotomy. If this pathway is used, is there the same danger of posterior perforation regarding the cricoid cartilage? The cricoid cartilage, located immediately above the beginning of the trachea, is a closed ring, which has a large cartilaginous plate posteriorly, the cricoid lamina, protecting the esophagus at this level against perforation.

Complications of tracheostomy

One of the most troublesome and occasionally fatal complications of tracheostomy, particularly when done under emergency conditions, is hemorrhage from veins and arteries. Because it is one of the prime requirements of an orderly tracheostomy to stay in the midline, the first question that arises is: Are there blood vessels of any size in the midline that may be endangered?

The following structures are noteworthy (Fig. 8-2):

1. The communication between the anterior jugular veins that crosses the midline within the suprasternal space has been mentioned previously.
2. The left brachiocephalic vein is apt to be located above the jugular notch in infants and children and may cause technical difficulties and severe complications in low tracehostomy.
3. The inferior thyroid vein, instead of being paired, may be unpaired, and the right and left veins may unite to form a single large vein that runs in the midline and generally drains into the left brachiocephalic vein.

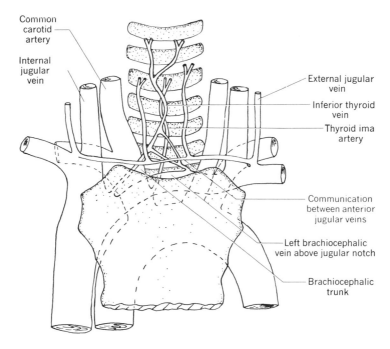

Common carotid artery

Internal jugular vein

External jugular vein

Inferior thyroid vein

Thyroid ima artery

Communication between anterior jugular veins

Left brachiocephalic vein above jugular notch

Brachiocephalic trunk

Figure 8-2. Potential sites of blood vessel injuries in tracheostomy as listed in text.

4. In 10 percent of all persons, an additional artery to the thyroid gland arises from either the brachiocephalic trunk, the arch of the aorta, or the right common carotid artery. It is named the lowest thyroid, or thyroid ima (lowest) artery, and it can be quite large. It may ascend in the midline in front of the trachea on its way to the thyroid gland and may complicate the operation.
5. Rarely, the brachiocephalic trunk may ascend above the jugular notch and be endangered in the operation.
6. It is difficult to conceive, and only understandable if emergency conditions in a very restless, suffocating child are visualized, that the common carotid artery, the internal jugular vein, or the recurrent laryngeal nerve may be injured. Such cases have been reported.

It should always be remembered that the brachiocephalic veins are cervical structures in infants and occupy a position of considerable danger, especially if they are distended as a result of intra-thoracic pathology. The cupola, dome of the cervical pleura, reaches upward above the clavicle and comes into the surgical field if the surgeon strays laterally from the midline. A resultant pneumothorax should be suspected when respiratory distress occurs after insertion of the tracheostomy tube.

What large muscle protects the common carotid artery and internal jugular vein in front and prevents their injury in tracheos-tomy? The sternocleidomastoid muscle overlies and protects the carotid sheath and its contents. It should, of course, be realized that under proper operating room conditions, venous hemorrhage and bleeding from an injured thyroid ima artery can be controlled by ligation of the damaged vessel without further consequences to the patient.

In infants a large thymus may protrude into the neck in front of the trachea and cause some operative difficulties in low tracheos-tomy. Moreover, the neck in infants is relatively short, and the trachea is softer, more mobile, and quite small (no larger than a pencil) so that the esophagus and adjacent blood vessels are readily endangered by the surgeon's knife.

If the skin is closed too tightly around the tracheostomy tube, expired air may be forced into the tissues of the neck, causing a subcutaneous accumulation of air (emphysema) in the loose tissue of the cervical region. It is anatomically possible for this air to leak gradually downward into the mediastinum and cause circulatory embarrassment by compressing the large vessels of the mediasti-num? The loose connective tissue of the neck continues into the mediastinum in so-called fascial spaces, which are spaces bound by the various layers of the deep cervical fascia, so that penetration of the air into the mediastinum is a frequent complication of cervical emphysema. If mediastinal emphysema is disregarded and remains untreated, the air may rupture into the pleural cavity and cause filling of the pleural sac (pneumothorax). If this happens on both sides, it may quickly become disastrous. Infection may likewise travel from the site of the tracheostomy down into the mediastinum and cause serious complications.

It should be realized that an emergency tracheostomy has up to five times as many complications as an elective procedure in the operating room and should be done only as a last-resort, life-saving measure. Cricothyrotomy is now preferred under such dire conditions. Even elective tracheostomy is done less frequently now and has been replaced in many cases by modern, more sophisticated procedures, such as nasopharyngeal catheterization of the trachea and endotracheal intubation.

9   Anatomy of Hanging

Thirty-five years ago, a murderer in the first degree was sentenced to death by hanging. After all legal appeals were exhausted, the murderer was taken to the gallows and prepared for hanging. His hands and feet were tightly secured. The knot of the noose was fixed in front of the angle of the left half of the mandible. The murderer dropped from the scaffold through a trap door. The torso and limbs convulsed violently for several minutes. The face could not be observed because it was covered by a hood. The pulse first slowed, then became weaker and faster and very irregular, until heart action stopped 13 min after the trap had been sprung. The prisoner was pronounced dead by the prison physician.

EXAMINATION

The autopsy showed fractures through the arch of the second cervical vertebra on both sides (Fig. 9-1). The body of the second vertebra was separated from that of the third vertebra and the disc between them had been torn. One could easily visualize that, with the weight of the body pulling at the site of the separated disk, there would be an inferior displacement of the remainder of the vertebral column. The spinal cord was severed at the same level as the fracture/dislocation. Other findings of significance were tears in the intima of the carotid arteries.

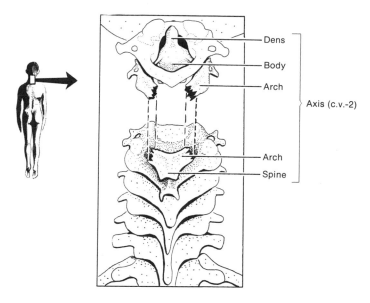

Figure 9-1. "Hangman's fracture," caused by a long drop. Note the fracture/dislocation of both sides of the arch of the second cervical vertebra with separation (up to 2½ inches) of the second vertebra from the third. Body and dens of the axis stay with the atlas and occiput, but the posterior portion of the arch and the spinous process of the axis are displaced inferiorly with the third cervical vertebra.

MEDICAL EXAMINER'S CONCLUSION

Death was by hanging and due to fracture/dislocation of the second cervical vertebra with severance of the spinal cord.

DISCUSSION

Severance of the spinal cord

To achieve quick death by snapping the vertebral column and cord and yet avoid decapitation, two things are of prime importance: the length of the drop and the position of the knot. The former depends on the weight of the person being hanged. The greater the weight, the shorter the drop. British sources recommend a minimum drop of

8 feet for a person of about 200 pounds, and this has been adopted in the United States; however, other sources recommend drops of 6 to 15 feet. At one time, German authorities preferred shorter drops, pointing out the chances of decapitation from long drops. The other equally important factor is the position of the knot, which should be on the left side of the jaw close to the chin. This location of the knot and the powerful pull of the weight of the body in conjunction with the long drop tend to thrust the head backward forcefully and abruptly. It results in a fracture/dislocation of the cervical part of the vertebral column, severing the spinal cord at the same time.

Just where along the cervical portion of the vertebral column does this fracture/dislocation usually take place? The common answer given in older textbooks of anatomy and forensic medicine is that death is due to rupture of the transverse ligament of the atlas. This rupture presumably allows the dens (odontoid process) of the axis to tilt backward and, in conjunction with the posterior dislocation of the atlas, to crush the spinal cord; however, this is now regarded as an "old wives' tale." The joints between the atlas and occiput and the atlas and axis are so strong that dislocation occurs infrequently at those levels. In addition, the cruciform (cruciate) ligament, of which the transverse ligament of the atlas is the strong horizontal part, and the tectorial membrane, an upward extension of the posterior longitudinal ligament, strengthen the previously mentioned joints.

Autopsy findings and radiographs of the victims of more modern judicial hanging show bilateral fractures of either the pedicles or the laminae of the arch of the second, third, or fourth cervical vertebra with dislocation of the second on the third or the third on the fourth vertebra. Accessory ligaments, including the anterior and posterior longitudinal ligaments, as well as the dura mater, are often torn at the level of fracture/dislocation.

Traffic accidents can cause a similar fracture of the vertebral column, described in the literature as "hangman's fracture." One difference is that, in the traffic victim, the cord may be only slightly damaged because there is little or no pull caused by the weight of the body. In the typical "hangman's fracture" of the axis, its body and dens remain attached to the intact atlas and occiput by ligaments. The separated posterior portion of the arch keeps its relationship to the third vertebra; however, it is often separated from the anterior fragment by a distance up to 2 1/2 inches (Fig. 9-1), which explains the severance of the cord at this level and may also be the cause of injury to the brain at a higher level, that is, between the medulla oblongata and pons. The dislocation part of this injury occurs most commonly in the joint between the bodies of the second and third cervical vertebrae.

Asphyxiation

Tearing of the spinal cord with the fracture/dislocation of cervical vertebrae is not the only cause of death in judicial hanging. Many cases have been described in the literature, particularly in Europe, in which death was brought about by asphyxiation resulting from occlusion of the air passages (Fig. 9-2). Asphyxiation is the principal cause of death in suicidal and accidental hanging and, although this case study is primarily concerned with judicial hanging, the anatomy of hanging in general is of considerable forensic importance.

Execution with a drop of less than 6 feet, in most cases, results in death due to asphyxia by strangulation. Interruption of the air passages in such cases is caused by fracture of the larynx, traumatic

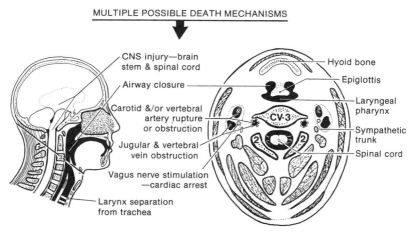

MULTIPLE POSSIBLE DEATH MECHANISMS

CNS injury—brain stem & spinal cord

Airway closure

Carotid &/or vertebral artery rupture or obstruction

Jugular & vertebral vein obstruction

Vagus nerve stimulation —cardiac arrest

Larynx separation from trachea

Hyoid bone

Epiglottis

Laryngeal pharynx

Sympathetic trunk

Spinal cord

CV-3

Figure 9-2. Oblique section through the hyoid bone and intervertebral disk between cervical vertebrae two and three, corresponding to the level of the noose in the short drop. Notice the position of the (1) laryngeal pharynx, (2) common carotid artery, (3) internal jugular vein, (4) vagus nerve, (5) sympathetic trunk, and (6) vertebral artery.

separation of the larynx from the trachea, or forceful separation of the upper portion of the trachea from the lower portion. In no reported case was there a fracture of the atlas or the dens of the axis. Fracture of other cervical vertebrae were rare exceptions; the spinal cord remained intact.

Midline placement of the strangling knot often causes occlusion of the pharynx by posterior displacement of the base of the tongue and soft palate against the posterior pharyngeal wall and vertebral column. This blocks the entrance of air into the larynx, trachea, and lungs, with death due to asphyxia.

Blocking of the arteries of the head

Death can also be caused by obstruction of the arterial flow to the brain by compression of the common carotid arteries within the carotid sheaths (Fig. 9-2), which leads to loss of consciousness within a few seconds as a result of anoxia of the brain. The autopsy in the present case study showed fine tears of the intima of the carotid arteries. In general, these tears are located just inferior to the division of the common carotid into its two terminal branches, the external and internal carotids. Injuries to the carotid arteries may include massive rupture with profuse hemorrhage into the adjacent tissues, including the cervical musculature. What are the other paired arteries that also conduct blood to the brain? The paired vertebral arteries also supply the brain after they enter the foramen magnum. They may be occluded or ruptured at the level of the cervical fracture in the hanging.

Obstruction of the veins of the head

Of the blood vessels draining the head, the internal jugular veins are the main channels transporting blood from the brain (Fig. 9-2). They lie lateral to the carotid arteries within the carotid sheaths and are rather thin-walled and easily compressed. Their obstruction may be responsible for the frequently observed edema of the brain and the fine petechiae (hemorrhages) within its substance. The other major pathways of venous drainage from the brain, the vertebral veins, may also be injured, particularly in the long drop when vertebral fracture and snapping of the spinal cord occur. Conjunctival petechiae, caused by obstruction of ophthalmic veins, have also been noted in autopsies of hanged people.

The importance of occlusion of the blood vessels as the cause of death is clearly evident in a case of suicide by hanging of a patient with a tracheostomy, in whom the air supply to the lungs obviously was not interfered with by the strangulating rope. At autopsy the blood vessels of the brain, including those to the vital centers, were found to be heavily engorged with blood.

Pressure on the nerves in the neck

The third important component within the carotid sheath, the vagus nerve, has also been implicated in death by hanging. The vagus nerve may be compressed by the sudden tightening of the noose (Fig. 9-2), which may cause inhibition of heart action accompanied by an instantaneous sharp drop in blood pressure and cardiac arrest; but this is not common. Tearing of the vagus occurs only if the long drop results in actual severance of the head from the neck, an accident that has happened on several occasions of judicial hanging. This case showed the often observed initial slowing of the heart beat, an indication of vagal irritation. The acceleration of the heart beat, as occurred next in this case, may have been due to vagal paralysis.

The site of placement of the noose coincides with the location of the carotid body and sinus, which are located at or close to the bifurcation of the common carotid artery. This neurovascular complex is formed mainly by afferent fibers from the glossopharyngeal nerve and by fibers from the vagus and the sympathetic system. Pressure on the sinus by the constricting noose causes slowing of the pulse rate and lowering of blood pressure. Just the pull of the carotid arteries by the drop of the body could activate the carotid sinus reflexes. Several authors have contended that these reflexes are frequently responsible for sudden cardiac arrest noted in some instances. Unevenness or narrowing of the pupils is frequently observed in hanged subjects, possibly resulting from pressure on the cervical sympathetic trunks, which traverse the neck behind the carotid sheaths posterior and lateral to the cervical viscera; in this location, they are as vulnerable as the contents of the sheath itself (Fig. 9-2).

Unconsciousness, convulsions, and time of death

We know by the continuing heart action of the condemned, after the drop from the gallows, that death does not occur immediately. One might ask whether the victim remains conscious. All authorities seem to agree that loss of consciousness—and therefore loss of sensitivity to pain—takes place instantaneously, probably due to shock of the brain caused by the sudden jolt of the head at the end of the long drop.

For how long is the executed person aware of painful stimuli, and when, as a rule, does death occur? The duration of physical suffering remains essentially a matter of conjecture, but all evidence indicates loss of consciousness is almost instantaneous.

Death, on the other hand, is delayed from 8 to 20 min after the trap has been sprung if death is defined as permanent cessation of heart action. Particularly upsetting and a source of great distress to witnesses are the signs of life and struggle in the executed person after unconsciousness has set in. Actions such as twitching, convulsions of limbs and trunk, and violent respiratory movements of the thorax are observed and are of reflex nature.

In suicidal and accidental hanging, the time that the victim is aware of painful stimuli and when death occurs must remain even more a matter of conjecture. In some instances, the body has not been fully suspended; the feet may be touching the floor or the victim may be leaning against a wall or lying in bed. In these situations death may be due to asphyxia, but it is more than likely caused by several contributing causes: blocking the carotids, obstructing the internal jugular veins, pressure on the vagus nerves, and pressure on the carotid bodies and sinuses. Therefore, physical suffering may be extended over many minutes, ending with loss of consciousness and death by suffocation.

ADDENDUM

Execution by hanging is an ancient practice. Methods of suspending the body have varied. After a noose is draped around the offender's neck, he may be forced to stand on a gallows and dropped through a trapdoor, to stand on a ladder that is jerked away by the executioner, or to stand on a cart that is then driven away. The latter method was employed in military hangings and in vigilante hangings of scoundrels depicted in movies of the "old American West." The term "kicked the bucket" comes from the suicidal hanging done by a person who kicks away a supporting bucket to achieve the drop.

At the end of 1992, four states—Montana, New Hampshire, Delaware, and Washington—still used hanging as an alternative to lethal injection for capital punishment. Presumably, all states originally used it because electrocution was developed as means of execution only in the nineteenth century.

10   Torticollis

A five-year-old girl is brought to the pediatrician by her mother with the complaint that since early childhood the right side of her neck has been twisted and deformed. On inquiry, the mother states that childbirth was prolonged and difficult and that delivery took place with buttocks presenting first (breech delivery). Within a few weeks after her daughter's birth, the mother noticed a spindle-shaped swelling over the right side of the infant's neck which was very tender on touch and on passive movement of the head. During the next few months the swelling and tenderness over the area gradually subsided. Later, when the child was about one year old, the large muscle at the right side of the neck appeared cordlike. Gradually and progressively, the neck became stiff and deformed with the head tilted toward the right side and the face turned toward the left. The face also became asymmetrical (Fig. 10-1).

EXAMINATION

On examination, the child appears somewhat underdeveloped and poorly nourished. On request the child is unable to straighten her head, even with the assistance of the examiner. In moving the head, the right sternocleidomastoid muscle appears contracted and transformed into a fibrous cord. The head is drawn toward the right shoulder; the chin is elevated and points toward the left. The facial asymmetry consists of shortening of the skull and face on the right

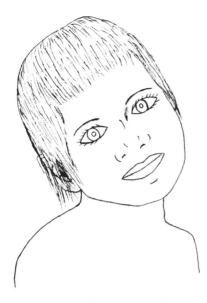

Figure 10-1. Right-sided torticollis in a young girl. Notice that the head is drawn toward the right shoulder, and the elevated chin points to the left.

side in an anteroposterior direction, a flattening of the lateral aspect of the face, and an uneven level of the eyes. Further examination and radiographs reveal that the patient has a left convex scoliosis in the lower cervical and upper thoracic regions and a compensatory right convex scoliosis in the middle and lower thoracic regions.

DIAGNOSIS

Congenital wry-neck or torticollis (twisted neck) is diagnosed.

THERAPY AND FURTHER COURSE

In view of the long duration of the condition, surgery is decided on. With the patient under general anesthesia, the platysma and the investing layer of the deep cervical fascia over the sterno-cleidomastoid muscle are divided. The muscle is seen to be transformed into a dense, fibrous band. The fibrotic muscle with its two heads is then excised, with attention given to avoiding injury to the underlying accessory nerve and the major vessels deep to the muscle. The head is gradually manipulated into the correct position. The investing fascia covering the posterior aspect of the muscle also appears taut and shortened. Portions of this layer are also excised. The wound is closed. The head is kept in a splinting harness for several weeks. Active and passive stretching exercises are then carried out. When the child is seen six months later, her head is in the normal position, and there is no obvious evidence of loss of motion of the head and neck.

DISCUSSION

We are dealing here with a congenital condition that has transformed the sternocleidomastoid muscle into a cordlike, nonfunctioning muscle. By its rigidity and shortening, this cord has distorted the position of the head and neck and has brought about alterations in the growth of the face. To understand this not uncommon entity of congenital torticollis, we must realize that it is primarily confined to the sternocleidomastoid muscle. All other deformities are secondary in character and result from the abnormal position of the head.

Normal function of the sternocleidomastoid muscle

What is the normal function of the sternocleidomastoid muscle or, to use a shorter term, the sternomastoid muscle? Its function is rather complex but can be deduced from its origin and insertion. The origin of the muscle is by two heads from the front of the manubrium of the sternum and the medial third of the clavicle. The sternal head is cylindrical and quite tendinous, the clavicular head broader. The muscle takes a spiral turn around the lateral side of the neck to its insertion into the mastoid process and into the lateral half of the superior nuchal line of the occiput. Notice that the muscle at its origin faces forward, at its insertion, laterally. Consequently, the course of the muscle from its origin to its insertion is directed obliquely upward, posteriorly and laterally. The effect of the shortening and scarring of the muscle on the position of the head in our case accurately simulates one-sided contraction of the normal muscle. The muscle tilts the same side of the head downward and rotates it in such a way that the chin points upward and to the opposite side

TORTICOLLIS 79

(Figs. 10-1 and 10-2). If the purpose of one-sided contraction is simple rotation in the atlantoaxial joint around a vertical axis, without lateral bending of the head toward the shoulder, part of the effect of sternomastoid contraction can be counteracted by activation of the opposite lateral flexors of the cervical vertebral column, such as the longus capitis, semispinalis capitis and cervicis, and splenius capitis as well as the scalenus medius.

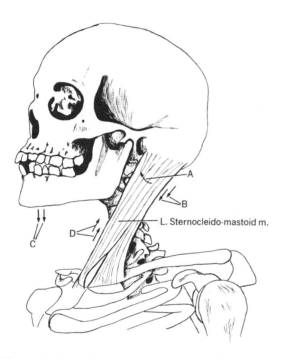

Figure 10-2. Action of sternocleidomastoid muscle. (Single arrow denotes one-sided contraction; double arrows indicate contraction of right and left muscles.) "A" refers to the motion of the left muscle in rotating the head to the right side with the chin pointing upward. In one-sided contraction, the head also is bent to the side of the muscle. "B" indicates extension of the head when both muscles are contracted. "C" indicates flexion of the head by sterocleidomastoid muscles in cooperation with flexors of the cervical spinal column. "D" shows muscles acting as accessory muscles of inspiration by raising the manubrium of the sternum when the head is fixed by other muscles.

Coming now to the combined action of both sternomastoids, it must be realized that the main portion of the insertion of the muscles is posterior to the transverse axis, passing through the two atlanto-occipital joints, and that contraction of the two muscles will therefore result in extension of the head, that is, a posterior tilt (Fig. 10-2). Other results of contraction of both muscles depend partly on the position of the head at the time of contraction and on combination with simultaneous contraction of other muscles. If, for example, the subject is lifting from the supine position, as in rising from a bed, the more anterior fibers of the muscle in front of the transverse axis will assist the flexors of the cervical vertebral column in flexing the head (Fig. 10-2). Bed-fast patients in a weakened condition are often unable to do this and need to be supported. In emaciated patients, the contracted sternomastoid muscles often stand out as they try to lift themselves from their beds.

Finally, the muscle should be regarded as an auxiliary muscle of inspiration if it acts from its insertion to the mastoid and superior nuchal line on its origin to the sternum and clavicle with the head being fixed by other muscles (Fig. 10-2). As an auxiliary muscle of inspiration, it draws the sternum and clavicle upward and with it, the ribs.

In trying to understand the action of an individual muscle, such as the sternomastoid, it must be realized that in living persons, no muscle ever contracts by itself. On the contrary, all movements, such as flexion, extension, rotation, and lateral bending of the head, require the cooperation of groups of muscles. Loss of function of one muscle is generally compensated for by the action of other muscles, which explains why our patient tolerated the excision of the muscle well. Similarly, the resection of the pectoralis major and minor muscles in radial surgery for cancer of the breast leads to surprisingly minor deficits of motion.

Nerve supply of the sternocleidomastoid muscle

The nerve supply to the sternocleidomastoid muscle originates essentially from the accessory nerve (XI) and in part also from the ventral rami of spinal nerves C2 and C3. Why must the accessory nerve be protected in surgery for torticollis if the muscle supplied by it is being excised? The accessory nerve also supplies the trapezius, which, of course, is preserved in this operation.

Causes of congenital torticollis

Various hypotheses address the cause of congenital torticollis. Many interesting applications of anatomy enter into this discussion.

Arterial supply of the muscle. A number of authors have ascribed the condition to arterial occlusion or partial interference with the arterial supply of the muscle during delivery, resulting in secondary scarring of the insufficiently nourished muscle. Actually, numerous arterial branches ramify in the muscle, and the blood supply is rather profuse. Whereas the arteries supplying the muscle show variations in their number and course, the following arteries have been given as a source of blood supply to the muscle: the posterior auricular, occipital, and superior thyroid arteries from the external carotid, a frequently mentioned direct muscular branch from the external carotid, and the transverse cervical and suprascapular arteries from the thyrocervical trunk of the subclavian artery. These arteries form a plexus within the substance of the muscle in such a way that the branches originating from the external carotid supply the superior and middle portions, and the vessels coming from the thyrocervical trunk carry blood to the lower part of the muscle. All these branches, however, communicate with each other along ascending and descending branches throughout the muscle belly. With the original sources of the arterial supply so widely separated, it is hardly conceivable that interference with one artery or a limited number of arteries during delivery can result in such widespread and diffuse degeneration.

Venous drainage of the muscle. A second cause given for congenital torticollis is venous occlusion during labor with resulting necrosis (cell death). Actually, the veins draining the muscle are even more numerous than the arteries supplying it. These veins are tributaries of all major neck veins and consist of veins accompanying the arteries mentioned previously and direct tributaries to the external, internal, and anterior jugular veins. There are broad communications between these veins, not only on the surface of the muscle but also by means of a well-developed intramuscular plexus so that the areas drained by these veins widely overlap. Other hypotheses pertaining to the cause of congenital torticollis have been offered but are similarly unconvincing.

Most plausible cause of congenital torticollis. It is interesting that about 50 percent of all cases of this disorder are breech deliveries. In light of this finding and convincing histologic changes in the muscle at the time of operation in early infancy, before maximal scarring of the muscle takes place, the most plausible explanation seems to be the following: The torticollis dates back to intrauterine malposition of the fetal head, which in a few cases has also been demonstrated in utero by imaging studies. This malposition subjects the muscle to undue pressure against the shoulder at a time when the muscle undergoes active growth and differentiation. The malposition also prevents normal entrance of the fetal head into the pelvis, resulting in breech presentation and other abnormal and prolonged types of delivery. Further trauma to the already deformed muscle at the time of birth ensues.

The later swelling of the muscle, observed in our and other cases, is the result of an inflammatory reaction to the prolonged birth trauma. Cases have been reported in the literature, however, describing torticollis as being present in infants delivered by cesarean section and thus not exposed to birth trauma.

11   Flexion-Extension
        Injury of the Neck

A 52-year-old female schoolteacher comes to her physician's office complaining of headaches, neck pain, and stiffness in the neck. These symptoms started four months ago after an automobile accident. Her car stopped at a traffic light and was struck from the rear by another car. She states that at the time of the accident she was badly shaken and developed immediate pain in the neck that radiated into both shoulders and gradually increased in intensity during the next few days. Since then, the shoulder pain has slowly diminished in intensity, but the other symptoms persist.

EXAMINATION

On examination, the patient's head is held rather rigid. Flexion, extension, and lateral rotation of head and neck cause pain and are resisted by the patient. There is some local tenderness on palpation, particularly over the area of the transverse processes of the fourth and fifth cervical vertebrae. A screening neurologic exam, including evaluation of deep tendon reflexes and plantar responses was normal. Thorough x-ray examination shows disappearance of the normal cervical lordosis. There are slight degenerative changes at the middle cervical vertebrae, with some bony spurs, particularly around the intervertebral foramina between C4 and C5; but the radiologist states that these alterations could be in keeping with the patient's age. The most important radiographic finding is the absence of any signs of fracture of the cervical vertebrae.

DIAGNOSIS

The patient has cervical syndrome due to hyperextension–hyper-flexion (whiplash) injury caused by a rear-end traffic collision.

THERAPY AND FURTHER COURSE

The patient is given a sponge rubberneck collar and told to wear it intermittently. Hot moist packs are to be applied by the patient herself at home. Muscle relaxants and sedation are prescribed, and she is cautioned not to drive her car in order to avoid sudden twisting motions of her head and neck. Under this treatment, the symptoms gradually improve, although some intermittent pain still remains but appears tolerable.

DISCUSSION

The term whiplash injury is an older term that refers to the mechanism of the trauma, not to the underlying lesion. Whiplash is used to indicate the rapid change in motion from hyperextension of the head and the upper part of the neck to hyperflexion in rear-end collisions and from extreme flexion to maximal extension in head-on collisions. The analogy to a whip refers to the more flexible upper part of the cervical spine acting as the lash, the more fixed lower portion as the handle of the whip.

The term "flexion-extension syndrome due to rear-end or head-on collision" is now preferred by most clinicians instead of whiplash injury of the neck. The broad spectrum of injuries to various tissues with possible involvement of muscles, ligaments, cartilage, bone, spinal cord, peripheral nerve structures, and blood vessels requires familiarity with the underlying anatomy.

In descending order of frequency, the tissue damage in the neck ranges from:

1. muscle strain or sprain of the cervical ligaments,
2. rupture of the ligaments and the intervertebral disks,
3. fractures of the vertebrae,
4. injury to the cervical spinal cord and emerging cervical nerves, and rarely,
5. damage of the vertebral artery with resulting interference with cerebral circulation.

Underlying anatomy of the condition

Muscular injuries.   Muscle strains in flexion–extension injuries of the neck involve the flexors of the head, such as the sternocleidomastoid, and perhaps to the rectus capitis anterior and longus capitis. Other flexors of the neck often injured are the longus colli and intertransverse muscles. Both groups of muscles lie along the anterior and anterolateral surfaces of the cervical vertebrae. The damage ranges in severity from minor tears of a few muscle fibers to partial or total avulsion (traumatic separation) of the muscular attachments to the cervical vertebrae. These injuries have been observed experimentally in anesthetized monkeys as well as clinically at the time of surgery or autopsy.

Ligamentous injuries.   Ligamentous sprains are the mildest form of neck injuries. What is a sprain? A sprain denotes a ligamentous injury with stretching of some of the fibers and tearing of others but with preservation of the continuity of the ligament. Which ligament connecting the vertebral bodies would be most likely to be sprained in forceful hyperextension of the neck and which in the opposite trauma of hyperflexion?

The thick anterior longitudinal ligament is a broad band that extends along the anterior surface of the vertebral column from the atlas to the front of the sacrum. Its more superficial fibers bridge several vertebrae, and its deeper portions extend from one vertebral body to the next. It is particularly these deeper portions of the ligament that may be stretched or torn in hyperextension injuries (Fig. 11-1).

Hyperflexion injuries may expose the posterior longitudinal ligament to undue traction. The posterior longitudinal ligament likewise extends over all vertebrae from the neck to the sacrum with its superficial fibers crossing several vertebrae and its deeper portions connecting adjacent vertebrae. The posterior longitudinal ligament attaches to the posterior aspect of the vertebral bodies in front of the spinal cord and checks extreme flexion. In this function it is assisted by the ligamenta flava, which connect the laminar portions of the vertebral arches, and the interspinal and supraspinal ligaments. The supraspinal ligaments are particularly well developed in the neck as ligamentum nuchae (ligament of the nape of the neck), which in humans forms a fibrous, intermuscular septum in the midline by

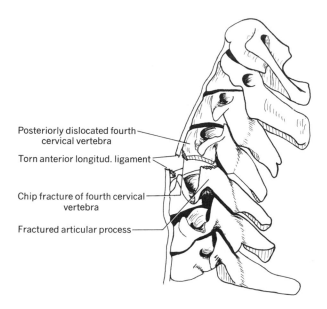

Posteriorly dislocated fourth
   cervical vertebra

Torn anterior longitud. ligament

Chip fracture of fourth cervical
   vertebra

Fractured articular process

Figure 11-1. Extensive hyperextension injury with tearing of the anterior longitudinal ligament, posterior dislocation of the fourth cervical vertebra with chip fracture of its body, and fracture of the articular process of the fifth cervical vertebra.

attaching to the bifid spinous processes. The posterior longitudinal ligament and the ligamenta flava may be stretched or torn in hyperflexion.

The reader is advised to obtain two or more adjacent cervical vertebrae and locate the anatomical structures in their proper relationship. As a substitute, the use of an anatomical atlas is recommended.

Intervertebral disk injuries.   Injury to the cervical disks in rear-end collisions is considered likely by many neurologists, although these disks are "preradiographic," generally appearing normal for some time. It is also likely that these flexion–extension injuries accelerate degenerative disk disease, which does not become apparent until new bone formation and calcification are seen years after repair of the injury.

What are the two parts of an intervertebral disk and the characteristic features of each portion? The outer ring, or the annulus fibrosus, consists of concentric layers of collagenous fiber bundles, which by their lamellar arrangement are able to withstand multidirectional strains. The centrally located nucleus pulposus consists of a soft, highly elastic, compressible, semigelatinous mass with a high water content. It acts as a shock absorber.

How does the uneven height of a given disk contribute to the normal cervical lordosis? The cervical disks are thicker anteriorly than posteriorly and thus are responsible for the forward convex curvature of the cervical vertebral column. Degenerative changes due to chronic trauma and age predispose the annulus fibrosus to rupture under severe compression and the nucleus pulposus to prolapse or herniate. This is particularly apt to occur in the neck at the level of the disks between cervical vertebrae 5 and 6 and vertebrae 7 and 8.

Spinal nerve and cord involvement. Keeping in mind that the intervertebral disk forms part of the anterior boundary of the intervertebral foramen, in what direction would the protrusion of a damaged annulus or a herniated nucleus pulposus have to occur to compress a cervical spinal nerve passing through this foramen? A posterolateral protrusion of the disk has this effect and explains the occurrence of nerve root symptoms such as shoulder pain and paresthesias (burning and tingling) in the affected dermatomes, which can be perceived as far distally as the fingers in involvement of C6 and C7. The commonly observed reflex spasm of the neck muscles with straightening of the normal curvature of the spine is another effect of nerve or nerve root irritation. Most serious is a protrusion of the disk in, or close to, the midline, leading to cervical cord compression.

Vertebral injuries and dislocation. There is a gradual transition in severity from the relatively harmless, common stretching of the anterior longitudinal ligament to its rupture, wrenching, and displacement of the disks and chip fracture of the anteroinferior corners of the vertebral bodies (Fig. 11-1). If the trauma is more destructive, the articular processes of the vertebrae may also fracture, and the upper part of the cervical vertebral column may be dislocated posteriorly with pressure on and damage to the cord. In these cases, open reduction by surgical means of is often required to remove pressure on the cord.

The intervertebral foramina and synovial joints. The intervertebral foramina in the cervical region have been called the "crossroads of neurological symptomatology." They are short canals that contain the ventral and dorsal roots and spinal ganglia within a meningeal sleeve, the recurrent meningeal nerves, the spinal arteries, and venous plexuses, all embedded in fat and connective tissue. The venous plexuses connecting the internal and external spinal veins allow blood to be expelled in movements of the cervical column, thus cushioning and protecting the nerve structures against pressure. The same holds true for the fat that is semifluid at body temperature.

Immediately posterior to the intervertebral foramina are the superior and inferior articular processes of adjacent vertebrae, forming synovial (facet) joints, which are surrounded by joint capsules (Fig. 11-2). Synovial joints are subject to many inflammatory arthritic and degenerative diseases that frequently lead to changes in joint configuration by narrowing the articulations, thickening the joint capsules, and bony spur formation (bone proliferation). These changes result in alterations in spatial relationship and encroachment on the intervertebral foramina and in hyperextension trauma expose the sensitive nerve structures within the foramina to stretching over preexisting abnormal bone formation. The presence of bony spurs adjacent to the intervertebral foramina between C4 and C5 was mentioned in this case and could partly explain the patient's symptoms.

Occasionally, a nerve root or parts of a nerve root may be caught, pincer-like, between deformed articular facets. It was mentioned previously that the intervertebral disks are an immediate anterior boundary of the intervertebral foramina and that protrusion of these disks as a result of trauma may explain the signs and symptoms of nerve involvement in disk degeneration (Fig. 11-2).

Uncovertebral joints. Another anatomical arrangement, typical only of the cervical area, has been the subject of extensive discussion in the clinical literature, although it is often ignored in anatomical texts, that is, the uncovertebral joints (lateral interbody joints, joints of Luschka). Although not true synovial joints, but apparently the result of degenerative processes starting in the cervical disks in childhood and adolescence, they give the appearance of joints. They are formed by the upward liplike projections on the superolateral

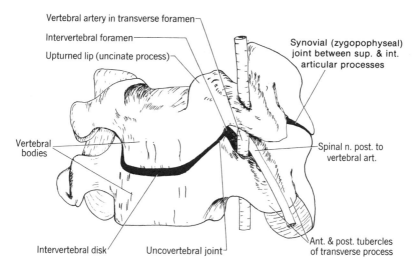

Figure 11-2. Oblique view of two articulated cervical vertebrae showing (1) anterior to the intervertebral foramen, the cartilaginous joint between vertebral bodies with the intervertebral disk and also the uncovertebral joint; and (2) posterior to the intervertebral foramen, the synovial joint between articular processes. Notice the vertebral artery passing through the transverse foramen in front of the cervical nerve that emerges from the intervertebral foramen.

surfaces of the cervical vertebral bodies (uncinate process) and corresponding beveled grooves on the inferolateral surfaces of the overlying vertebrae. These bony areas are covered with cartilage and surrounded by synovial-like capsules. The presence of these joints predisposes to disk collapse and arthritic changes with bone proliferation. They are part of the anterior boundary of the intervertebral foramina and lie in close relationship to their nerve root contents, (Fig. 11-2). Again, as with other degenerative and proliferative joint changes, superimposed trauma on these joints leads to or aggravates the clinical condition of nerve root compression.

In summary, the nerve structures within the intervertebral foramina are bounded anteriorly by the cartilaginous joints between vertebral bodies (intervertebral disks), anterolaterally by the uncovertebral joints, and posteriorly by the intervertebral synovial (facet) joints. All these articulations alter their configuration during flexion, extension, and torsion of the cervical spine and thereby encroach on the intervertebral foramina and their contents. This is particularly true in hyperextension and more so if the joints are already deformed by degenerative or proliferative bone changes. It is easily realized that the emergence of spinal nerves from the spinal canal through foramina that are bounded anteriorly and posteriorly by movable joints is conducive to injury of these nerves. How does this compare with the emergence of the cranial nerves from the skull? Here the nerves leave the cranial cavity through bony foramina that are not exposed to changing contours of their boundaries. What spinal nerves have an arrangement similar to that of the cranial nerves? The sacral nerves leave the spinal canal through sacral foramina bounded by solid bone.

Vertebral artery injury. An unusual and sometimes quite serious complication of hyperextension injury is compression of the vertebral artery as it runs through the neck. What is its course in the neck? It is the first branch of the subclavian artery and ascends through the transverse foramina of the cervical vertebrae, starting with C6 and leaving through the transverse foramen of the atlas, to enter the cranial cavity through the foramen magnum. It joins with its partner of the opposite side to form the basilar artery, which supplies the cerebellum, posterior portion of the cerebrum, and much of the brain stem. As the vertebral artery passes through the transverse foramina it lies in front of the emerging nerve roots. Hyperextension injury may occasionally traumatize the intima of the artery, particularly if its walls have become atherosclerotic and rigid, which may lead to vascular insufficiency of the posterior portions of the brain caused by a dissecting aneurysm and secondary thromboembolism. Bizarre clinical pictures, such as vertigo, ataxia (loss of muscular coordination), disturbances of vision and hearing, and temporary loss of consciousness, may result.

   Fortunately for the patient, her symptoms were transitory. They can probably be explained by a ligamentous sprain with resulting muscle spasm and some temporary injury to the cervical nerves, which may have been stretched over existing bone proliferations at levels C4 and C5.

   For more information on the vertebral artery and its collateral circulation in case of atherosclerotic obstruction, see the case study on subclavian steal syndrome (Chap. 40).

12   Central Venous Catheterization

A 45-year-old man in shock has been transferred from another hospital to the emergency department. He is experiencing epigastric pain that radiates to his back and has had protracted nausea and vomiting.

EXAMINATION

The patient appears pale and delirious. His extremities are cool, his temperature is 38.5° C, blood pressure is 70/40, heart rate is 135 beats per/min, and respiratory rate is 24/min. His lungs are clear and his heart sounds are normal except for the tachycardia. Abdominal examination reveals an absence of bowel sounds (paralysis of the intestine) and epigastric tenderness with guarding when palpated.

A plain radiograph of the abdomen shows multiple air and fluid levels within dilated loops (sentinel loops) of the small intestine overlying the splenic flexure. The patient's hemoglobin is low (12 g/dl), and his white cell count is high, 22,000//mm³). Laboratory tests show markedly elevated amylase (1,110 IU) and lipase (850 IU), normal values are 35 to 85 for amylase and 100 to 500 for lipase.

DIAGNOSIS

The patient's condition is diagnosed as hemorrhagic pancreatitis, possibly a result of a small gallstone's blockage of the main pancreatic duct where it enters the hepatopancreatic ampulla, which is the dilatation at the junction of the common bile duct and the main pancreatic duct in the medial wall of the descending part of the duodenum. Clinicians commonly call the hepatopancreatic ampulla by its eponym, ampulla of Vater.

THERAPY AND FURTHER COURSE

The emergency department physician rapidly adminsters intravenous (i.v.) fluid through a catheter placed in the right internal jugular vein, which is effective in combating the patient's hypovolemia (abnormal reduction in circulating blood volume). Central venous catheterization is chosen because the blood volume depletion had collapsed the peripheral veins. What other sites for placing catheters into the central veins are commonly used? The left internal jugular and the left and right subclavian veins are equally satisfactory for the infusion of fluids. The choice is usually based on physician's previous experience.

In the first hour the patient receives 3 L of fluid. A nurse inserts a bladder catheter, and urine output is soon adequate. The vital signs improve: blood pressure rises to 110/70, heart rate falls to 90 beats/min, and respiratory rate diminishes to 18/minute.

Cultures of blood and urine are taken. Precautionary broad spectrum antibiotics are administered through the internal jugular line. A nasogastric tube is placed and slow suction started. A computed tomograph (CT) of the abdomen demonstrates a large edematous pancreas with moderately dilated extra hepatic and intrahepatic biliary ducts. A sonogram of the right upper quadrant of the abdomen corroborates the CT findings and also shows numerous small gallstones in the gallbladder. The patient is admitted to the hospital for observation and supportive care.

The patient's condition improves the next day, but he is still experiencing epigastric pain and bloating. Bowel sounds remain absent and his amylase and lipase levels continue to be elevated. Because his course of therapy is likely to be protracted, total parenteral nutrition (TPN), the infusion of essential nutrients, is initiated. To minimize the chance of infection from the i.v. catheter (central venous line) placed by the emergency department physician, it is removed and a second central line placed in the right subclavian vein under aseptic conditions by an internist trained in central venous catheterization procedures.

The patient's health improves during the next week of hospitalization. On the fourth day, bowel sounds returned (resumption of motility) and the patient tolerates liquids administered orally. By the end of the week, he is able to eat solid food. The patient is then discharged and told that a cholecystectomy will probably be necessary in the near future to avoid recurrence of the episode from gallstone blockage of the main pancreatic duct.

DISCUSSION

The patient underwent successful treatment for shock by infusion of fluid. The pancreatitis resolved spontaneously after the presumed passage of the gallstone into the duodenum. Intravenous feeding and antibiotics also aided the patient's recovery.

The elevated amylase and lipase levels in the blood represented responses of autolytic injury to the exocrine portion of the pancreas caused by blockage of main pancreatic duct. In this case the blockage took place where the main pancreatic duct empties into the hepatopancreatic ampulla.

What caused the paralysis of the small intestine revealed by the lack of bowel sounds and the multiple air and fluid levels revealed in the abdominal films? The best explanation is that neurotoxic inflammatory products from the pancreas cross the peritoneum covering the pancreas to enter the wall of the small intestine that is in contact with the pancreas and produce a localized ileus. The radiographic finding of loops of the small intestine that are filled with air and fluid, with the fluid occupying the gravity dependent part of the loops (sentinel loops of the small intestine), is often encountered with pancreatitis, but the finding is not specific.

Central venous catheterization allows invasive hemodynamic monitoring, temporary cardiac pacing, and safe delivery of a wide variety of drugs and hypertonic solutions that irritate peripheral veins. Central venous catheters are also vital in providing i.v. fluids, drugs, and total parenteral nutrition in patients with diminished peripheral venous access sites, as in this case. Quick, skillful placement of central venous catheters minimizes the patient's risk and discomfort.

Anatomy of Central Venous Catheterization

Subclavian vein. A standard anatomy atlas can be consulted to review the venous anatomy of the axilla and root of the neck by those learning or reviewing internal jugular or subclavian central venous catheterization. The osteology of the upper chest and clavicle is especially relevant to these procedures because it provides important topographical landmarks for guiding the catheters accurately. In reviewing the clavicle, one should pay particular attention to its S-shaped form, which divides it into thirds with medial, middle, and lateral components. The junction between the medial and middle thirds (commonly referred to as the *break* of the clavicle) is emphasized because it serves as the landmark for subclavian vein cannulation. The sternoclavicular joint should be located because the brachiocephalic vein, which is formed by the union of the internal jugular and subclavian veins, lies directly behind it.

The subclavian vein travels medially from the axilla toward the brachiocephalic vein in the narrow space between the clavicle and the first rib. It passes over the first rib just in front of the insertion of the anterior scalene muscle, behind the medial part of the clavicle. After crossing the inner border of the first rib, it lies upon the cupula of the lung. The adventitia of the subclavian vein is directly attached to the periosteum of the posterior surface of the medial third of the clavicle, the costoclavicular ligament, and the fasciae of the subclavius and anterior scalene muscles. What is the significance of the connective tissues that surround the external surface of the subclavian vein? The tethering of the subclavian vein to surrounding connective tissues has great clinical importance because it prevents the subclavian vein from collapsing, even in the case of hypovolemia or hypotension, so that catheterization of this vein is more successful that of any other veins.

The operator is now ready to perform the procedure by selecting the skin entry site for subclavian venipuncture. This site is located 1 cm inferior and one cm lateral to the convex bend (the break) between the medial and middle thirds of the clavicle. An 18-gauge "finder" needle, 2 1/2 inches long, is inserted into the skin at the entry site and is aimed toward the tip of the index finger of the opposite hand, which is placed deeply in the patient's suprasternal notch. This trajectory aligns the needle with the longitudinal axis of the subclavian vein as it courses posterior to the medial third of the clavicle (Fig. 12-1). The operator should be aware that doing so keeps the directed horizontally in a coronal plane, thereby minimizing the risk of puncturing either the lung or subclavian artery. In some patients the shoulders jut so far forward that it is difficult to direct the needle horizontally. In these patients, it may be necessary to move the shoulders posteriorly by placing a rolled towel between the shoulder blades.

During needle advancement, the operator should apply slight back pressure on the plunger of the syringe to provide continuous

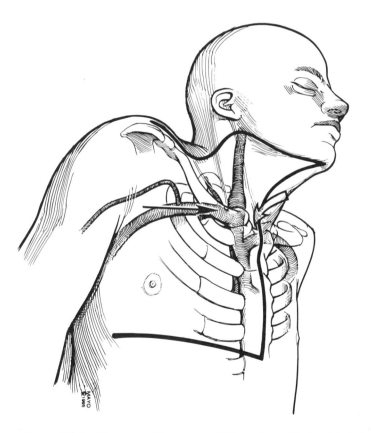

Figure 12-1. Diagrammatic representation of a catheter (straight arrow) within the subclavian vein directed toward the suprasternal notch (curved arrow). It is emphasized that the catheter enters the vein deep to the medial third of the clavicle in the direction indicated by the arrow.

negative pressure. Confirmation of needle entry into the vein is made when venous blood (dark colored) is aspirated into the syringe. The syringe is removed, and venous entry is further confirmed by noting the absence of arterial pulsations. A guidewire is inserted into the bore of the needle into the vein. The needle is removed, leaving the guidewire in place. A small incision is made in the skin along the wire. Next the operator feeds a dilator down the wire to expand the tissue to the size of the catheter. The dilator is removed and the catheter is inserted into the vein.

Different points of resistance are usually encountered with the finder needle in seeking the subclavian vein. The points of resistance vary according to the laterality of the entry site. When the entry site is more medially placed, the points of resistance are (1) the skin and superficial fascia, (2) the subclavius muscle, (3) the costoclavicular ligament, and (4) the posterolateral surface of the bulky medial end of the clavicle if the needle pass is too shallow. When the entry sites are more laterally placed, the subclavius muscle and the costoclavicular ligament may not be encountered. Entry sites too close to the costoclavicular angle have been implicated in the fracture of pacemaker leads and the kinking and obstruction of indwelling catheters.

Internal jugular vein. The surface anatomy used to locate the skin entry site for successful catheterization of the internal jugular vein can be reviewed by examining the lower part of the sternocleidomastoid muscle either on a volunteer or on oneself while looking in a mirror. To examine the right sternocleidomastoid, the head should be rotated downward toward the left shoulder and vice versa for the left sternocleidomastoid. This action will bring the sternocleidomastoid muscle into relief, so that the cordlike form of the sternal head contrasts with the less-defined, thinner, flat clavicular head. In practice, the operator will ask the patient to lift his or her head off the table to define further the two heads of the sternocleidomastoid. The legs of the triangle, brought into relief by this action, are formed by the superior aspect of the medial third of the clavicle, the lateral border of the sternal head, and the medial border of the clavicular head of the sternocleidomastoid.

The apex of this triangle, located about 2 inches above the clavicle, serves as the skin entry site for the central approach to internal jugular vein catheterization. Experienced practitioners know that the internal jugular vein (within the carotid sheath) lies against the deep surface of the sternocleidomastoid requiring a penetration depth by the finder needle of only 10 to 15 mm from the skin surface before it enters into the vein. In less experienced hands, the finder needle is frequently inserted too far resulting in penetration of the lung apex. What structures separate the internal jugular from the skin surface of the neck? What is the approximate thicknesses of each? The structures are the skin (2 mm), the superficial fascia containing the thin platysma muscle (3–6 mm), and the sternocleidomastoid (5–6 mm). The internal jugular vein is a shallow structure.

Three other anatomic points help to ensure safe central venous catheterization via the internal jugular vein. First, the internal jugular vein lies on the anterior surface of the cupula covering the apex of the lung. This relationship makes the lung vulnerable to accidental puncture when the needle is pushed through the vein, as mentioned above. Second, the easy collapsibility of the vein may complicate entry into the lumen (interior of the vessel). When the needle encounters the anterior wall of the vein, the external pressure from the advancing needle may exceed the distending pressure of the vein, which is low in patients suffering shock. In this case the needle may press the anterior wall of the vein against its posterior wall. As the needle advances, it may pass through both walls without entering a patent (open) lumen. If no blood rushes into the syringe, at a depth of about 2 to 2.5 cm, the needle should be slowly withdrawn while maintaining back pressure on the syringe. This action is intended to draw the anterior wall of the vein away from the posterior wall and to create a lumen, allowing blood to enter the needle. Third, the trajectory for catheterization of the internal jugular veins is critical to the success of the procedure. The method described here is to enter the skin at the apex of the central triangle of the sternocleidomastoid while aiming the needle at a downward angle of 45 to 60 degrees to the horizontal plane in a parasternal direction. Keeping the needle parallel to the sternal border accurately directs it down the central axis of the vein.

Complications of Central Venous Catheterization

As we have seen, the juxtaposition of the apex of the lung to the subclavian and internal jugular veins poses a risk for lung puncture by misdirected needles and this can lead to pneumothorax (collapsed lung). What are the boundaries of the cupula, the dome of the pleural cavity which houses the lung apex, and what important relationships does the cupula have to the subclavian vein and internal jugular veins? The cupula is at the level of the first rib posteriorly, but the first rib slopes downward and forward. Thus, the cupula and apex of the lung extend above the level of the anterior part of the first rib and above the thoracic inlet into the root of the neck. They lie behind the sternocleidomastoid muscle, 3 cm above the level of the medial third of the clavicle. The important anterior relationships of the cupula are with (1) the apex of the lung and the subclavian artery and its branches, anterior to which lies the anterior scalene muscle with the phrenic nerve crossing it anteriorly; and (2) the internal jugular and subclavian veins passing anterior to the insertion of the anterior scalene muscle onto the first rib.

The incidence of pneumothorax is reported to be between 0.06 and 6.0% for subclavian vein catheterization but lower for the internal jugular vein. An adequate explanation of the lower incidence of internal jugular complications is lacking. Because an estimated three million central venous catheter procedures are performed annually in the United States, a great number of people suffer pneumothorax as a complication of central venous catheterization procedures.

Pneumothorax is caused by creating a bronchopleural fistula (an abnormal communication between two normally unconnected structures). This fistula is between the bronchial tree and the pleural space. The injury to the visceral pleura and lung from the penetrating catheter allows atmospheric air within the bronchial tree to enter the pleural space. This breaks the "suction effect" (surface tension) between the parietal and visceral pleurae, allowing the natural tendency of the chest wall, lined with parietal pleura, to expand outward, and of the lung, covered by visceral pleura, to retract inward upon itself. In essence, the normal negative pressure in the pleural space, which keeps the lungs inflated against the parietal pleura, is lost. The lung retracts upon itself toward the lung root because of the pull of its elastic tissues and smooth muscle; thus, it becomes ineffective in respiration. Less threatening, but still of concern, is accidental puncture of the arteries that travel alongside the veins: the subclavian artery located just behind the subclavian vein and the common carotid artery lying medial to the internal jugular vein.

II   BACK

13   Prolapse of an
        Intervertebral Disk

A 43-year-old college professor tried to push his car, which was caught in a snowdrift, and immediately suffered sudden and severe pain in the lower back. He felt as if something "snapped" in the lower part of his spine. Later, his pain extended down the posterior aspect of his right thigh and leg. He also noticed some numbness and tingling over the lateral part of his right leg, foot, and little toe. He reports that for several years past he has had episodes of "bad back," particularly after lifting heavy objects from a stooping position.

EXAMINATION

During the history taking, the patient complains that he has a dull ache in the lower back and that the pain goes down his leg when he is straining and coughing. There is a diminution in the spinal lumbar curve and a tilt of the trunk to the left side. Because of his pain, he has marked limitation of movement in the lumbar vertebral column. Raising his right extended leg is quite painful. On further examination, tenderness to palpation along the course of the sciatic nerve in the right thigh is noted, and there is some weakness in plantar flexion of his right foot as well as some loss of sensory perception over the dorsal side of the right fourth and fifth toes.

An MRI (magnetic resonance image) and a CT-myelogram (computed tomogram after injection of contrast medium into the subarachnoid space) of the lower back were ordered (Fig. 13-1).

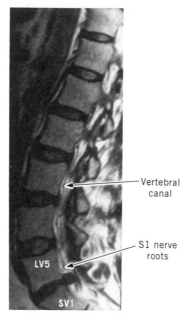

Figure 13-1. A sagittal MRI of the vertebral column from the level of thoracic vertebra 12 downward through sacral vertebra 1 showing the herniated LV5–SV1 disk as it protrudes posteriorly into the vertebral canal, where is impinges on the nerve roots of the first sacral nerve.

DIAGNOSIS

This patient has a rupture of the intervertebral disk between the fifth lumbar and first sacral vertebrae with protrusion of the nucleus pulposus and nerve root involvement of the first sacral nerve (slipped disk).

THERAPY AND FURTHER COURSE

Under conservative treatment and bed rest for two days on a reinforced hard mattress, the patient improves sufficiently to start a set of exercises recommended to strengthen the flexor and extensors of the vertebral column.

DISCUSSION

The combination of low back pain and pain along the course of the sciatic nerve aggravated by straining is rather typical of a disk lesion.

What is the function of the intervertebral disk and what are its two components? The intervertebral disks act as shock absorbers; each consists of an outer firm fibrocartilaginous ring, the annulus fibrosus, and an inner softer, more pliable, gelatinous center, the nucleus pulposus. Chronic trauma, particularly in the middle-aged or older patient with degenerative changes in the intervertebral disk, leads to a posterior tear in the annulus fibrosus at the site of greatest mechanical stress. A later consequence, particularly in conjunction with further acute or chronic trauma, is protrusion or herniation of the nucleus pulposus into the (spinal) canal. Usually the herniation takes place to one side of the midline because of the ligamentous reinforcement in the midline. What is the name of the ligament that runs along the posterior aspect of the bodies of the vertebrae from the atlas to the sacrum and is intimately blended with the disks? The posterior longitudinal ligament attaches to the occiput above and extends all the way down into the sacral canal. It narrows behind each vertebral body but broadens over the disks.

The "snap" that the patient felt may have been caused by the annular tear, with partial expulsion of the nucleus pulposus. The lower lumbar disks, being among the most flexible areas of the vertebral column, are the most common sites of herniation. The disappearance of the normal lumbar concavity, or lordosis, is due to exaggerated contraction of what group of muscles responsible for motions of the vertebral column? The disappearance of the normal lumbar concavity is due to exaggerated contraction of the flexors. Pain in disk lesions is usually greatest when sitting and leaning forward. What are its main flexors? The chief flexors of the lumbar vertebral column are the rectus abdominis and the iliopsoas muscles.

Cauda equina and subarachnoid space

Is the spinal cord subjected to pressure at the level indicated? What is the lowest extent of the cord in terms of vertebral level? Is the area involved within the extent of the subarachnoid space? Remember that the cord in the adult ends approximately at the level of the second lumbar vertebra or the disk between LV_{1-2}, and the subarachnoid space ends at the level of the second sacral vertebra. What are the contents of the subarachnoid space (thecal, meningeal sac) below the level of the cord? The contents inferior to the conus medullaris are cerebrospinal fluid, the cauda equina, and the filum terminale. Does the cauda equina consist of spinal nerves or nerve roots? The cauda equina consists of dorsal and ventral nerve roots that continue downward in the vertebral canal within the meningeal sac, approximately to the level of emergence from their intervertebral foramina, and are covered by meningeal sleeves as far as the spinal ganglia. Here the meningeal membranes are continuous with the epineurium.

Posterolateral herniation of the nucleus pulposus may readily impinge on the nerve roots within the vertebral canal as they course diagonally downward toward their exit (Fig. 13-2). The prolapse is particularly apt to compress the roots of the next lower spinal nerve. Thus herniation of the disk between the fifth lumbar and the first sacral vertebrae involves most commonly the roots of the first sacral nerve, as in the case presented here (Figs. 13-2 and 13-3). The fifth

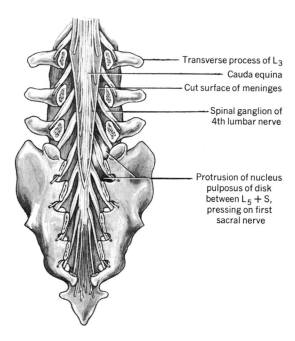

Transverse process of L₃
Cauda equina
Cut surface of meninges

Spinal ganglion of
4th lumbar nerve

Protrusion of nucleus
pulposus of disk
between L₅ + S,
pressing on first
sacral nerve

Figure 13-2. Vertebral arches have been removed and the spinal canal has been exposed. The dura and arachnoid have been cut and reflected. The oblique course of spinal nerves is shown. Observe the prolapsed nucleus pulposus pressing on the first sacral nerve and ganglion.

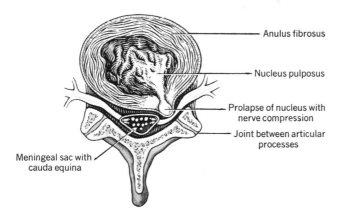

Figure 13-3. Cross section of intervertebral disk and spinal canal. Observe the ruptured anulus fibrosus with posterior protrusion of nucleus pulposus and compression of the spinal nerve on the right.

lumbar nerve leaves the vertebral canal above the fifth lumbar disc, and the first sacral nerve crosses this disc in its course to the first sacral foramina (pelvic and dorsal).

What is the expanation for the aggravation of pain by straining and coughing? These actions, by increasing intravenous pressure, also increase the pressure of the cerebrospinal fluid, which adds to the pressure on the involved nerve roots. On the other hand, tilting of the trunk away from the compressed roots decreases the pressure on them and lessens the pain.

Sciatic nerve and its roots

The roots of the first spinal sacral nerve represent one of the important components of the sciatic nerve. What are its other components? The sciatic nerve takes origin from the fourth and fifth lumbar and the first three sacral nerves. Raising the extended leg of the patient in the recumbent position puts the sciatic nerve on the stretch and is painful in cases of sciatic nerve root compression, as is direct pressure on the sciatic nerve itself in its course along the thigh. Where in the thigh is the nerve readily subjected to pressure? Remember, the nerve runs almost vertically down the thigh midway between the great trochanter and the ischial tuberosity.

Weakness of plantar flexion of the right foot is a sign of involvement of the motor root of the first sacral nerve. Clinical experience shows that the branch of the tibial nerve supplying the main plantar flexor, the gastrocnemius muscle, does not contain fibers from all five motor roots of the sciatic nerve but mainly fibers from the first and second sacral nerves. The sensory area of the skin supplied by the first sacral nerve (dermatome) varies somewhat. The most typical area of disturbed sensation in involvement of the first sacral nerve comprises the lateral aspect of the leg below the knee and the lateral-most toes. These are also the areas involved in this patient.

Conservative treatment will usually suffice, but if objective signs (such as atrophy of the calf muscles and reflex anomalies with sensory deficiencies) persist, surgical treatment is indicated. One operation consists of laminectomy (removal of the posterior portion of one or more vertebral arches) and surgical excision of the prolapsed disk. A more recent, less radical type of surgery, called microlumbar discetomy, may be performed. In this operation, only the herniated part of the disk is removed, and this is accomplished through the use of microsurgical instruments and a surgical microscope. The results are the same as with standard discectomy. The advantage is that the incision is smaller, resulting in less surgical trauma. The disadvantages are the possibility of insufficient exposure leading to inadequate decompression in cases of coexistent spinal stenosis (narrowing of the spinal canal).

14   Lumbar Puncture

A 15-year-old boy is referred to the hospital by his family physician for symptoms of sneezing and coughing, severe headache, stiffness of the neck, and high fever.

EXAMINATION

On physical examination the boy, although in good nutritional state, appears to be quite ill and restless. He is drowsy and responds to questions rather hesitatingly, as though he has difficulty orienting himself. His reaction to physical stimuli is slow. His temperature is 104° F, and his pulse rate is accelerated. He displays all signs of an upper respiratory infection, but the lungs are clear. He complains of severe headache, which extends into the neck and is symmetrical on both sides of the head. On forward bending of the head and neck (flexion), the neck appears rather stiff. This movement is painful and is actively resisted by the patient.

Neurologic examination does not reveal any specific defect in the central nervous system. Functions of the cranial and spinal nerves are intact. Examination of the fundus of the eye (eye grounds) with the ophthalmoscope shows the interior of the eye to be normal. There is no swelling of the optic disc, the site of entrance of the optic nerve into the eyeball; increased intracranial pressure is therefore unlikely. To confirm or exclude the diagnosis of infectious meningitis, a lumbar puncture is done. Although the cerebrospinal fluid pressure is somewhat elevated, the fluid itself is clear, colorless, and of normal protein and cell content. Consequently, infectious meningitis can be ruled out.

DIAGNOSIS

Febrile upper respiratory infection with meningeal irritation (meningismus) is diagnosed.

THERAPY AND FURTHER COURSE

The patient is given antibiotic treatment to avoid spread of the infection to the lungs. Aspirin and sedatives are prescribed for the fever, headache, and general discomfort. His fever is further reduced by frequent sponging with tap water and alcohol solution. Ice bags are applied to the patient's head.

During the next few days, the patient continues to complain of headache, but his fever, general malaise, and upper respiratory symptoms gradually subside. The patient is discharged from the hospital after 10 days. Follow-up shows that he has completely recovered.

DISCUSSION

What is lumbar puncture?

Lumbar puncture (LP) is the tapping of the subarachnoid space in the lumbar region for the removal of cerebrospinal fluid (CSF) or for the introduction of drugs, such as antibiotics or anesthetics. It was introduced into our diagnostic and therapeutic armamentarium more than 80 years ago and has proved to of unforeseen value as a sensitive diagnostic procedure and therapeutic tool. Why should edema (papilledema) of the optic papilla, a sign of increased intracranial pressure, be excluded before LP can be undertaken? Sudden pressure reduction in the subarachnoid space by LP in the presence of elevated intracranial pressure may lead to herniation of the tonsils of the cerebellum through the foramen magnum into the spinal canal or to prolapse of portions of the temporal lobe through the tentorial notch. The result in either case may be a serious or fatal compression of vital portions of the brain.

Site of lumbar puncture

What is the optimal site of LP? It is done in the lower part of the lumbar spinal column between vertebrae L3 and L4 or L4 and L5, generally to the exclusion of higher levels of the column. Is there an external landmark available for the proper site of entrance of the LP needle? A horizontal line connecting the highest points of the iliac crests, as seen from the posterior aspect, crosses the midline at about the level of the spinous process of L4. The adjacent inter-spinous spaces above or below are then chosen as the site of LP. Does the direction of the lumbar spinous processes facilitate entrance of the needle into the spinal canal? In the lumbar area there is a wide space between adjacent, horizontally directed spinous processes; this space allows easy access to the spinal canal (Fig. 14-1). Is the same true in other areas of the vertebral column? Entrance into the canal between thoracic spinous processes is impossible because they are directed inferiorly in a sharp angle and overlap each other so much that there is very little area in the midline that is free of bone.

What movement of the lumbar vertebral column widens the space between adjacent spinous processes and is therefore used in positioning of the patient for LP? Maximal flexion of the vertebral column (arching of the back) is applied either in the sitting or lateral horizontal position, with the patient's knees drawn as close to the chin as possible.

Lowest extent of the spinal cord in the infant and adult

Why are more superiorly located areas of the vertebral column excluded as puncture sites? Obviously, needle puncture of the spinal cord with resulting injury to the central nervous system must be avoided. The problem then focuses on the question of what lowest extent of the spinal cord is in terms of vertebral landmarks. Is there any variation in the inferior extent of the cord? In the adult the lowest point of the cord is the tip of the conus medullaris, located at the lower border of the first lumbar vertebra or at the level of the body of the second lumbar vertebra. How do you explain that in the newborn and infant the terminal point of the cord is lower than the levels given for the adult? In the young fetus, the spinal cord extends through the whole length of the spinal canal down to the

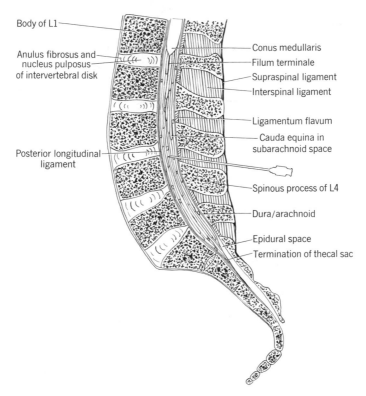

Body of L1

Anulus fibrosus and
nucleus pulposus
of intervertebral disk

Posterior longitudinal
ligament

Conus medullaris

Filum terminale

Supraspinal ligament

Interspinal ligament

Ligamentum flavum

Cauda equina in
subarachnoid space

Spinous process of L4

Dura/arachnoid

Epidural space

Termination of thecal sac

Figure 14-1. Midsagittal section through the lumbar spinal column with spinal puncture needle in place between the spinous processes of L3 and L4. Notice the slightly ascending direction of the needle. The needle has pierced three ligaments and the dura/arachnoid and is in the subarachnoid space.

coccyx. As development progresses, the growth of the spinal cord does not keep pace with the longitudinal growth of the vertebral column (differential growth). Already at birth considerable discrepancy exists between the length of the cord and the column, with the cord ending at the inferior border of the third lumbar vertebra. Ultimately, the disproportion in length becomes even greater so that in adults the end of the cord is generally two vertebrae higher, that is, at the lower border of the first lumbar vertebra.

Subarachnoid space and cauda equina

Between what meningeal layers is the spinal fluid located, and what is the lowest extent of the subarachnoid space (meningeal, thecal) sac containing this fluid? The CSF fills the subarachnoid space between arachnoid and pia mater. The lowest extent of the subarachnoid space is at the level of the second sacral vertebra. Why, then, is spinal puncture not undertaken at lower levels than the typical sites, for example, in the upper region of the sacrum? The solid bony mass of the posterior boundary of the sacral canal prevents entrance into this part of the subarachnoid space. Are there any nerve structures contained in the subarachnoid space that may be injured by LP below the level of the cord? The cauda equina (horse's tail) is a collection of spinal nerve roots (sensory and motor) that descend from the lowest part of the cord to their exit as spinal nerves through the lumbar intervertebral and sacral foramina. If students were asked approximately how many "hairs" make up the "horse's tail" just below the conus medullaris with a choice of 10, 20, 30, or 40 as an answer, most would probably choose 20, counting four lumbar, five sacral, and one coccygeal nerves on each side. The answer is twice that, because the spinal nerves have not yet formed, and the contents of the subarachnoid space are the ventral and dorsal roots rather than the nerves. The filum terminale that is essentially made up of pia mater may be considered one of the strands of hair of the "horse's tail." Is injury to one of the nerve roots by the tip of the needle a danger in LP? If one of the roots is touched by the needle, it generally escapes injury, being easily displaced in the fluid medium; however, in case of contact with a sensory root, the patient may perceive a shooting pain in the lower extremity on that side, and the needle should be withdrawn slightly. It may be helpful for students to think of the analogy provided by a straw broom and its bristles to the spinal cord and the cauda equina wherein it would be easy to stick a needle into the handle of a broom (spinal cord) but nearly impossible to stick it into one of the bristles (dorsal or ventral root).

Ligaments of the spine

What are the ligaments involved in LP? In the typical midline puncture, three ligaments must be traversed by the needle; identify them. They are the supraspinous and interspinous ligaments and the ligamentum flavum (Fig. 14-1). Although the ligamenta flava are frequently described as not being continuous across the midline, they often are, and because the needle often strays from the theoretical midline, they must be considered structures encountered by the needle. After the needle has pierced the skin and superficial fascia, these ligaments are encountered in the order given.

The length of the needle is adjusted to the amount of fat in the subcutaneous tissue and to the size of the patient. The supraspinous ligaments connect the tips of the spinous processes; the interspinous ligaments join the superior and inferior borders of adjacent spinous processes and are fairly well developed in the lumbar area. The ligamenta flava are strong plate-like membranes, composed of yellow elastic fibers, that in the lumbar area may reach a thickness of 1 cm. They offer a noticeable resistance to the entering needle, and their penetration is felt as a "snap" or "click." They interconnect adjacent laminae and run from the anterior-inferior border of the lamina of the higher vertebra to the posterior-superior aspect of the lamina of the adjacent lower vertebra. Thus, they cover the interlaminary space between two vertebrae, which on inspection of the skeleton and on the x-ray appears to be quite large in this area. The ligamenta flava fuse laterally with the capsules of the joints formed by the articular processes and blend posteriorly with the interspinous ligaments in the midline. It is the function of the ligaments flava to assist the erector spinae muscle in sustaining the upright position. They are put on the stretch in flexion and their elastic pull helps to restore the upright (extended) posture. Because flexion is the position assumed by the patient in LP, the ligaments are stretched and more easily traversed by the needle than when the patient is in an extended position.

Epidural space and epidural anesthesia

Identify the potential space that the needle enters once it has penetrated the ligamentum flavum. It is the epidural (extradural) space, which extends from the foramen magnum to the sacral hiatus and communicates through the intervertebral foramina with the space outside the vertebral column. The epidural space surrounds the spinal meninges and separates the dura mater from the wall of the vertebral canal (Fig. 14-1). Its contents are the ventral and dorsal nerve roots, enveloped by their meningeal sleeves, and fatty tissue, in which a fair-sized vertebral plexus of veins, small arteries, and lymphatics is embedded. The practical importance of the epidural space and its contents for LP lies in the possibility of inadvertently puncturing the venous plexus resulting in a bloody tap. Striking the roots of a spinal nerve is another mishap that may lead to long-lasting paresthesias.

The epidural space is commonly used as the site of anesthesia of the spinal nerves. This procedure should not be confused with spinal anesthesia in which the anesthetizing fluid is injected into the subarachnoid space. In caudal anesthesia, the needle is inserted through the sacral hiatus into the distal part of the sacral canal without penetrating the dural sac, which ends at the second sacral vertebra. It is a useful method of obtaining analgesia of the perineum in obstetrics.

Subdural and subarachnoid spaces

The next step in LP, after the ligamentum flavum has been penetrated and the epidural space passed, is the piercing of the dura and arachnoid, which again may be perceived as a "snap." The needle is now in the subarachnoid space, and under normal conditions CSF will appear at the hub of the needle (Figs. 14-1 and 14-2). The pressure of the CSF should be determined and its clearness, color, cell and protein count investigated. Fluid for bacterial cultures also should be collected. Is there a subdural space between dura and arachnoid? There is a capillary interval containing a minimal amount of fluid for lubrication of the contiguous aspects of the two membranes.

Lateral approach

In older people or patients with metabolic disease, the supraspinous ligament may be ossified or calcified, and perforation by the puncture needle may become difficult. Such a calcified ligament may also deflect the needle from its intended course so that it strikes the bony lamina above or below the puncture site. In this case a slightly lateral approach to one side of the midline may be chosen (Fig. 14-2). The needle is directed slightly superiorly to miss the lamina of the lower vertebra and slightly medially to compensate for the lat-

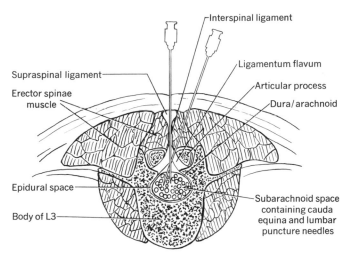

Figure 14-2. Horizontal section through the body of L3. Notice two puncture needles in the subarachnoid space. The median one is in the midline
corresponding to the position in Figure 14-1. The lateral exemplifies the
lateral approach, which avoids the occasionally calcified supraspinal ligament. Notice the lateral needle piercing the intrinsic musculature of the
back and only one ligament, the ligamentum flavum.

eral point of entrance. In this approach the needle passes through
skin, a variable amount of superficial fascia and fat, the dense posterior layer of the thoracolumbar fascia, and the erector spinae muscles. The needle must now penetrate only the ligamentum flavum
(the supraspinous and interspinous ligaments have been bypassed),
the epidural space, and the dura-arachnoid before CSF escapes.

Side effects and complications

One of the side effects has already been mentioned: a bloody tap due
to puncture of the epidural venous plexus. Acute root pain or longer
lasting neuralgia of a spinal nerve may be caused by contact with the
needle if it is misdirected in the lateral approach. A serious, often
fatal complication is prolapse of the temporal lobe or cerebellum
with compression of the vital centers of the brain stem in patients
with increased intracranial pressure as a result of sudden release of
the pressure; this condition has been discussed previously. If the
needle passes through an infected area or if a faulty, nonsterile

technique is employed, septic meningitis may result. Other incidents include puncture of the posterior longitudinal ligament and the annulus fibrosus, resulting in prolapse of the nucleus pulposus of the intervertebral disk. One author compiled 57 cases of this type of injury from the literature and his own experience. Surprisingly, the literature also reports the presence of bone marrow cells in the CSF caused by penetration of the vertebral body by the puncture needle.

Post-puncture headache

The most frequent side effect is post-puncture headache, which is slow in starting, and takes two to three days to reach its peak. The pain is caused by leakage of CSF at the site of puncture of the dura, resulting in decreased hydrostatic pressure in the subarachnoid space, which leads to slight dislodgment of the brain and traction on pain-sensitive blood vessels and intracranial dura. The surface of the brain does not contain pain fibers. The headache is increased when the patient is in the erect position and in temporarily relieved by a second LP with injection of saline solution. A horizontal position, with the patient's head flat and unsupported by pillows, alleviates the pain. The headache generally lasts only a few days. It is obvious that small-gauge puncture needles and avoidance of multiple punctures will relieve many of the side effects and prevent post-puncture headache.

III THORAX

15   Cancer of the Breast

A 51-year-old homemaker comes to the clinic because one month earlier she had noticed a lump in her right breast. Since then she has felt occasional dull aches in her breast. She has applied iodine but received no benefit. Her personal physician diagnosed cancer. She has always been in good health and never consulted a physician except at childbirths, of which she has had three. She reached menopause three years ago.

EXAMINATION

The patient has been in the best of health. As she sits in the chair, the right nipple is a good half inch higher than the left. The upper outer quadrant of the right breast contains a reddened area two inches in diameter, the borders of which gradually shade into the surrounding skin. This area is flatter in contour than the same area of the left breast, and the skin over the area seems dimpled. As the patient is turned from side to side and bent forward, the right breast remains more rigid and does not respond to the action of gravity as does the other breast. The axilla of the right side seems fuller than on the left.

   On palpation the reddened area is found to be hard and boardlike. The whole breast moves freely over the pectoral fascia, but the skin in the involved quadrant is firmly fixed and has the hard, rough corrugated feel of an orange peel. The right nipple is retracted and fixed and does not respond to traction, whereas the left does. The right axilla is occupied by a solid tumor that is freely movable on the surrounding tissues. No supraclavicular nodes are palpable. Both the mass in the breast and the tumor in the axilla are sensitive to firm pressure. All other examinations are negative.

DIAGNOSIS

Adenocarcinoma of the breast with axillary metastasis is diagnosed.

THERAPY AND FURTHER COURSE

A radical mastectomy is done with removal of the breast, pectoralis major and minor muscles, axillary tumor, axillary lymph nodes, and axillary fat. The tributaries of the axillary vein in the operative field are also removed, but the long thoracic and thoracodorsal nerves are identified and preserved. Microscopic study of the breast and axillary nodes confirm the diagnosis of cancer.

The patient's postoperative recovery is typical, but she has some swelling of her arm, which is treated with physical therapy. Six months later she has a recurrence in the axilla and dies of lung metastasis nine months after surgery.

DISCUSSION

The physical findings of a large mass in the right breast, the dimpling and fixation of the skin in the involved quadrant, the retracted and fixed nipple, and the mass in the axilla leave no doubt as to the advanced stage of the cancer.

Anatomical signs of spread

What is the reason for the reddening of the skin in the area of the cancer? The reddening of the skin over the tumor is due to increased flow of blood to and from the area. The blood supply to the breast is derived mainly from the internal thoracic, lateral thoracic, posterior intercostal, thoracoacromial arteries, and anterior intercostal arteries (Fig. 15-1A and B). Veins essentially follow the course of the arteries.

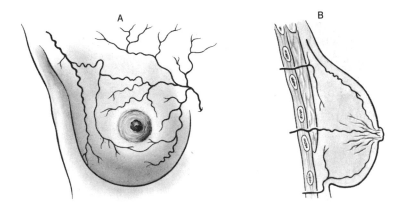

Figure 15-1. A.—Front view of the arterial supply to the breast showing medial and lateral mammary branches from the internal thoracic and lateral thoracic arteries, respectively. Other lateral mammary branches originate from the thoracoacromial and intercostal arteries. Medial and lateral mammary branches communicate around the nipple. B.—Parasagittal section of breast showing, in addition to the arteries visualized, in A, deep (perforating) mammary branches passing through the intercoastal spaces.

How do you explain the fixation of the skin to the tumor and the orange-peel appearance of the skin? The dimpling and fixation of the skin to the tumor imply cancerous invasion of the suspensory ligaments (of Cooper) that anchor the gland to the skin (Fig. 15-2). The orange-peel appearance of the skin indicates cancerous obstruction of the lymphatics draining the skin; the hair follicles and cutaneous glands, which are more firmly attached to the subcutaneous tissue, withstand the expansion caused by lymph blockage and therefore appear as pits or depressions (Fig. 15-2).

What do the elevation, retraction, and fixation of the nipple mean in anatomical terms? These conditions are explained on the basis of cancerous involvement and subsequent scarring of the lactiferous ducts (Fig. 15-2). What is the explanation for the mass in the axilla? The axillary tumor is a typical sign of metastasis to the axillary lymph nodes, the site of the principal lymph drainage of the breast.

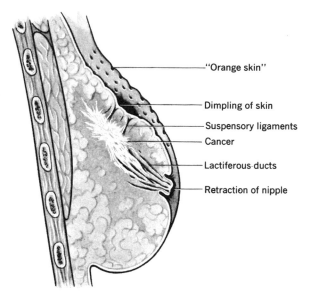

Figure 15-2. Dimpling and orange-peel-like appearance of the skin, retraction and elevation of the nipple, and signs of cancerous spread to suspensory ligaments of the breast, obstruction of the cutaneous lymphatics, and involvement of the lactiferous ducts.

Axillary lymph nodes

The term axillary nodes applies to a large aggregation of nodes located within the axilla. Their separation into individual groups is somewhat artificial, but it facilitates the understanding of regional lymphatic drainage and helps to clarify the location of the nodes. It should be understood, however, that the axillary nodes are subject to great variations in location, size, and number and that the groups have a rich system of interconnecting anastomoses.

There are five groups of nodes, the first three of which can be regarded as peripheral outposts, whereas the other two groups are more centrally located within the axillary fossa and toward its apex. The following are the five groups of nodes:

1. the lateral set along the upper part of the humerus in the medial bicipital groove in relation to the axillary vein;

2. the subscapular set following the posterior axillary fold along the lateral border of the scapula in relation to the thoracodorsal and subscapular veins;

3. the pectoral set beneath the anterior axillary fold in relation to the lateral thoracic veins;

4. the central set formed by rather large and fairly numerous nodes in the fat of the axilla, which receives the preceding three outlying groups;

5. the apical set behind the costocoracoid membrane in relation to the more proximal part of the axillary vein which receives the efferent vessels from all other groups.

The axillary nodes, taken as a whole, receive two streams of lymph, one from the upper extremity, the other from the adjacent thoracic wall, particularly from the breast. The two currents meet and fuse within the central and apical chains. The lymph from the arm drains into the outlying lateral nodes, and the lymph from the breast is filtered mainly by the pectoral nodes, in which the lymph trunks from the breast terminate. The efferent vessels from the pectoral nodes go to the central set that drains into the apical nodes. From there, the lymph empties by way of the subclavian trunk into the junction of the subclavian and internal jugular veins, or it may terminate on the right side in the right lymphatic duct and on the left side in the thoracic duct, being in part filtered through the supraclavicular (inferior deep cervical) nodes.

Thus, we have the following lymph nodes interposed in the pathway of cancerous emboli from the breast before they reach the venous bloodstream: pectoral, central, apical, and possibly supraclavicular nodes. Shortcuts that bypass one, two, or even three of the more peripheral lymphatic stations may occur; hence direct drainage from the breast into the central or apical or even the supraclavicular set can take place. In the last case, we have the clinical picture of enlarged supraclavicular nodes without involvement of the axillary nodes, a condition that most surgeons regard as inoperable. A direct lymphatic channel from the deeper superior portions of the mammary gland to the apical nodes is well known. It passes around the inferior border or through the substance of the pectoralis major and ascends on the surface of or deep to the pectoralis minor to the apical nodes. Small interpectoral nodes may be interposed in this pathway. The possible presence of this channel explains the need to remove of both pectoral muscles in radical mastectomy. As stated, anastomoses between the outlying pectoral, lateral, and subscapular chains exist so that the latter two may likewise, although rarely, be affected in cancer of the breast.

Accessory lymphatic channels

Additional lymph vessels connect the breast, particularly its medial half, with the parasternal nodes. These vessels traverse the pectoralis major and intercostal muscles and follow in their course the anterior intercostal branches of the internal thoracic vessels. They terminate in parasternal nodes located in the upper intercostal spaces in relation to the internal thoracic vessels close to the lateral margin of the sternum. These nodes tend to atrophy in old age. Their efferents go to the supraclavicular nodes and lymph trunks in the neck. Direct lymphatic connections to the opposite breast and opposite axilla have also been postulated on the basis of occasional metastasis in breast cancer. In this discussion on lymphatic drainage of the breast and lymphatic spread of cancerous emboli, it must be realized that obstruction of the normal lymph current by metastatic growth in the lymph nodes may lead to reversal of the lymph flow and to involvement of lymph nodes in atypical locations, for example, the inguinal region.

Vulnerable nerves in mastectomy

What important motor nerves should be identified and preserved, as done in our case? What muscles do they supply, and what is the effect of injury to either nerve? The long thoracic nerve supplies the important serratus anterior, whose paralysis results in "winged scapula" and a severely compromised ability to rotate the scapula upward so that the glenoid cavity is turned up. Patients suffering winged scapula have difficulty in raising their hand as in brushing their hair or reaching to retrieve items from an overhead shelf. Injury to the thoracodorsal nerve leads to loss of function of the latissimus dorsi and therefore to difficulties in extension, adduction, and medial rotation of the humerus. The latter two motions are already compromised by the removal of the pectoralis major.

Anatomy of edema

What is the cause of the postoperative swelling (edema) of the upper limb? It is presumed to be due to a combination of lymphatic and venous obstruction. The former results from the severance and removal of most of the lymphatic channels that drain the arm, and the latter is caused by the frequently occurring thrombosis of the axillary vein, which is the consequence of the necessary surgical handling and endothelial injury of the vein. Delicate dissection at the time of surgery with massage and physical therapy postoperatively will alleviate the swelling.

PROGNOSIS

With what stage of the cancer are we dealing in this case? The attachment of the skin to the tumor, the reddening and swelling of the skin over the tumor, the fixation of the nipple, and particularly the pronounced axillary involvement are all signs of a fairly advanced cancer of the breast.

What anatomical findings are favorable to the patient? The location in the upper outer quadrant of the breast is the most common and, according to many authors, the most favorable site of cancer. The mobility of the breast over the pectoral fascia is a sign of noninvolvement of the underlying fascia and muscle and is therefore advantageous to the patient. The absence of palpable supraclavicular lymph nodes is also a relatively favorable sign.

In view of the short history and the relatively advanced state of the breast cancer in this patient, the prognosis on admission would have to be guarded despite the technical operability of the tumor and its axillary metastasis. On average, survival in such cases is less than two years.

Comments on present-day treatment

Breast cancer at the more advanced stage presented in this case still occurs, and the operation described here (radical mastectomy of Halsted) is still employed in selected cases. During recent years, alternative, less radical approaches have become common. They range from simple removal of the tumor (lumpectomy), to removal of the tumor plus a surrounding area of normal tissue (partial mastectomy), to removal of the whole breast (modified radical mastectomy) leaving the pectoralis muscles intact but removing the entire breast and axillary lymph nodes with better cosmetic and functional results.

Today such an advanced cancer would be regarded as a systemic disease and be treated with less extensive surgery combined with radiation and chemotherapy. Chemotherapy following surgery and radiation reduces the incidence of cancer recurrence.

Agreement prevails that early diagnostic measures, including the application of x-ray mammography, are of great value; however, in women younger than 50, mammography misses existing cancers nearly half the time. This is especially so in women whose breasts contain more glandular and fibrous tissue and less fat than is typical. This structure makes their breasts prone to scatter x-rays, rendering the images cloudy and preventing physicians from seeing the subtle architectural distortion indicative of cancer. The use of MRI for the screening of breast cancer is not used widely at this time, but it may become more common because it is superior to radiographs for imaging soft tissues (Sci. Am., 1995).

REFERENCES

Hertzier, A. E. *Clinical Surgery by Case Histories,* vol. 1, St. Louis: C. V. Mosby, 1921, p 317.
"Changing the image." *Scientific American,* April 1995, p 42.

16   **Segmental Abscess of the Lung**

A 16-year-old boy comes to the hospital because of cough and foul expectoration. He complains of great weakness, a continual cough with expectoration of a dark yellow, foul-smelling mucous substance, and pain along the right upper chest wall, particularly under the right scapula. His trouble began two days after he underwent a tonsillectomy while under general anesthesia five weeks earlier. It started as a sharp pain in the chest, worsened by deep inspiration. The cough did not begin until about two weeks after the first attack of pain. About the time he began to cough, he thought he had a fever.

EXAMINATION

On examination his temperature is 105° F and he has a leukocytosis. Radiographic examination in anteroposterior (AP) and lateral views shows an abscess cavity with fluid in the right posterior upper area of the chest (Fig. 16-1). Visibility of the oblique and horizontal fissures on lateral x-ray view makes it possible to locate the abscess in the posterior bronchopulmonary segment of the upper lobe.

DIAGNOSIS

Segmental abscess of the lung is diagnosed.

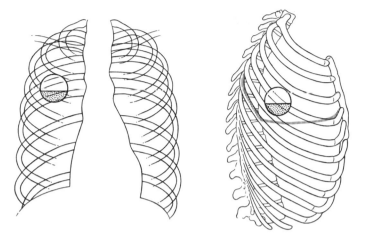

Figure 16-1. Abscess cavity with fluid level in the posterior segment of the right upper lobe on front and side views.

THERAPY AND FURTHER COURSE

The abscess completely clears under vigorous antibiotic therapy. Three months later the healing is complete and the patient is free of symptoms.

DISCUSSION

Tonsillectomy not infrequently leads to inhalation of infected material from the throat during general anesthesia, resulting in lung abscess. Segmental abscess as well as pneumonia is also frequently caused by aspiration of various foreign substances that lodge themselves in bronchi.

Definition of a bronchopulmonary segment

As a result of intensive anatomic study during the 1930s, bronchopulmonary segmentation was defined as the part of a lobe supplied by a direct branch of a lobar bronchus. In addition to its own bronchus, a bronchopulmonary segment has its own artery of supply and is generally separated from adjacent segments by a thin connective tissue septum. A segment must be visualized as a pyramidal or cone-shaped portion of lung tissue with the apex pointing toward the hilum, where bronchus and artery enter, and with the base directed toward the pleural surface of the lung. Subsequent studies from the 1950s through the 1960s were concerned with the distribution and variability of segmental and subsegmental bronchi, arteries, and veins; the location and constancy of intersegmental septa; and the air exchange across segmental boundaries (collateral ventilation).

For the names and location of bronchopulmonary segments, see anatomical texts and atlases.

Clinical pathology and surgery of pulmonary segments

Pneumonia may start in a segment and remain confined there or spread to involve the whole lobe. Bronchiectasis (chronic dilatation and inflammation of large or small bronchi and bronchioles) has a predilection for the basal segments of both lower lobes, the right middle lobe, and the lingula of the left upper lobe. Tuberculosis of the adult type may initially be confined to the posterior bronchopulmonary segment of the upper lobes. Other segments often involved in isolated tuberculous cavitation or breakdown are the apical segments of the upper and lower lobes of both lungs. Segmental collapse is due to pressure of enlarged lymph nodes, intrabronchial malignancies, or scarring bronchitis. Favored locations of segmental pulmonary abscess are given in the discussion of this case history to follow.

Pulmonary segments as surgical units

Historically, surgery has advanced from pneumonectomy (resection of a whole lung) to lobectomy and finally segmentectomy (segmental resection). This advance has resulted in the preservation of vital respiratory tissue. Veins located in the intersegmental planes serve as landmarks for the surgeon.

Accessory lobes

Accessory lobes are segments that have gained greater independence by having a visceral pleural septum separating the segment from adjacent lobes. An exception to this definition is the lobe of the azygos vein. The arch of the azygos vein partially bisects the apex of the right lung into a lateral part, and a medial part that is termed the lobe of the azygos vein. The arch of the azygos vein runs through the cleft separating the two parts.

Anatomy of segmental abscess

In the supine position of the body during and after surgery, the posterior segments of the lungs are particularly endangered; indeed, the posterior bronchopulmonary segment of the upper lobes is the most common site of pulmonary abscess. What posterior segments of the lower lobes may also be involved? The superior and posterior basal segments of the lower lobes could readily be infected in the supine position of the body.

If surgery becomes necessary, from what region would the thorax (thoracotomy) be entered, keeping in mind that the involved segment should be attacked from its pleural aspect without proceeding through uninvolved segments? The posterior approach would best fulfill these requirements. It is important to realize that, as in this case, the upper lobes may reach inferiorly on the posterior chest wall as far down as the sixth rib. Is that in keeping with textbook diagrams? Textbook figures, based on the cadaveric position of the lungs in maximal expiration, generally show the oblique fissures being projected on the posterior thoracic wall at the level of the fourth rib or fourth interspace because the diaphragm relaxes and rises superiorly after death. Thus, the thoracic viscera are higher after death whether the body is in the recumbent or erect posture. In living persons, the oblique fissure follows the sixth rib. It can also be located by tracing along the vertebral border of the scapula when the patient's hand is placed on his or her head.

Pleural pain

Since the lung and visceral pleura themselves are insensitive to pain, how is the patient's severe pain explained? In contrast to the visceral pleura, the parietal pleura, particularly in its costal portion, is extremely sensitive to pain, which may be intensified by spasms in the overlying muscles of the chest wall. What nerves transmit this pain from the parietal pleura? The costal and peripheral parts of the diaphragmatic pleura are supplied with sensory fibers from the intercostal and subcostal nerves. The central portion of the diaphragmatic pleura and the mediastinal pleura receive their sensory supply from the phrenic nerve. This pain is often referred to the neck and shoulder.

17   Middle Lobe Syndrome

A 32-year-old homemaker comes to the chest clinic with a history of chronic cough and blood-tinged sputum. The symptoms began eight months earlier when she had an acute flulike respiratory infection. Since that time she has suffered from bouts of fever that occur every two to three weeks. These episodes are accompanied by right-sided chest pain and production of a large amount of purulent and frequently blood-tinged sputum. She has lost 18 pounds, feels tired, and is hardly able to do her work. The patient is admitted to the hospital for diagnosis.

EXAMINATION

On examination the chest findings are minimal. On auscultation some abnormal breath sounds are found over the lower anterior portion of the right chest. Her temperature is 98.8° F. The sputum is negative for tubercle bacilli. Films of the chest in PA (posteroanterior) and lateral views reveal infiltration and partial collapse of the right middle lobe (Fig. 17-1). Examination of the right lung with a bronchoscope shows narrowing and inflammation of the mucosa of the middle lobe bronchus, which exudes a purulent secretion. Computed tomography (CT) shows partial obliteration of the middle lobe bronchus, which prevents distinct filling of its branches, areas of atelectasis (airlessness) and bronchiectasis (bronchial dilation). These findings lead to a tentative diagnosis of obstruction of the middle-lobe bronchus.

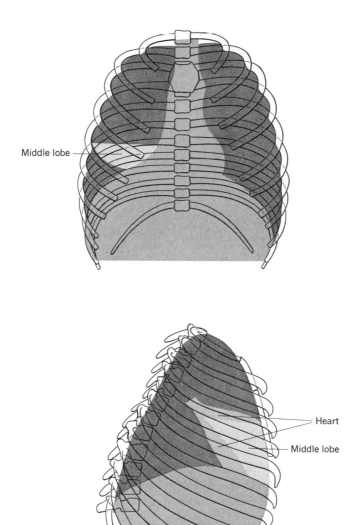

Figure 17-1. Partially atelectatic and infiltrated middle lobe as it appears on posteroanterior and lateral radiographs.

DIAGNOSIS

We are dealing here with an interesting clinical and pathological entity that has become known as the middle lobe syndrome.

THERAPY AND FURTHER COURSE

After the diagnostic workup is completed, the patient is admitted to the thoracic surgical service for operation. Right-sided thoracotomy is performed. The thorax is opened through the right fifth intercostal space with the patient in a semilateral position. The middle lobe is partially collapsed and consolidated. Numerous enlarged lymph nodes surround the middle lobe bronchus. The middle lobe is resected, after its bronchus and artery and the veins draining it have been ligated. Study of the excised lobe reveals that the lobe is the site of chronic infection with many inflammatory changes. The lobe also shows numerous dilated bronchi (bronchiectasis).

The postoperative course is uneventful, and the patient is discharged 10 days after operation. Repeated examinations at three-month intervals show that the patient is relieved of all her symptoms and has regained her previous weight.

DISCUSSION

The sequence of events generally starts with a bacterial infection of the lung, which then spreads along lymphatic channels to regional lymph nodes at the root of the lung. These nodes become inflamed and enlarged. Later, the nodes, which have increased in size, may harden or even become calcified and compress the middle lobe bronchus.

Lymphatic channels

What is the chain of lymph nodes that drains the lung, bronchi, and visceral pleura? A few lymph nodes, called pulmonary nodes, are located within the substance of the lung along the larger bronchi near the hilus. They drain into bronchopulmonary nodes at the hilus of the lung. Their lymph is received by the superior and inferior tracheobronchial nodes, with the former lying in the angle between the trachea and main bronchi and the latter within the bifurcation of the trachea. In turn, their efferent vessels transport lymph into a group of nodes distributed along each side of the trachea, called paratracheal nodes (Fig. 17-2). Efferent lymph vessels of the paratracheal nodes and direct lymph channels from the tracheobronchial nodes join lymphatics from nodes that drain mediastinal organs to form the right and left bronchomediastinal trunks. These commonly open into the venous angle formed by the internal jugular and subclavian veins. Less frequently, the right trunk may drain into the right lymphatic duct and the left into the thoracic duct.

Obstruction of the middle-lobe bronchus

Compression of a lobar bronchus by enlarged lymph nodes, leading to bronchostenosis, may occur at the site of any lobar bronchus but is most common at the middle-lobe bronchus. Are there any features in the anatomy of the middle-lobe bronchus that make it particularly susceptible to stenosis and compression by enlarged lymph nodes? The answer is yes. The stem of the middle-lobe bronchus descends

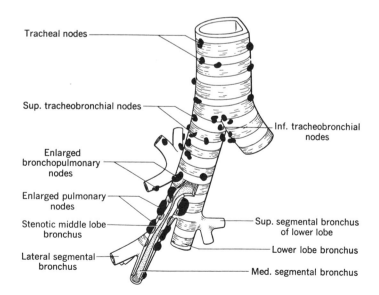

Figure 17-2. Opened middle lobe bronchus partially obstructed by the enlarged lymph nodes and the chains of lymph nodes associated with the trachea and bronchi. The tracheobronchial tree is rotated to the right.

forward and downward before it divides, and during this course it is
encircled by a group of pulmonary lymph nodes that, when enlarged, may reach the size of a cherry (Fig. 17-2). Other lobar bronchi do not enter into such close relationship with nodes and are
therefore not as likely to be compressed.

Do these nodes that surround the middle lobe bronchus drain
the middle lobe exclusively? Lymphatic drainage does not strictly
follow a lobar pattern. Each lung can be subdivided into three
zones of lymphatic drainage that do not coincide with the lobar
boundaries. Thus, the lymph nodes around the middle-lobe bronchus receive lymph not only from the middle lobe but also from
adjacent portions of the lower lobe. It is therefore conceivable that a
primary infection of the lower lobe may lead to enlargement of
lymph nodes, which then compress and obstruct the middle-lobe
bronchus with the typical consequences of chronic stenosis of this
bronchus.

Partial occlusion of the middle lobe bronchus may allow air to
enter but prevent it from leaving, as inspiratory forces are stronger
and the airway tends to collapse on expiration. Overdistention of the
air spaces (emphysema) in the middle lobe, is the result. On the
other hand, if the obstruction is complete, the air is absorbed by
the capillaries of the lung and the lumen collapses (atelectasis). If
infection enters a lobe that is supplied by a partially obstructed
bronchus, a vicious circle is set up, consisting of pulmonary infection
followed by further lymph node enlargement and an increase in the
bronchostenosis, which prevents drainage of the accumulated pus
from the involved lobe. Destructive changes in the lung parenchyma follow, leading to chronic suppuration and tissue breakdown, is accompanied by dilatation of the bronchi (bronchiectasis)
whose walls are damaged by the infection. Lung abscesses and
pleurisy may also be part of the clinical picture. Our case
shows many of the signs mentioned, particularly infection of the
middle-lobe parenchyma, bronchiectasis, and pleurisy. The last of
these could be predicted from the preoperatively present pleural
pain, the others from the fever, malaise, weight loss, and the large
amount of purulent and sometimes bloody sputum expectorated
from the middle lobe. Frequently, particularly in children, enlargement of the lymph nodes compressing the middle lobe bronchus
may be due to tuberculosis, which has a predilection for lymphatic
spread.

Applied anatomy of the middle lobe and its bronchi

Is the direction of the middle lobe bronchus conducive to easy drainage from the infected lobe? The middle-lobe bronchus originates from the bronchus known clinically as the intermediate bronchus, which is about 2 cm long, and located distal to the upper lobe bronchus. It gives rise to both the middle and lower lobe bronchi. The middle-lobe bronchus originates at a rather acute angle and takes a distinctly inferior direction, which makes drainage more difficult. Some observers call attention to the length and pliability of the bronchus, which facilitates compression by encircling nodes. How long is the middle-lobe bronchus? Name the segmental bronchi into which it divides. The middle-lobe bronchus has an average length of about 1.8 cm, after which course it divides into its two segmental branches, the medial and lateral bronchi. The medial bronchus runs downward and forward, the lateral bronchus downward, forward, and laterally. The course of these segmental bronchi is important, as is the shape of the segments supplied by them, because these segments may be the site of isolated collapse resulting from compression of the segmental bronchi by enlarged lymph nodes. Identification of the involved segments can be made from PA and lateral x-ray films; but it may be helpful to visualize these segments as located anteromedially and posterolaterally, realizing that the terms "anterior" and "posterior" apply only to their relation to each other within the lobe. Both segments are, of course, located in front of the oblique fissure, as is the whole middle lobe.

How are the medial and lateral segments approached surgically? Would the posterior chest wall be entered? The medial segment is best approached from the front just below the level of the horizontal fissure, which approximately coincides with the fourth costal cartilage. The lateral segment is reached surgically from the axillary region, where it lies in front of the lower part of the oblique fissure, the level of which roughly coincides with the course of the sixth rib.

What segmental bronchus of the lower lobe has its origin almost directly opposite the origin of the middle-lobe bronchus? The superior bronchus of the lower lobe arises opposite the middle-lobe bronchus. If the superior bronchus is diseased, infected material may readily enter the middle-lobe bronchus and lead to secondary involvement of the middle lobe. Pus and infected sputum from the superior (apical) segment of the lower lobe are particularly likely to enter the middle-lobe bronchus if the patient with an apical abscess of the lower lobe is placed in the prone position (chest down) for purposes of drainage of this abscess.

Keeping in mind that the middle lobe is bound by the horizontal fissure superiorly and the oblique fissure posterolaterally, what would be the shape of an infected lobe on PA and lateral radiographs? The PA view may reveal only subtle changes in right middle-lobe syndrome, often showing a shadow or infiltrate abutting the right heart border with a sharp upper horizontal boundary corresponding to the horizontal fissure. The shadow fades laterally and inferiorly because it is overlapped by normal air-containing lung. The lateral film, which is more revealing of the middle lobe, displays a triangular shadow, the apex of which points posteriorly, and its superior and posterolateral boundaries are formed by the horizontal and oblique fissures bordering on normal air-containing lung tissue of the upper and lower lobes (Fig. 17-1).

18   Lung Cancer with Metastasis

A 56-year-old systems analyst is referred to the hospital by his family physician. His symptoms consist of persistent cough producing blood-tinged sputum and discomfort in the left chest. He also complains of respiratory wheezing and some shortness of breath. The symptoms started about six months ago and have gradually worsened. His cough keeps him awake at night. His appetite is greatly diminished and he has lost twenty pounds.

EXAMINATION

Physical examination of this rather emaciated, weak-appearing patient showed dullness on percussion over the lower posterior portions of the left lung and absence of breath sounds over the same area on auscultation. An imaging study of his chest revealed collapse of the left lower lobe. There was widening of the upper right mediastinum, which was bound toward the lung by a lobulated margin. It was assumed that this widening was caused by a cluster of enlarged paratracheal lymph nodes. Direct bronchoscopy revealed an intraluminal obstruction of the left lower lobe bronchus (Fig. 18-1) and afforded an opportunity for removal of a biopsy specimen, which revealed a squamous cell carcinoma.

DIAGNOSIS

The diagnosis is bronchogenic carcinoma in the left lower bronchus with bronchial obstruction and collapse of the lower left lobe.

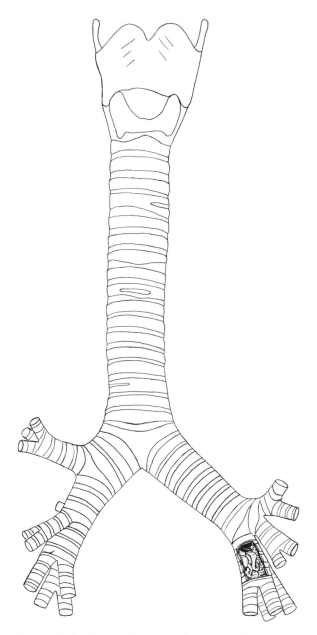

Figure 18-1. Obstructive tumor in the left lower lobe bronchus.

THERAPY AND FURTHER COURSE

During the next two weeks, the patient developed a spiking fever that was probably caused by a superimposed infection in the collapsed lobe. The amount of sputum increased, and he was put on antibiotics. In view of the probable cancerous involvement of the mediastinal lymph nodes on the contralateral side, radical surgery, consisting of removal of the left lung and all accessible lymph nodes, did not seem to offer a good chance for cure. Biopsy of the scalene (supraclavicular) nodes on both sides was undertaken to assess the prognosis for this patient by determining the presence or absence of cancerous invasion of these nodes. They were found to be involved on both sides. Thus, radical resection of the left lung was ruled out and radiation treatment was given. Under this treatment the patient improved temporarily. Inquiry, however, revealed that he died six months later at another hospital. At autopsy, a large tumor was found that occluded the left lower-lobe bronchus (Fig. 18-1). It penetrated the bronchial wall and invaded the surrounding lung parenchyma. The rest of the lobe was collapsed and showed signs of infection and scarring. Numerous cancerous lymph nodes were found in both hilar regions and on both sides of the trachea. There also was metastatic involvement of the brain and suprarenal (adrenal) glands.

DISCUSSION

Anatomy and results of surgical treatment of bronchogenic cancer

We are dealing here with a bronchogenic cancer, which, in those who smoke heavily, is the most common cancer. In only a third of patients with lung cancer is surgical treatment possible and with it the chance of a cure. In the other two thirds, treatment, including radiation therapy, can only be palliative, designed to relieve suffering and make death easier. In operable patients, removal of a whole lung (pneumonectomy) rather than of only a lobe (lobectomy) is the rule. By its nature, pneumonectomy includes ligation and subsequent division of the pulmonary artery, two pulmonary veins, and a main bronchus. In addition, all accessible regional lymph nodes are excised. A more radical version of this operation includes block dissection in one piece of the bifurcation nodes, the paratracheal nodes on both sides, and as many mediastinal nodes of the opposite side as possible. Lobectomy, on the other hand, is resorted to as a curative procedure for tumors of limited extent with minimal involvement of the regional nodes or, in more advanced cases, as a palliative measure in patients with poor respiratory or cardiac reserve. The main danger of both operations is leakage of the bronchial stump, that is, a bronchopleural fistula and infection of the pleural cavity. The five-year survival rate of all patients with pulmonary cancer, including inoperable cases, is 6 to 8 percent; however, 21 to 30 percent of the patients who underwent surgery were alive after five years.

Pulmonary lymphatic system in cancer spread

The pulmonary lymphatic system is the most important channel of spread of lung cancer. It has been said that the surgery of malignant disease is not so much the surgery of the involved organs, but more so of the lymphatic system draining these organs. This statement applies particularly well to cancer of the lung, where the chance for cure and survival is essentially dependent on the anatomy of lymphatic cancer spread. Cancerous involvement of the lymph vessels and subsequent dissemination via these channels to the hilar and mediastinal nodes are the most important modes of cancer dispersal (metastasis). Direction of the lymph stream, along with lymphatic drainage of various regions of the lung, is a fixed and inherited characteristic that does not follow a strict lobar pattern. It allows us to predict with fair accuracy that lymph and abnormal contents of the lymph stream, such as clusters of cancer cells (cancerous emboli), will be carried to specific lymph nodes. In addition, however, more variable pathways exist, which, through anastomoses with the typical lymphatic channels, may conduct some of the lymph as well as cancerous emboli into different sets of lymph nodes. For the lung the typical channels are well established and are discussed in the literature. They comprise the pulmonary, bronchopulmonary, tracheobronchial, and paratracheal nodes, listed in the order in which the lymph stream traverses them. The subsidiary or collateral lymphatic pathways, which represent additional channels of lymph drainage of various lung regions, however, are not as well known and are more variable. They are particularly likely to play a role in cancer spread if the typical regional lymph nodes are

blocked by cancerous growth. In this case small anatomically preformed or newly formed lymph vessels may open up to bypass the
obstructed nodes. Reversal of lymph flow may also occur as well as
crossing of the midline by lymph vessels that connect with nodes on
the opposite side.

The original breakthrough of cancer of the bronchial mucosa
occurs into peribronchial and perivascular lymphatics. From there,
the spread is generally discontinuous with small masses of cancer
cells (emboli) carried in the lymph stream to regional lymph nodes.
The typical number of lymph nodes concerned with drainage of the
lung is about 50 to 60 nodes.

Because the incidence of regional lymph node involvement
(metastasis) at autopsy of lung cancer patients is as high as 95 percent
and in surgical specimen amounts to more than 70 percent, interest
is naturally focused on the path and sequence of intrathoracic lymph
node involvement. The following eight questions and answers may
summarize recent findings on this topic.

1. In cancer of the right upper and middle lobes, which nodes
   among the bronchopulmonary chain are preferentially involved?
   The bronchopulmonary nodes located in the angle between right
   upper and middle lobe bronchi (Fig. 18-2A).
2. As the cancer metastasizes, which group among the tracheobronchial nodes is favored by lymphatic spread from upper or
   middle lobe cancer? The inferior tracheobronchial (subcarinal or
   bifurcation) nodes (Fig. 18-2B).
3. Does bypassing of bronchopulmonary nodes and direct spread to
   tracheobronchial or tracheal nodes occur? It does and is one of
   the characteristic features of lymphatic spread of pulmonary cancer, regardless of the lobe involved.
4. Are cancers of the right upper lobe likely to spread to bronchopulmonary nodes inferior to the middle lobe bronchus? This
   is unlikely.
5. Which of the bronchopulmonary nodes are commonly involved
   in cancer of the left upper lobe? Nodes in the angle between the
   left upper and lower lobe bronchi (Fig. 18-2C).
6. Which accessory lymph channel and nodes often become cancerous in spread from the left upper lobe? An anterior mediastinal channel and subaortic nodes adjacent to the ligamentum arteriosum and the recurrent laryngeal nerve (Fig. 18-2D).

7. Which nodes are typically affected in cancer spread from the right or left lower lobes? Bronchopulmonary nodes between middle and lower lobe bronchi on the right (Fig. 18-2E) and upper and lower lobe bronchi on the left (Fig. 18-2C) as well as nodes between upper and middle lobe bronchi on the right (Fig. 18-2A) and above the upper lobe bronchus on the left. Further drainage takes place into superior (Fig. 18-2F) and inferior tracheobronchial nodes (Fig. 18-2B) and also to nodes in the pulmonary ligament and posterior mediastinal nodes (not shown in figure).

8. Is there a difference in the lymphatic drainage of the right and left lower lobes? Contralateral spread to the right paratracheal nodes in cancer of the left lower lobe is a common occurrence, whereas spread to left nodes in right-sided lung cancer seems infrequent.

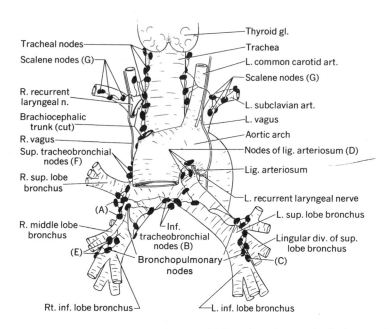

Figure 18-2. Tracheobronchial tree with lymph nodes particularly apt to be involved in the spread of bronchogenic malignancies. For explanation and identification of nodes marked by symbols, see text.

The latter point is well exemplified by our case of cancer in the left lower-lobe bronchus displaying spread to contralateral paratracheal lymph nodes on the imaging study. The autopsy findings in our patient showed involvement of most of the lymph nodes in the right and left hilar and paratracheal areas. The finding is fairly typical in fatal cases.

Scalene node biopsy

Our case history mentions that a scalene node biopsy was done and that the finding of cancer cells in these nodes precluded radical surgery. How is this diagnostic procedure performed? What are its dangers and its rationale? Scalene node biopsy for diagnosis of cancer spread from the lung and even from abdominal viscera was initiated about 50 years ago, paralleling the increasing interest in radical pulmonary surgery. The operation, which is done with the patient under local anesthesia, consists of removal of the inferior deep cervical lymph nodes, known clinically as scalene (also supraclavicular) nodes because of their relationship to the anterior scalene muscle. After division of skin, platysma, and the appropriate layers of deep cervical fascia, and after medial retraction of the sternocleidomastoid muscle, a pad of fat and embedded lymph vessels and nodes superficial to the scalene muscles are removed in toto. The territory involved is bound by the posterior belly of the omohyoid laterally, the internal jugular vein medially, and the subclavian vein inferiorly. The operation may require ligation of the external jugular vein and the transverse cervical and suprascapular vessels. Care must be taken not to injure the dome of the parietal pleura (cupola), the internal jugular vein, the subclavian vein, the phrenic nerve, the brachial plexus, and the thoracic duct on the left side. Identify these structures on atlas pictures and remember that the phrenic nerve lies on the anterior scalene muscle deep to the prevertebral fascia. The operation is frequently extended into the upper mediastinum with the aim of removing some of the paratracheal nodes as well. Is the scalene node removal always done on the side of the suspected malignancy? Because the lymph from the left lower lobe drains at least in part into the right paratracheal nodes and also because lymphatic communications across the midline have been demonstrated as subsidiary channels, particularly in the presence of obstruction of the lymph stream, bilateral scalene node biopsy is probably the operation of choice, more so when the tumor is in the left lower-lung region.

What is the rationale for scalene node biopsy? The lungs and trachea, including the cervical part of the trachea, drain into the scalene nodes (Fig. 18-2G). How often does this cancerous involvement of the scalene nodes occur? Carcinoma of the lungs yields a positive diagnosis in about 40 percent of all scalene node biopsies. If such metastasis has occurred, the case is regarded as inoperable, and opening of the thorax becomes unnecessary. It is worth mentioning that scalene node biopsy is done also in cases of other lung diseases, such as sarcoidosis and tumors of the lymphatic system.

Usually the nodes receiving drainage from the lungs are grayish and mottled with black material. What is the reason for their darkened coloration? How is this black coloration useful to the surgeon and pathologist? The blackened appearance of the nodes is termed anthracosis (anthraco-coal) and is due to the presence of carbon filtered and collected in the nodes draining the lungs. Most of the carbon that enters the body comes from dust or smoke that is inhaled.

Mediastinal complications in lung cancer

Mediastinal lymph node involvement may lead to some noteworthy complications. Mention has been made of spread to a lymph node or nodes in the vicinity of the left recurrent laryngeal nerve. What clinical complications would occur with pressure on this nerve? It would result in hoarseness due to paralysis of the left vocal cord (Fig. 18-2D). One side of the diaphragm may be paralyzed by pressure on the phrenic nerve in the case of enlarged and cancerous mediastinal lymph nodes. The latter may also displace the esophagus and cause difficulty in swallowing (dysphagia), which is easily demonstrated by a radiographic examination, with the patient swallowing an opaque medium. A chest film or coronal magnetic resonance imaging scan may also reveal widening of the angle of bifurcation caused by enlarged inferior tracheobronchial lymph nodes. The superior vena cava may be obstructed by tumors of the right upper lobe or cancerous invasion of the regional lymph nodes.

Vascular spread of lung cancer

In addition to involvement of the lymphatics, erosion of the pulmonary veins in bronchial carcinoma is quite common and carries serious consequences because it leads to dispersal of cancerous emboli through the bloodstream. Describe the pathway along which such emboli from the lung must travel to reach distant organs throughout the body. After the pulmonary veins have been invaded by cancer, the emboli pass through the left atrium, the left ventricle, and by way of the aorta into the arterial circulation until they are arrested in the capillary filters of various organs. Such hematogenous metastases are most frequent in the suprarenal glands, brain, bone, liver, and kidneys.

19   Mediastinal Pleurisy

An eight-month-old infant boy is brought into the outpatient department by his mother because of a history of irritability and restlessness for the preceding two months. The mother reports that three months earlier her son had a middle-ear infection that required lancing of the eardrum (myringotomy) and drainage of the middle ear. She also states that he has been coughing for some time and that his breathing has become noisy and wheezing, particularly at night. The baby is admitted to the hospital.

EXAMINATION

Examination shows that the infant is well developed but slightly underweight. His upper respiratory tract is moderately inflamed. He has the physical signs of a bronchitis and a low-grade fever.

Radiographic examination of the chest reveals a homogeneous, laterally well-defined shadow paralleling the right cardiac margin (Fig. 19-1). On further study with the patient in various positions, this abnormal radiographic finding is interpreted as an encapsulated effusion, located anteriorly in the lower part of the right pleural cavity between visceral and mediastinal pleurae.

DIAGNOSIS

Right-sided anterior-inferior mediastinal pleurisy with exudate is diagnosed.

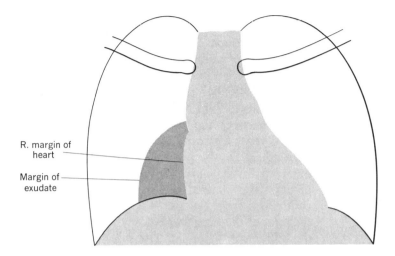

R. margin of
heart

Margin of
exudate

Figure 19-1. Roentgenogram of the chest show a homogeneous, laterally sharply defined shadow paralleling the right cardiac margin caused by right-sided anterior-inferior mediastinal pleurisy with exudate.

THERAPY AND FURTHER COURSE

The pleural cavity was tapped through the anterior thoracic wall, and 250 ml of clear fluid was removed. Although no pathogenic organisms could be identified in the fluid, the patient was put on antibiotic and antifebrile medication. During the next two weeks, his breathing improved and cough and fever subsided. The subsequent radiographic study showed disappearance of the previously described shadow. The patient was discharged from the hospital.

DISCUSSION

Pleural effusions as a concomitant or result of upper respiratory infections are not an uncommon finding in infants. What is the content of the normal pleural cavity? This cavity is only a potential space containing a thin film of lubricating fluid that facilitates sliding respiratory motion between the two layers of pleura. What are these two layers, and at what location are they continuous with each other? Do the pleural cavities of the two sides communicate? What are the subdivisions of the parietal pleura? The visceral pleura that covers each lung is continuous with the parietal pleura as a sleeve around the hilus of the lung and below the hilus as a pleural fold, the pulmonary ligament. The subdivisions of the parietal pleura, which line the thoracic walls and reach into the neck above the anterior portion of the first rib, are the cervical, costal, diaphragmatic, and the mediastinal pleuras. The pleural cavities of the two sides do not communicate.

Location of pleural exudates

Exudates as a result of pleural inflammation may collect in the pleural cavity between the previously named parts of the parietal pleura and the visceral pleura. If sufficiently large, the exudate may completely envelop the pleura-ensheathed lung laterally, anteriorly, posteriorly, medially, superiorly, and inferiorly. Frequently, however, with time, broad adhesions between parietal and visceral pleurae are formed that localize the exudate in one or more areas. Such encapsulated effusions may, for example, be found between the base of the lung and the diaphragmatic pleura.

Are all pleural exudates fluid collections between parietal and visceral pleuras? No. Interlobar pleurisy results in accumulation of fluid between two layers of visceral pleura in the horizontal and oblique fissures.

Anatomy of mediastinal pleurisy

In infants with respiratory infection, encapsulated fluid collections between mediastinal and visceral pleurae are quite common and are identified as a mediastinal pleurisy. Is this exudate in the mediastinum? The mediastinum is the space between right and left mediastinal pleurae and is not involved in this case. The fluid collection is located on the right side of the mediastinum.

To understand the topography of a mediastinal pleurisy, it is necessary to visualize the difference in the extent of the mediastinal pleural space at the hilus, both superior and inferior to it. What is the difference in the cross-sectional arrangement of the pleural space at these three levels (Fig. 19-2)? Above the hilus of the lung, the mediastinal pleural space extends without interruption from the sternum to the vertebral column. By contrast, at the hilus and below it, the pleural sleeve around the root of the lung and the pulmonary

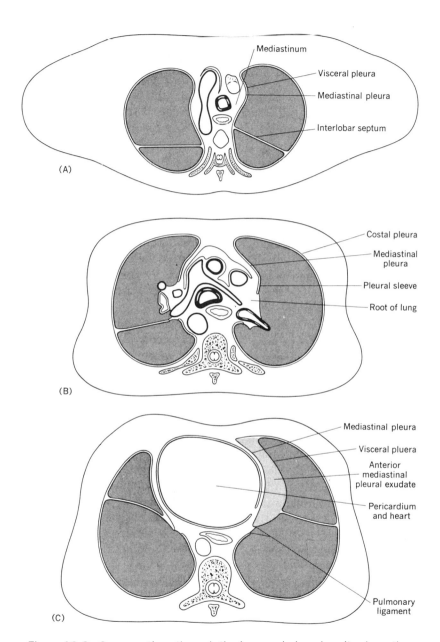

Figure 19-2. Cross sections through the lung and pleural cavity above the root of the lung (A), at the root of the lung (B), and caudal to the root of the lung at the level of pulmonary ligament (C). Note exudate in C in anterior pleuromediastinal space.

ligament inferior to the root divide the space into anterior and posterior compartments.

Where would effusions between mediastinal and visceral pleurae more commonly occupy the whole anteroposterior extent of the pleural space, above or below the root of the lung? Although adhesions between the mediastinal portion of the parietal and the visceral pleurae may confine the extent of the fluid in an anterior or posterior location, for anatomical reasons, fluid collections superior to the hilus are frequently more extensive in a sagittal (anteroposterior) plane than are exudates located more inferiorly. Can you give the boundaries of the fluid collection in the case under discussion (Fig. 19-2C)? The exudate here is confined by adhesions and normal anatomical boundaries to a part of the right pleural cavity that is bound anteriorly by the sternum and costal cartilages, medially by the lower part of the right mediastinal pleura, inferiorly by the diaphragmatic pleura, laterally by the medial anterior aspect of the visceral pleura covering the mediastinal surface of the lung, and posteriorly by the pulmonary ligament. The exudate was large enough to displace the right lung laterally to a considerable extent.

Prognosis

In general, this type of pleurisy can be regarded as a benign disease whose symptoms gradually disappear under treatment, but that quite often leaves pleural adhesions obliterating the involved part of the pleural cavity.

20   Angina Pectoris

A 59-year-old physician who is 30 pounds overweight enters the hospital with a history of attacks of pain that started two years earlier. The pain is located in the left shoulder, radiating from there to the sternum and to the pit of the stomach. These attacks of pain came at lengthy intervals until the preceding two weeks, when they began to occur every day, forcing him to stop work. The pain is not severe and is always relieved by rest. His left arm feels weak, especially after an attack of pain.

EXAMINATION

On physical examination, involvement of the joints, muscles, periosteum, and peripheral nerves must be considered. The shoulder joint shows no objective abnormality and movements are free. Myalgia, an aching condition of the skeletal muscles, should be considered, particularly in this age group, whenever unusual physical exercise precedes the attack of pain. What muscle located in the painful area would likely cause a similar distribution of pain? By what motion can a check be done for noninvolvement of this muscle in putting its fibers on the stretch? The fibers of the pectoralis major would be stretched in abduction and lateral rotation of the arm. An absence of pain in performing these motions would rule out inflammation of this muscle.

An inflammatory lesion in the richly innervated periosteum

over the ribs can be excluded by the absence of tenderness. Neuralgia of the intercostal nerves can be ruled out by the absence of pressure pain along the course of the intercostal nerves. How can the cause of such pain be discovered by physical examination, keeping in mind the course of the intercostal nerves in the area involved? In case of neuralgia of one or more intercostal nerves, there would be localized tenderness on pressure along the costal groove and inferior margin of the corresponding ribs.

Further examination shows that the heart is slightly enlarged but otherwise negative. Palpation reveals radial and brachial arteries that are markedly thickened and tortuous. With reference to the patient's complaint, we note that the pain comes in attacks that are relieved by rest and that it has very wide radiation.

Angiography confirmed the preliminary diagnosis of coronary artery disease. The right coronary artery was 85% blocked and the anterior interventricular artery (left anterior descending or LAD) 70% blocked.

DIAGNOSIS

Pain of the type described in a man aged 59 years suggests angina pectoris.

THERAPY AND FURTHER COURSE

The patient's pain is relieved by the administration of nitrates which dilate the coronary arteries. Coronary bypass is suggested to the patient, and he is referred to a cardiologist for further care.

Two weeks later, a team of cardiovascular surgeons perform a double bypass using saphenous vein graphs. The surgery goes well and after two days in the intensive coronary care unit (ICCU) and four days of bed rest, including a consultation with a dietitian and exercise physiologist, the patient is discharged for further recovery at home. He is put on aspirin and a low-fat diet and, six weeks later, a program of regular exercise.

DISCUSSION

Angina pectoris is characterized by attacks of moderate to severe chest pain originating in the heart. The attacks are usually precipitated by exertion, excitement, or a heavy meal and are relieved or diminished by rest. The pain is felt beneath the sternum and radiates most commonly to the neck, left shoulder, or arm. The pain is customarily explained on the basis of *ischemia*, or an insufficient supply of oxygen to the heart muscle as a result of arteriosclerotic narrowing of the coronary arteries, particularly when the heart is required to perform increased amounts of work.

Pain pathways in angina pectoris

What are the anatomical pathways for pain impulses from the heart? Do all cervical cardiac nerves participate in the transmission of pain? Are the cervical cardiac nerves the only pathway for cardiac pain? Is the vagus important in the transmission of pain impulses from the heart? Where are the cell bodies of the pain fibers located? Do pain fibers return to spinal nerves via gray or white rami communicantes?

The answers to the preceding questions can be arrived at by knowledge of the anatomy of cardiac sensation. Stimuli are received by free nerve endings in the cardiac connective tissue and the adventitia of the cardiac blood vessels. From there, they travel in visceral sensory fibers through the cardiac plexus and through the middle and inferior cervical cardiac and thoracic cardiac nerves to the sympathetic chain ganglia of the neck and upper thorax. From the middle and inferior cervical chain ganglia, these fibers descend without synapse in the chain to upper thoracic ganglia, where other pain pathways arrive directly via thoracic cardiac nerves. From the upper four or five thoracic chain ganglia, the fibers continue, again without synapse, via white rami communicantes, to spinal nerves T1 to T5 and their corresponding dorsal roots and ganglia. Here their cell bodies are located. Central fibers from these dorsal root ganglia go to the upper thoracic cord segments (Fig. 20-1). The superior cervical cardiac nerves probably do not contain any afferent fibers, and the sensory components of the vagus nerve apparently do not transmit any pain impulses from the heart but participate in reflex actions (typical of parasympathetic sensory fibers) that lower blood pressure and slow the heart rate.

The correctness of these cardiac pain pathways is confirmed by successful surgical attack of cardiac pain. The latter can be eradicated by division of the upper five thoracic dorsal spinal nerve roots on both sides. The same result will be obtained if the upper four or five thoracic chain ganglia or the white rami communicantes are

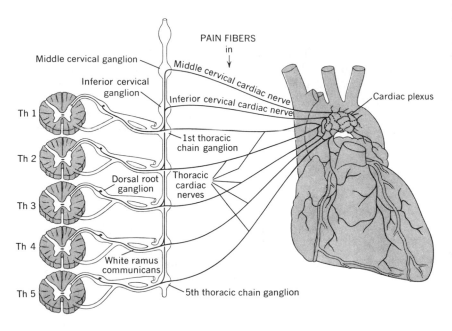

Figure 20-1. Pathways of cardiac pain.

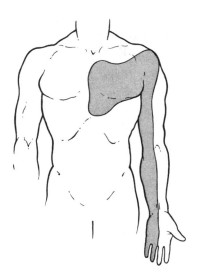

Figure 20-2. Typical area of pain referral in angina pectoris.

removed or chemically blocked on both sides (Fig. 20-1). Surgery or blockage on the left side may occasionally suffice.

The details of referred pain remain incompletely understood; however, cardiac pain is referred to areas of the body surface that send sensory impulses to the same segments of the spinal cord that receive cardiac sensory impulses, that is, mainly cervical 8 to thoracic 5. A preponderance of the pain occurs on the left side. The highest two segments listed are responsible for pain along the medial side of the arm and forearm (Fig. 20-2). In addition to the often occurring sensation of retrosternal pressure and constriction, cardiac pain may atypically be referred to the side of the neck, ear, lower jaw, and back of the chest, particularly the interscapular area. This type of pain referral is hard to explain on an anatomical basis.

21   Myocardial Infarction

A 52-year-old insurance adjuster is brought to the hospital in an ambulance. His wife, who accompanied him, states that during dinner he started to complain of excruciating chest pain in the region of the sternum. These symptoms were accompanied by nausea, vomiting, and severe shortness of breath. She also points out that for several years the patient has been suffering from chest pain that radiated into the left arm, particularly after physical effort or emotional upsets.

EXAMINATION AND FURTHER COURSE

On admission the patient appears to be in shock. His skin is ashen gray with some cyanosis (bluish tinge) and is cold and clammy. His blood pressure is low, his pulse is quite weak, and his pulse rate is 110 beats per minute. His respirations are noisy and gasping. On auscultation of the lungs, abnormal breath sounds are heard. His heart sounds are feeble and arrhythmic. Despite oxygen application, intravenous injection of circulatory stimulants, electric defibrillation, and cardiac massage, the patient dies within 2 h after admission.

    At autopsy marked narrowing of both coronary arteries and many of their branches, is found, a result of atherosclerosis of the vessel wall. There is an old occlusion in the first portion of the right coronary artery and a fresh intimal hemorrhage in the anterior interventricular branch (left anterior descending, LAD) near its origin from the left coronary artery. This, in combination with a fresh blood clot, has completely occluded the anterior interventricular branch.

DIAGNOSIS

Sudden death is caused by coronary occlusion due to atherosclerosis of the coronary arteries (myocardial infarction).

DISCUSSION

Ischemic heart disease, that is, heart disease caused by insufficient blood supply to the heart muscle, is one of the most frequent conditions encountered in patients aged older than 40 years. It is the leading cause of death in the United States.

The function of the coronary arteries is to carry blood to the myocardium and thus maintain its nutrition. When the lumen of a coronary artery becomes narrowed or obliterated by atherosclerosis of the intima, the portion of the myocardium supplied by the affected artery suffers from lack of oxygen (hypoxia) and becomes damaged. This myocardial hypoxia may result in rapid death, as happened in our patient, and generally brings about ventricular fibrillation. The latter condition is a cardiac arrhythmia leading to completely disorganized ventricular excitation and ineffective contraction resulting in circulatory failure and, frequently, death.

Anatomy of the coronary arteries

The decisive factor in the life of individuals with coronary artherosclerosis is the state of the coronary circulation. Identify the arterial supply to the heart and give the origin of these arteries. The right and left coronary arteries are middle-sized muscular arteries that arise from the right and left aortic sinuses of the ascending aorta just distal to the aortic semilunar valves. The main arteries run in the epicardial fat of the atrioventricular and interventricular grooves; they are partly concealed by fat and in some locations also by thin layers of ventricular myocardium, so that dissection becomes necessary for their demonstration.

To what extent does the statement that the right coronary artery supplies the right side of the heart, and the left coronary artery the left heart, require qualification? Typically, the right coronary artery supplies the right atrium and the right ventricle with the exception of the left part of the sternocostal surface of the right ventricle, which is supplied by the left coronary artery. The left coronary artery supplies the left atrium and left ventricle with the exception of the left auricle, the posterior surface of the left atrium, and the right part of the diaphragmatic aspect of the left ventricle, which are supplied by the right coronary artery. What is the blood supply to the interatrial and interventricular septa, where important parts of the conducting system are located? Whereas the interatrial septum is usually supplied from the right coronary artery, both the right and left coronary vessels participate in the arterial supply of the interventricular septum through their interventricular branches, with the left commonly carrying the greater share (Fig. 21-1).

Are coronary arteries end arteries?

Are coronary arteries end arteries? What is your definition of an end artery? End arteries are arteries that do not anastomose (communicate) with other arteries or arterial branches of the same artery. Obstruction of such an end artery interferes with the blood supply to that part of the organ supplied by the artery and leads to necrosis (tissue death) of that segment of the organ.

What are some vital organs that are supplied by end arteries? The retina, inner ear, brain, liver, and kidney are nourished by arteries that do not anastomose or anastomose only to a degree insufficient to keep the segment viable that is supplied by the obstructed artery. The area of necrosis is known as an infarct. From the frequent occurrence of cardiac infarction, we can deduce that a collateral circulation is absent or inadequate in these cases; however, the branches of the coronary arteries are not true end arteries, because numerous anastomoses take place either between the right and left coronary arteries (intercoronary anastomoses) or between branches of the same artery (intracoronary anastomoses).

Intracardiac collateral circulation

What are some of the common sites of anastomosis between the two coronary arteries? The coronary sulcus, the posterior interventricular sulcus, the area of the apex, and the interventricular septum are

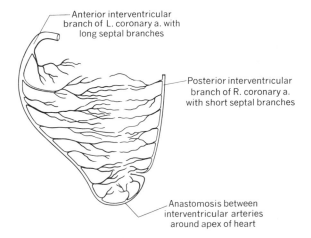

Anterior interventricular
branch of L. coronary a. with
long septal branches

Posterior interventricular
branch of R. coronary a.
with short septal branches

Anastomosis between
interventricular arteries
around apex of heart

Figure 21-1. (modified after James and Burch)—Arterial supply of the
interventricular septum. Notice that in this type the anterior two thirds of
the septum are supplied by the anterior interventricular branch of the left
coronary and the posterior third by the posterior interventricular branch of
the right coronary. Observe the site of anastomosis between the two interventricular branches of the coronary arteries around the apex of the heart
and the communications of the septal branches.

locations where arterial anastomoses can frequently be demonstrated (Figs. 21-1 and 21-2).

Give an example of an intracoronary anastomosis. The two main
branches of the left coronary artery, the anterior interventricular
and the circumflex, can often be seen to communicate around
the left (obtuse) border of the heart. Commonly, however, these
communications, although anatomically patent, are small and func-
tionally inactive. Thus, we can speak of the coronary arteries as
physiologic end arteries. In other words, the collateral circulation in
the normal is usually ineffective in preventing an infarction in case of
sudden interruption of the circulation. Depending on the degree of
obstruction and the order and size of the obstructed arterial branch,
interference with the coronary circulation may result in functional
insufficiency, leading to angina pectoris, that is, cardiac pain, or
myocardial necrosis of variable extent. If, however, the occlusion of
a coronary branch is slow and gradual, anastomoses may enlarge and
carry an adequate circulation to the heart muscle.

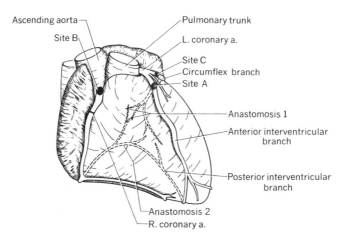

Figure 21-2. Location of two typical intercoronary anastomoses and three sites of predilection of coronary occlusion. Anastomosis (1) depicts the communication in the posterior part of the coronary sulcus between the right coronary artery and circumflex branch of the left coronary artery. Anastomosis (2) shows the communication in the posterior interventricular sulcus between the posterior and anterior interventricular branches of the right and left coronary arteries. Notice the three most common locations of coronary occlusion. They are, in descending order of frequency, the anterior interventricular branch of the left coronary (site A), the right coronary (site B), and the circumflex branch of the left coronary (site C). Occlusion occurs in all three sites, most commonly close to the origin of the vessels.

Why can a patient who has cardiac ischemia, as indicated by angina pectoris, and who survives a cardiac infarction, be relieved of his pain afterwards? The reason for this clinically well-known phenomenon is that the patient has now developed a more efficient collateral circulation than before the attack.

Sites of coronary occlusion

What are some of the sites of predilection of coronary occlusion? The most common location for coronary occlusion is the anterior interventricular branch of the left coronary (about 70 percent of all cases). Next in frequency comes the right coronary, then the circumflex branch of the left coronary artery. In the vast majority of cases, the occlusion involves only the proximal portion of the involved blood vessels (Fig. 21-2).

Variations in dominance of coronary arteries

Of great practical importance is the variation in the pattern of coronary arterial distribution from individual to individual. Identify the three types of distribution in terms of the dominance of one or the other of the coronary arteries. What is their respective frequency? In about 50 percent, the right coronary artery is the preponderant vessel, which, with its posterior interventricular branch, supplies most of the diaphragmatic surface of both ventricles and part of the interventricular septum. In about 20 percent, the left coronary artery predominates, with the posterior interventricular branch essentially derived from the circumflex branch of the left coronary. In the remaining approximately 30 percent there exists a balanced circulation.

Given an atherosclerotic obstruction of the left circumflex artery, which of the three types just described would be least desirable? In this case the left preponderant type would present the greatest risk. The area of infarction would be larger than in the other types, the heart would have the least chance for development of a satisfactory collateral circulation, and the prognosis would be poorer. On the other hand, ischemic involvement of a nondominant artery would offer the best chance for development of compensatory channels.

Intramural circulation

Does all blood carried in the coronary arteries pass through the capillary bed into the cardiac veins? It is a peculiarity of the cardiac circulation that there are channels that pass from coronary arterioles, from the capillary bed, and from the cardiac veins directly into the lumen of the heart. Irregular thin-walled channels larger than capillary size, called myocardial sinusoids, also receive blood from the coronary arterioles or the capillary bed and communicate with the smallest cardiac veins (Thebesian veins) that open directly into the chambers of the heart, particularly into the atria. It has been assumed that the stream in these veins can be reversed and thus help to nourish the ischemic myocardium in case of coronary obstruction. Some of these openings in the cardiac cavity can be seen with the naked eye by inspection of the endocardial lining. They vary from pinpoint size to almost 1 mm in diameter.

Heart surgeons have taken advantage of the reversed flow phenomenon in cases of multiple coronary obstructions by carrying out retrograde cardioplegia of the right ventricle during open heart surgery. In this procedure cold hyperkalemic blood is infused into the coronary sinus, which arrests the heart and reduces energy demand.

With the exception of the smallest cardiac veins, do all cardiac veins drain into the coronary sinus? The anterior cardiac veins are several smaller veins that drain part of the sternocostal surface of the right ventricle and open directly into the right atrium.

Extracardiac anastomoses

Does the coronary arterial system enter into communications with other arteries in the neighborhood and, if so, how do these arteries reach the heart? How important are they for the supply of the ischemic myocardium? Anastomoses do exist between the coronary circulation and extracardiac arteries. These communications are small branches of the pericardiacophrenic and musculophrenic arteries given off by the internal thoracic artery and of the posterior intercostal, superior phrenic, bronchial, and esophageal arteries from the thoracic aorta. They enter by way of the pericardial reflections around the major veins and arteries entering and leaving the heart. Rarely are they large enough to serve as a significant source of supply for collateral circulation in case of coronary stenosis or obstruction.

Surgical procedures used to produce a collateral circulation

What surgical measures have been undertaken to increase the blood supply to the ischemic heart? In the past, experimental and clinical attempts were made to increase the normally present and just mentioned extracardiac anastomoses of the coronary bed by obliterating the pericardial cavity through irritants inserted into the pericardial sac or by scarifying the epicardial surface of the heart with the expectation that new outside vessels will invade the myocardium. Those procedures are now obsolete. Other sources of additional blood supply that are currently used include implantation of the pectoralis major or the latissimus dorsi muscles onto the ischemic myocardium.

Bypass operations are much more common. A great saphenous vein autograft (graft from the same person) can be used to connect the ascending aorta with portions of the right or left coronary artery distal to the occlusion(s), thus bypassing the diseased section of the artery. This approach provides instant perfusion of aortic blood into the peripheral distribution area of the coronary arteries. An equally popular method of bypassing the area of blockage makes use of the internal thoracic artery (frequently called the internal mammary artery by clinicians). The artery is dissected from the anterior chest wall in sufficient length to reach beyond the occluded coronary artery. It is left attached proximally at its origin from the subclavian artery, and its anterior intercostal branches are ligated. Its severed end is implanted into the diseased coronary artery distal to the blockage.

The technique of dilating a blocked vessel by the insertion of a small balloon (balloon angioplasty) into the stenosed area has also become commonplace. Known as percutaneous transluminal coronary angioplasty (PTCA), this is a nonsurgical technique in which a balloon-tipped catheter that has a double-lumen is inserted percutaneously into an artery and advanced under radiographic control until the catheter tip has passed into the narrowed region. At this point the balloon is inflated, forcing the vessel stenosed (narrowed) with atherosclerotic plaque to open.

Although the various methods of revascularization of the ischemic myocardium, including laser angioplasty are still under trial, surgical treatment for coronary artery disease is an accepted method. It has a low mortality and offers hope of a better quality of life and increased life expectancy in patients with coronary artery disease.

22   Coarctation of the Aorta

A 28-year-old construction worker comes to the outpatient department with complaints of headache, nosebleed, occasional dizziness, and palpitations. For the past five months, he also has increasing shortness of breath on exertion that, to a certain extent, has interfered with his working capacity. On examination six years earlier, he was told that his blood pressure was elevated.

EXAMINATION

On physical examination the patient appears normally developed, in good nutritional state, and in no apparent distress. Significant findings are the following. There is considerable elevation of pressure in the brachial arteries but diminished pressure in the popliteal arteries. The pulse in both femoral arteries appears quite weak and delayed compared with the radial pulse. On percussion the left ventricle appears enlarged. On auscultation there is a systolic murmur over the heart that is also demonstrable in the interscapular area to the left of the midline. Radiographic examination of the thorax shows normal lungs, but the left ventricle is hypertrophic and moderately enlarged. The aortic knob, the transitional area between the arch and descending aorta, is not clearly visualized, and there is a definite bilateral notching and erosion of the inferior margins of the posterolateral portions of ribs four to nine. The patient is admitted to the hospital.

On reexamination, previous findings are confirmed, and the following evidence of collateral arterial circulation of the thorax is elicited. There are pulsations visible and palpable in the interscapular area and inferior to both scapulae. Similar pulsations can be demonstrated adjacent to the clavicle and along both sides of the sternum in the area of the internal thoracic artery. On close inspection, tortuous and enlarged blood vessels can be seen under the skin of the back and sides of the thorax.

On the basis of a history of hypertension and the findings of elevated blood pressure in the upper extremities and diminished pressure in the lower extremities, the weak femoral pulse, the presence of demonstrable collateral arterial circulation over the thorax, and the typical radiographic findings, a tentative diagnosis of stenosis or constriction at the isthmus of the aorta (coarctation) is made. In view of the poor prognosis in this condition if left untreated, surgery is taken under advisement.

A preoperative aortogram of the thoracic aorta is decided on to obtain a clear picture of the anatomical condition, particularly the site, width, and length of the aortic constriction. Although an MRI (magnetic resonance imaging) study would provide much of this information without the use of contrast medium, the traditional aortogram was selected because it also provides valuable information, unavailable by MRI, about the intercostal arteries soon to be encountered in the thoracotomy.

A catheter is introduced into the radial artery against the direction of the bloodstream and pushed under fluoroscopic control as far as the ascending aorta. An x-ray opaque medium is rapidly injected, and multiple radiographs are taken after injection, which show a circumscribed stenosis at the typical site of the aortic isthmus beyond the origin of the left subclavian artery. The prestenotic segment of the aorta is somewhat wider than normal; the brachiocephalic trunk and the left common carotid and left subclavian arteries are moderately enlarged. The poststenotic segment is also enlarged, proving that the obstruction of the aorta is incomplete. The following greatly widened and tortuous arteries are demonstrated by an aortogram as part of the collateral circulation. Branches of the right and left internal thoracic arteries anastomose with the inferior epigastric arteries. An enlarged subscapular artery and a few tortuous posterior intercostal arteries are also visualized.

DIAGNOSIS

Circumscribed stenosis of the aortic isthmus with well-developed collateral circulation (aortic coarctation) is diagnosed.

THERAPY AND FURTHER COURSE

In view of the anatomical findings of a circumscribed obstruction at the typical site, grafting or the utilization of a vascular prosthesis is ruled out, and an end-to-end anastomosis after resection of the stenotic portion is planned.

Under general endotracheal anesthesia the aorta is approached from the left side of the chest, where the fourth rib is removed and the thorax is entered through the bed of the resected rib. Several enlarged and tortuous vessels of the chest wall are encountered and doubly ligated. The aorta is mobilized above and below the stenosed area, starting just distal to the left subclavian artery. Here several dilated and fragile posterior intercostal arteries are seen and ligated. The ligamentum arteriosum is ligated and divided. After the aorta is sufficiently freed, it is clamped on either side of the constricted portion, and the area of coarctation is excised. Enough vascular tissue is resected to provide for normal caliber at the site of the anastomosis. Then the cut ends of the aorta are approximated, evened, and sutured together so that the interior of the vessel is covered everywhere by intima. The clamps are slowly opened and the suture lines checked for leaks. The chest wall is closed, leaving a catheter behind for drainage.

The excised specimen shows that the lumen of the aorta at the constricted site consists only of a small opening not more than 2 mm in diameter and narrower than expected from the outside appearance of the aorta. The obstruction in the interior of the aorta is due to a diaphragm-like infolding of the media with some secondary intimal thickening. The aortic end of the ligamentum arteriosum, which was removed with the narrowed segment of the aorta, is nonpatent.

During the operation and postoperatively, the patient is given blood transfusions. Postoperatively, he has some fever and is given antibiotics, after which his temperature slowly returns to normal. The patient is gradually allowed to become physically active. He is dismissed from the hospital three weeks after the operation. During this period pulsations in the femoral artery gradually increase in intensity, and there is also a gradual diminution of blood pressure in the upper extremity and a concomitant increase to normal in the lower. The patient is seen in six months and again one year after the operation. He is well satisfied with the result and has returned to his former work. His blood pressure in the upper and lower extremities remains normal.

DISCUSSION

We are dealing here with a congenital cardiovascular anomaly, which is seen with a frequency of about one in 2000 of all autopsies. It is four or five times more common in males than in females. Coarctation (L coarctare, to constrict) is a pathologic condition in which the lumen of the aortic arch or of the descending aorta just beyond the arch is significantly constricted on a congenital basis.

Define the term "isthmus of the aorta." It is that portion of the aortic arch between the left subclavian artery and the ductus arteriosus. It is normally constricted at birth but enlarges soon thereafter as the ductus arteriosus becomes obliterated. This is also the typical site of a diffuse type of coarctation of the aorta in the infant, in which case the ductus arteriosus often remains patent. More common is the type in which clinical signs and symptoms become apparent only during adult life and in which the constriction is more circumscribed and located at or just beyond the point of entrance of the ductus arteriosus (or ligament), as in our case (Fig. 22-1). Other variants also occur, although rarely, for example, an aortic stenosis proximal (not distal) to the origin of the left subclavian artery.

Cause of coarctation

What is the explanation for the occurrence of congenital coarctation of the aorta? The cause of the condition was thought to be an extension into the aorta of the obliterative process that occludes the ductus arteriosus. This view seems hardly tenable if one realizes that coarctation frequently occurs in the absence of obliteration of the duct. Other explanations offered are traction on the aortic wall with infolding of the media caused by the pull of the ductus arteriosus, the dimensions of which do not keep step with the growth of the aorta. The mode of genesis of the malformation remains obscure, although it is probably related to the involution of the ductus arte-

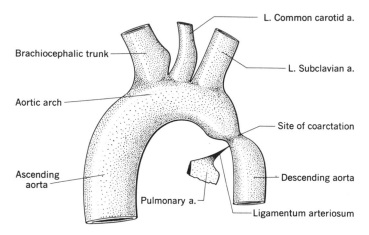

Figure 22-1. Coarctation of the aorta beyond the origin of the left subclavian artery at the site of attachment of the ligamentum arteriosum. Aortic
arch and its branches are dilated.

riosus. From what primitive aortic arch is the latter derived? The
ductus arteriosus represents the dorsal part of the left sixth arch.

Explanation of signs and symptoms

How do you explain the clinical symptoms of the patient, consisting
of headache, nosebleed, and dizziness, in light of the anatomical
picture of a circumscribed stenosis of the aorta? His complaints are
due to increased blood pressure in the prestenotic portion of the
aorta and its branches, most likely caused by the additional resistance offered to the propulsion of the blood at the site of the stenosis.
It is also borne out by the objective finding of hypertension in both
brachial arteries present in the patient. As a result of the greatly
increased arterial pressure in the prestenotic portion of the aorta,
the aortic arch and its branches are enlarged and the left ventricle
becomes hypertrophied and dilated, leading to gradual failure of the
heart with respiratory distress on exertion (also present in our patient). Are there clinical signs of decreased pressure in the poststenotic part of the aorta and its branches? Hypotension was demonstrated in the popliteal artery and was also indicated by the
weakened pulse in the femoral artery. Where do you normally feel

the pulse of the femoral artery? The pulse is elicited by palpating rather deeply inferior to the inguinal ligament, midway between anterior superior iliac spine and symphysis pubis.

Collateral circulation

What features in the clinical picture of the patient demonstrate the presence of a collateral circulation that allows blood to bypass the constriction, and what can the survival of the patient be ascribed to (Fig. 22-2)? In addition to the direct radiographic evidence of enlarged and tortuous vessels in the region of the thoracic wall, we find visible and palpable pulsations in the interscapular area and all along the thoracic wall, particularly at both sides of the sternum. On close inspection, dilated arteries can also be seen under the skin of the

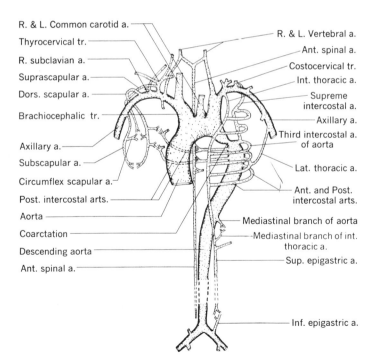

Figure 22-2. Various sites of collateral circulation in a case of aortic coarctation.

thorax. Is there evidence that coarctation in our case is not complete? Direct opacification of the thoracic aorta demonstrates immediate but faint filling of the poststenotic area.

These, then, are the sources of arterial blood in the poststenotic portion of the aorta and its branches: direct filling through a narrowed aperture in the aorta at the constricted site and an indirect discharge of blood into the peripheral distribution area of the aorta distal to the coarctation through well-developed collateral arterial channels. Fortunately for the patient, in this location of the arterial obstruction ample communicating channels are available that permit the development of a collateral flow around the partial occlusion.

What are these vessels? For purposes of classification, they can be divided into four groups:

1. The *scapular and cervical anastomosis:* Scapular and cervical branches from the subclavian and axillary arteries carry blood from above the obstruction to posterior intercostal arteries coming off the aorta below the obstruction. Identify these branches. They are the transverse cervical, deep cervical, suprascapular, and dorsal scapular arteries derived directly or indirectly from the subclavian artery and the subscapular artery and its circumflex scapular branch of the axillary artery. Some of these channels could be seen or their pulsation felt in the patient.

2. The *internal thoracic anastomosis:* This was clearly demonstrated in this case on the aortogram of the aortic circulation. The internal thoracic artery, a branch of the subclavian artery, anastomoses by way of its anterior intercostal arteries with the posterior intercostal aortic branches, and its musculophrenic and mediastinal branches communicate with phrenic and mediastinal branches of the descending aorta. Finally, one of its two important terminal branches, the superior epigastric artery, anastomoses with the inferior epigastric from the external iliac, thus bypassing the coarcted area of the aorta.

3. The *intercostal anastomosis:* This has already been referred to in relation to the communications between the anterior and posterior intercostal branches of the internal thoracic artery and aorta respectively. It also includes the communications between the supreme (highest) intercostal artery from the costocervical trunk of the subclavian artery and the posterior intercostal artery for the first, second and third spaces.

4. The *spinal anastomosis:* The anterior spinal artery derived from the vertebral artery, a branch of the subclavian, communicates with segmental spinal branches of the posterior intercostals from the descending aorta and the lumbar and lateral sacral arteries and thus establishes a further collateral channel in coarctation of the aorta. Here it is often dilated and tortuous.

One radiographic finding demonstrable on routine chest films is caused by the development of the just described collateral circulation and remains as the single most important radiologic sign of aortic coarctation. Identify it. It is the notching and erosion of the bodies of the ribs in the area of the costal grooves and is caused by the sometimes greatly enlarged posterior intercostal arteries. These dilated arteries may occasionally cause difficulties for the surgeon because they often become quite friable; some may have to be ligated and excised, as in this case.

What is the clinical significance of the delayed appearance of the femoral pulse in our case? It proves that the major portion of the blood coursing through the femoral artery arrived in the artery by way of devious collateral channels rather than directly through the stenotic area. Does the presence of a clearly demonstrable pulse in the more inferiorly located arterial channels in the leg, such as the posterior tibial artery at the medial side of the ankle or in the dorsalis pedis artery, rule out aortic coarctation? It does not prove the absence of aortic obstruction because a well-developed collateral circulation may keep these arteries well supplied with blood. How can the systolic murmur demonstrable over the cardiac and left interscapular areas be explained? It is due to obstruction to the free flow of blood across the coarctation, creating a high-velocity jet during midsystole.

Causes of fatal outcome in untreated cases

A final question needs to be discussed. Why is dangerous surgery, which may on occasion be fatal, indicated in this case, when the clinical complaints of the patient are relatively insignificant? If left unoperated, three fourths of these patients will die before the age of 40. The average life expectancy of all patients with coarctation is 35 years. What is the cause of death in these cases? The harmful effects of coarctation are derived from the hypertension in the upper part of the body, which may eventually lead to cardiac failure and death. The prestenotic area of the aorta will dilate and may rupture. Cerebral vessels derived from vertebral and internal carotid arteries likewise dilate as a result of the hypertension and may also rupture, leading to fatal cerebral hemorrhage. Finally, bacterial infection may occur at the site of coarctation or at the aortic valve, a complication that is a frequent accompaniment of aortic coarctation.

23   Obstruction of the Superior Vena Cava

A 57-year-old man is admitted to the hospital for recurrent nose-bleed and progressive shortness of breath. The bleeding from the nose started 3½ months earlier and required two admissions to the hospital. The shortness of breath began three years before admission and was particularly noticeable on exertion. Chronic cough gradually developed.

For the past 24 years, the patient has noticed a gradual appearance of distended tortuous veins over the anterior part of the chest wall and has been increasingly aware of dizziness, especially on rising and bending over. His face appears puffy with a bluish hue (cyanosis), which becomes worse when he reclines or bends forward. His collar size has increased, although he has not gained weight. The patient recalls that before development of these veins he had many had furuncles (boils) on the trunk and in both axillae.

EXAMINATION

On examination the patient shows cyanosis of the face and neck. With the patient in the supine position, the cyanosis deepens. The eyes are prominent and the eyelids slightly swollen. There are numerous prominent tortuous superficial veins over the neck, both arms, axillae, and anterior chest wall. Numerous veins cross the anterior costal margins and continue down over the abdomen toward the pubic area. The entire trunk is covered with large acne-type skin eruptions and numerous old, healed scars of previous skin lesions. In contrast to the upper extremities, the skin of the lower extremities is of normal color.

Further physical examination reveals signs of chronic pulmonary emphysema (overdistention of air); otherwise, the internal organs are normal. Radiographic study of the chest shows a widening of the mediastinal shadow in the region of the right upper mediastinum and a group of heavily calcified lymph nodes lying against the right side of the trachea down to the level of the bifurcation. Radiographs of the chest following injection of a contrast medium into the cubital vein reveal that the widening of the upper mediastinum is caused mainly by abnormal veins. The termination of the right subclavian vein appears to be constricted and accompanied by numerous collateral channels. Complete obstruction is present in the right brachiocephalic vein inferior to its formation by the confluence of internal jugular and subclavian veins. No contrast medium enters the heart during the x-ray exposure but is diverted to maximally dilated and tortuous collateral veins in and over the upper part of the thorax. The medium is seen to enter an enlarged internal thoracic vein that descends and joins with greatly dilated abdominal veins. There is no filling of the terminal portion of the azygos vein. Studies of venous pressure show three times the normal pressure in the veins of the upper extremities, although the pressure in the veins of the lower extremities is normal.

DIAGNOSIS

Obstruction of superior vena cava is diagnosed.

THERAPY AND FURTHER COURSE

Chronic bronchitis and emphysema improve with drug treatment and respiratory exercises. The venous obstruction continues to cause mild symptoms.

DISCUSSION

The progressive shortness of breath and the cough of the patient can be ascribed to pulmonary emphysema, resulting from chronic bronchitis and degenerative changes in the lungs. These symptoms are apparently not connected with the other outstanding findings.

The swelling of the face, bleeding from the nose, cyanosis, and increased pressure in the veins of the upper extremity, as well as the distention and tortuosity of the veins of neck, arms, and upper trunk, are due to an obstruction of the venous channels that drain the blood from the upper part of the body. Because the obstruction is of such long standing (25 years) and the clinical findings and radiographic studies do not prove otherwise, a benign cause is be assumed. In view of the history of severe skin infections of the chest wall extending over several years, the obstruction can reasonably be ascribed to thrombosis (clotting of blood) in mediastinal veins originating from an inflammation of these veins. What main veins are involved? The right brachiocephalic vein and the superior vena cava are definitely involved. Why does distention of the visible veins increase when the patient is in the supine position or bending forward? Keep in mind the direction of the blood flow and that the absence of valves in the veins of the mediastinum allows blood to accumulate in the most gravity-dependent locations. Bending forward increases intrathoracic pressure, which impedes venous return, causing distention of peripheral veins.

Calcification of mediastinal lymph nodes in the area of the obstructed veins, furthermore, suggests the presence of inflammatory changes in these nodes caused by infection of the adjacent areas. Thus, the combination of chronic inflammation of the mediastinal lymph nodes with scarring and compression of the veins of the mediastinum and of clotting inside these veins resulted in obstruction of the right brachiocephalic vein and the superior vena cava. Clinical tests and radiographic studies also indicate obstruction of the azygos vein at the site of its termination (Fig. 23-1).

The most common cause of obstruction of the superior vena cava, in addition to the two factors effective here, are neoplasms, either pressing on or invading the superior vena cava. Circumscribed enlargement (aneurysm) of what large artery in the neighborhood of the superior vena cava would also be likely to compress the vein? An aneurysm of the ascending aorta could easily lead to compression of the superior vena cava.

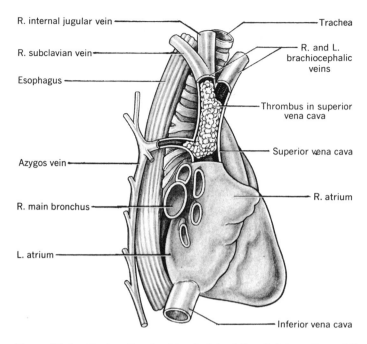

R. internal jugular vein ——————————————— Trachea

R. subclavian vein———

Esophagus ——

R. and L. brachiocephalic veins

Thrombus in superior vena cava

Superior vena cava

Azygos vein ——

R. atrium

R. main bronchus ——

L. atrium ——

Inferior vena cava

Figure 23-1. Obstruction by blood clot of the distal portion of the right brachiocephalic vein, the superior vena cava, and the terminal part of the azygos vein.

Collateral venous pathways in obstruction of the superior vena cava

What collateral venous channels are available in this case where the proximal portion of the right brachiocephalic vein, the superior vena cava, and the termination of the azygos vein are obstructed? How is the return of venous blood to the right atrium from the upper part of the body accomplished? Keep in mind that in this case, in which the termination of the azygos vein is also obstructed, all blood that normally drains into the superior vena cava must return to the heart by way of the inferior vena cava (Fig. 23-2).

The visible dilatation and tortuosity of the superficial veins of the neck, arms, and trunk indicate that these channels are involved in the bypass from the superior vena cava to the inferior vena cava.

They comprise anastomoses between the veins of the thoracic wall, which normally drain into the axillary and internal thoracic veins, and tributaries of the femoral vein. One of the numerous veins belonging to this group is designated the thoracoepigastric vein. What named veins that eventually drain into the superior and inferior vena cava, respectively, does this vein connect? It connects the lateral thoracic vein with the superficial epigastric vein. The lateral thoracic vein drains into the axillary vein, and the superficial epigastric vein drains into the great saphenous and through it into the femoral vein (Fig. 23-2). Veins belonging to this group are par-

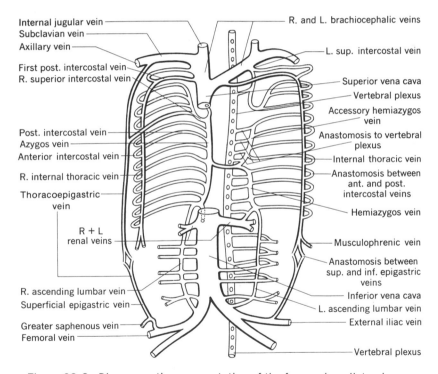

Figure 23-2. Diagrammatic representation of the four main collateral systems effective in obstruction to the superior vena cava. Notice (1) the superficial venous system, represented by the thoracoepigastric vein, (2) the internal thoracic system with the anastomosis between the superior and inferior epigastric veins, (3) the vertebral plexus, and (4) the azygos route and its anastomoses with other systems.

ticularly involved in the bypass if the termination of the azygos vein
is also obstructed, as in our case.

A second collateral system bypassing the obstruction is represented by the internal thoracic venous system. Here again, reversal
of blood flow is facilitated by the absence or scarcity of valves.
Named communicating vessels of this system are represented by the
superior epigastric vein, musculophrenic vein, anterior intercostal
veins, and perforating cutaneous branches. With which named veins
belonging to the inferior caval system do these veins anastomose?
These veins, all tributaries of the internal thoracic vein, anastomose
directly or indirectly with the inferior epigastric vein draining into
the external iliac vein (Fig. 23-2).

A third channel is represented by the vertebral plexus of veins.
Where in relation to the vertebral column is this plexus located? Do
the veins draining into this plexus anastomose with previously listed
veins? What anatomical feature in this plexus would facilitate reversal of the bloodstream? The vertebral plexus of veins comprises an
aggregate of veins extending from the head to the sacrum on the
outside of the spinal column anteriorly and posteriorly (external
plexus) as well as inside the vertebral canal (internal plexus). These
veins are characterized not only by rich anastomoses with segmental
veins, such as the intercostals, but also by longitudinal anastomoses
and by cross-communications between right and left across the midline and by anastomoses from inside the vertebral canal to the outside. Reversal of the blood flow is facilitated by the absence of valves
in this plexus (Fig. 23-2).

Azygos route

The azygos route, although its normal drainage into the superior
vena cava is blocked, can contribute to the collateral circulation
through reversal of its blood flow and by virtue of the fact that it
receives important segmental tributaries from the thoracic wall and
from the other bypassing systems, mentioned previously. What are
these segmental tributaries? How is the azygos vein formed? Locate
its anastomoses with the internal thoracic and vertebral routes. Usually the azygos vein is formed by the confluence of the right ascending lumbar and subcostal veins. It frequently also connects directly
with the inferior vena cava. It receives its segmental venous contributions through the lower right posterior intercostal veins directly

and through the right superior intercostal vein indirectly and also commonly receives left segmental contributions through the hemiazygos and accessory hemiazygos veins. All these intercostal veins are the channels of anastomosis with the internal thoracic and vertebral routes (Fig. 23-2).

What additional collateral channels would be available if the superior vena cava were obstructed above the point of entrance of the azygos vein? One must realize that in case of patency (openness) of the azygos vein, the latter would be capable of carrying blood to the lower part of the superior vena cava, in addition to the previously mentioned bypasses to the inferior vena cava.

If, instead of the superior vena cava, the inferior vena cava were obstructed, could the same veins also be employed to channel blood to the superior vena cava? This would be possible by simple reversal of the blood flow in the previously listed channels.

24   Cancer of the Esophagus

A 53-year-old carpenter is admitted to the hospital as an emergency. He has severe shortness of breath (dyspnea) and great difficulty in swallowing (dysphagia). The patient states that for the past six months he has suffered increasing difficulty and pain in swallowing. He has had to subsist on a liquid diet and has lost 30 pounds. His shortness of breath has been present for the past three months. From time to time, he has severe coughing spells, his sputum is blood-tinged, and occasionally he brings up as much as a cupful of blood. He states that for the last few weeks he has become quite hoarse. He has also noticed a swelling on his right collar bone, which is painful on motion.

EXAMINATION

On examination the patient appears quite emaciated and in great distress. Laryngoscopic examination reveals the left vocal fold in a semiabducted position on respiration and phonation. His face is dark purple and he suffers from labored respiration. His pulse is rapid and his temperature is 101° F.

Radiographic examination of the chest shows widening of the mediastinum with destruction of the lateral half of the right clavicle corresponding to the soft tissue tumor in this area (Fig. 24-1). Brief fluoroscopic examination of the esophagus with radiopaque barium demonstrates an obstruction at the level of the bifurcation of the trachea.

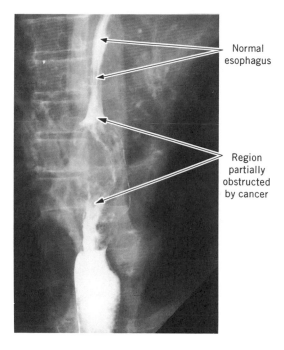

Normal
esophagus

Region
partially
obstructed
by cancer

Figure 24-1. X-ray of the esophagus with swallowed barium coating the mucosal lining. Notice the poorly filled irregular region that indicates cancer of the esophagus.

DIAGNOSIS

Cancer of the esophagus with obstruction and perforation into the trachea is diagnosed.

TREATMENT AND FURTHER COURSE

The patient is put on oxygen and narcotics and given intravenous fluids. On the fourth day, he became comatose and died.

At autopsy, a large cauliflower-like tumor was found in the esophagus that obstructed the lumen of the esophagus. The esophagus above the obstruction was greatly dilated. At the level of the tracheal bifurcation, the mass had perforated the trachea, which showed an ulcerous communication with the esophagus (Figs. 24-2 and 24-3). The tumor mass surrounded and compressed the trachea

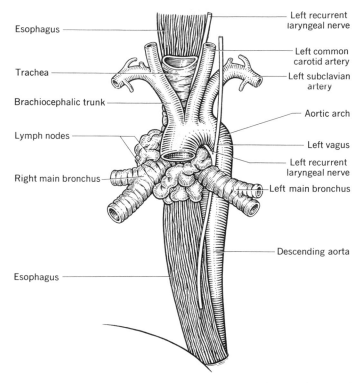

Esophagus

Trachea

Brachiocephalic trunk

Lymph nodes

Right main bronchus

Esophagus

Left recurrent
laryngeal nerve

Left common
carotid artery

Left subclavian
artery

Aortic arch

Left vagus

Left recurrent
laryngeal nerve

Left main bronchus

Descending aorta

Figure 24-2. Anterior view of the esophagus, trachea, and aorta showing the changing relationship of the aorta to the esophagus and the course of the left recurrent laryngeal nerve in relation to the aorta, trachea, and esophagus. Notice the enlarged and cancerous lymph nodes and the dilatation of the upper thoracic portion of the esophagus.

over a 3-cm long area. The left recurrent laryngeal nerve was likewise embedded in the mass. The mediastinal lymph nodes, particularly in the posterior mediastinum, were greatly enlarged and adhered to each other. The dependent portions of both lungs showed signs of bronchopneumonia. There were nodular metastases of varying size in both lungs and scattered over the visceral pleura. There also were round tumors in the liver. On microscopic examination, the area of destruction of the right clavicle was found to be a cancerous metastasis.

DISCUSSION

We are dealing here with the terminal course of an esophageal cancer that has obstructed the esophagus at one of its most common sites: the level of the tracheal bifurcation. The common sites of esophageal cancer correspond to the physiologic constrictions of the esophagus. Where are these located? One is found at the beginning of the organ in the neck at the level of the cricoid cartilage. The second is at the level of the bifurcation of the trachea and the third at

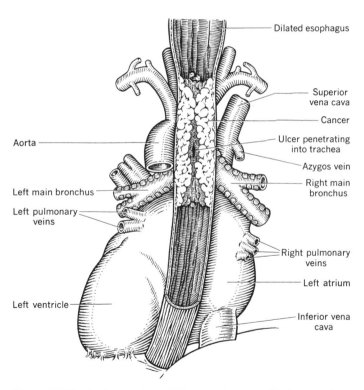

Figure 24-3. Posterior view of the esophagus with the esophagus partly opened. The extensive obstructing cancer is shown as well as the erosion into the trachea and the enlargement of the esophagus above the obstruction. Notice the close relationship of the esophagus to the left atrium.

the site of the esophageal passage through the diaphragm. Other narrowings are often described at the level of the aortic arch and just below the bifurcation where the left bronchus crosses the esophagus. Dilatation of the esophagus above the obstruction, which is found in this case, is common in cases of esophageal stenosis and represents the result of mechanical stretching of the organ by the ingested food and liquid above the site of the impasse.

Topographic anatomy of the esophagus as applied to cancer

The complications of the esophageal cancer caused by invasion of organs and structures in its neighborhood are exemplified in this case by the compression of and breakthrough into the trachea and the paralysis of the left recurrent laryngeal nerve. What coat is lacking in the wall of the esophagus that in most other portions of the gastrointestinal tract serves as at least a temporary barrier to cancerous invasion of the neighborhood? The esophagus does not have a serosal coat and is separated from the trachea by only a small amount of areolar tissue, explaining the frequent involvement of the trachea in esophageal cancer. The compression of the trachea by the tumor mass explains the severe dyspnea and cyanosis (purple discoloration due to deficient oxygenation of the blood by the lungs) of the patient. The invasion and ulcerous penetration of the trachea caused the bronchopneumonia, the tracheal hemorrhages, and the blood-tinged sputum. What arteries supply the trachea and esophagus at the level of the bifurcation, branches of which were eroded by the cancer in this case? Tracheal and esophageal branches of the thoracic aorta are responsible for the blood supply of the two tubes.

How do you explain the paralysis of the left recurrent laryngeal nerve, which resulted in the hoarseness and change in position of the left vocal fold as revealed by laryngoscopic examination? The left recurrent laryngeal nerve arises from the vagus, where the latter passes over the left (lateral) aspect of the aortic arch. It then winds behind the ligamentum arteriosum, below the arch and from there runs upward in a gutterlike groove on the left side of the trachea and esophagus (Fig. 24-2). As frequently occurs in esophageal cancer, the mass compressed the nerve. What is the function of the recurrent laryngeal nerves in the larynx? They supply all laryngeal muscles, with the exception of the cricothyroid muscle. Blockage of the nerve immobilizes the vocal fold of that side and puts it in a semiabducted position. Does the recurrent laryngeal nerve also send sensory fibers to the larynx? It supplies the mucous membrane of the larynx below the vocal folds. Why is the left recurrent laryngeal nerve more frequently paralyzed than the right in cancer of the esophagus? This is due to the difference in the course of the two nerves, with the right entering into relationship only with the cervical portion of the esophagus.

Knowledge of the anatomical relations of the thoracic esophagus will allow us to identify other structures and organs frequently penetrated by the growing cancer. Thus, in addition to the trachea and main bronchi, the pleural cavity, lungs, aorta, and pericardium and heart may be invaded. Because of the closer relationship of the left bronchus to the esophagus, this bronchus is more frequently involved than the right. On the other hand, it is the right mediastinal pleura that is more likely to insinuate itself between the esophagus and aorta, forming a retroesophageal recess. It is therefore more commonly affected than the left in the pleural spread of esophageal cancer. Perforation into the aorta may lead to immediate fatal hemorrhage. Remember, in the posterior mediastinum, the aorta is at first on the left side and then posterior to the esophagus. "The thickness of the pericardium and esophagus is all that intervenes between the wall of the left atrium and the food you swallow" (Grant). Consequently, the left atrium is the chamber of the heart that may be infiltrated by cancerous growth from the esophagus (Fig. 24-3).

Lymphatic spread of esophageal cancer

Cancer does not spread only by invasive growth to the surrounding tissues and organs. More important even for the final outcome is penetration of the lymphatic and vascular channels that disseminate clusters of tumor cells (tumor emboli) to all parts of the body. This dissemination is well exemplified in this case. The patient had large masses of cancerous lymph nodes in the posterior mediastinum that were demonstrable on the x-ray film. These, together with periesophageal lymph nodes adjacent to the organ and tracheobronchial nodes, represent the area of regional lymph drainage from the middle portions of the esophagus. We must visualize that the primary tumor invaded the lymph capillaries in the mucosa and spread from there by way of the lymph vessels in the esophageal musculature to the regional lymph nodes. Lymphatic metastases from the esophageal cancer may reach these regional lymph nodes first and then, because of rich lymphatic anastomoses, may spread to nodes located at considerable distance, ascending as far as the neck or descending to lymph nodes in the abdomen around the celiac artery.

The common involvement of lungs and pleura, also present in our case, might be explained on the basis of direct spread of the primary cancer. More likely, though, is retrograde dissemination of the cancer through the lymphatics of lung and pleura from the cancerous tracheobronchial lymph nodes. It should also be kept in mind that all lymph, and with it cancerous emboli, finally reach the venous circulation through the termination of the thoracic and right lymphatic ducts in the venous angles of the neck. Thus, lymphatic spread, if not arrested by surgery or radiation, in the end will bring cancerous fragments into the venous circulation and from there to the lungs, a common site of metastasis.

Venous spread of esophageal cancer

Invasion of the esophageal veins at the site of the tumor must also be assumed to have taken place and with it spread of cancerous emboli along venous channels. Where do the veins of the esophagus drain? The wall of the esophagus is an important site of anastomoses between systemic veins that drain blood by way of the azygos and hemiazygos veins into the superior vena cava and veins that are tributaries of the portal system, such as the lower esophageal veins. The latter drain into the left gastric vein. Cancerous invasion of and spread via the lower esophageal veins explains the metastatic involvement of the liver in our case.

If some of these cancerous emboli were small enough to be transported by way of the portal vein and its branches through the sinusoids of the liver, how would they ultimately arrive in the capillary bed of the lung? They would pass through hepatic veins into the inferior vena cava and the right atrium and ventricle and from there through the pulmonary arteries into the pulmonary circulation. On the other hand, how would spread via the esophageal veins draining into the azygos vein reach the lungs? The azygos vein empties into the superior vena cava, which drains into the right heart. Thus, dissemination of the cancer through superior and inferior venae cavae might readily be an additional explanation of metastatic involvement of the lungs.

Arterial spread of esophageal cancer

The final pathway for metastasis from and through the lung is the general arterial circulation. Is this terminal phase of cancerous spread exemplified in our case? The involvement of the right clavicle can be explained only on the basis of an arterial metastasis. How did the cancer, which in one way or other had reached the venous circulation, locate in the nutritional artery of the clavicle? After breaking into the tributaries of the pulmonary veins, clusters of cancer cells must have passed to and through the left heart, aorta, and its branches to the nutritional vessel of the clavicle.

In summarizing, we see that, as is so often the case in terminal cancer, the neoplasm in this patient used all available channels for dissemination through the body: direct invasion of structures in the neighborhood, such as the trachea and recurrent laryngeal nerve; lymphatic spread to regional lymph nodes and lungs; venous spread to the liver and possibly lungs and pleura; and arterial dissemination to the clavicle.

IV   ABDOMEN

25 Indirect Inguinal Hernia

A 10-year-old boy comes to the outpatient department with the complaint that occasionally, particularly when he stands or strains, a "bulge" appears in his right groin. Off and on, he has moderate pain in this area that is increased by lifting a heavy object or straining hard during a bowel movement.

EXAMINATION

On inspection with the patient in the upright position, a walnut-sized bulge is noticeable in the right inguinal area that increases in volume on coughing or nose blowing. On palpation, the swelling seems to extend upward into the inguinal canal; however, its upper end cannot be felt. With the patient in the horizontal position, the lump disappears. When the examiner invaginates the skin of the scrotum and inserts his little finger into the superficial inguinal ring, he feels a definite impact on coughing. On straining, the bulge again becomes demonstrable and is noticeable also when the boy is in a horizontal position. It can be reduced by the examiner; when his fingers are pressed firmly over the area of the deep inguinal ring, the mass does not descend into the inguinal canal. Examination of the left side does not reveal any abnormality.

DIAGNOSIS

Right-sided, complete, reducible, indirect inguinal hernia is diagnosed.

THERAPY AND FURTHER COURSE

The treatment of choice of inguinal hernia in a boy aged 10 years is surgery, as spontaneous obliteration of the hernial sac at this age does not occur. The patient is operated on one week later.

With the patient under general anesthesia, the skin and superficial fascia are divided by an incision above and parallel to the inguinal ligament down to the aponeurosis of the external oblique muscle. Blood vessels encountered in the superficial fascia are clamped and ligated.

The inguinal canal is opened by incising the aponeurosis of the external oblique muscle. This incision extends the length of the canal and includes the superficial inguinal ring. The ilioinguinal nerve is identified and carefully displaced. Both portions of the divided external oblique aponeurosis are reflected by blunt dissection. With reflection of the anterior wall of the canal, the spermatic cord and hernial sac within the coverings of the cord are visualized. By blunt dissection the coverings of the cord are removed from the hernial sac, and the sac is isolated. The walls of the sac are then carefully incised without injury to its contents. The contents in this case consist of a loop of small intestine (Fig. 25-1). The intestine is gently replaced into the peritoneal cavity. The sac is then separated by dissection from the structures of the cord, which lie lateral and posterior to the sac. After the sac has been widely opened and carefully inspected for any further contents, it is ligated at its proximal end and excised. The spermatic cord is replaced in its normal position, and the divided portions of the external oblique aponeurosis, including the superficial inguinal ring, are reunited. The superficial fascia and skin incisions are closed in layers.

The patient is out of bed for short periods on the first postoperative day and leaves the hospital three days later. The parents are told to restrict physical activities of the boy for six weeks. On reexamination he shows no signs of recurrence and has no complaints.

DISCUSSION

We are dealing here with a complete, right-sided, reducible, indirect inguinal hernia. Define indirect inguinal hernia.

An indirect inguinal hernia is a hernia in which an outpouching of the peritoneal sac enters the inguinal canal at the deep inguinal

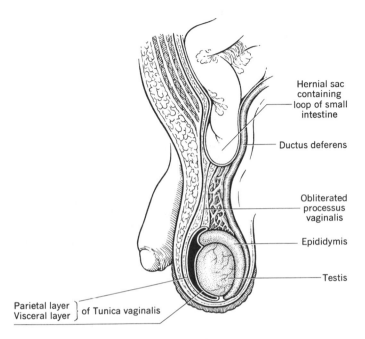

Hernial sac
containing
loop of small
intestine

Ductus deferens

Obliterated
processus
vaginalis

Epididymis

Testis

Parietal layer ⎫
Visceral layer ⎭ of Tunica vaginalis

Figure 25-1. Section through an indirect inguinal hernia with the hernial sac containing a loop of small intestine. Notice the partial obliteration of the processus vaginalis.

ring and, if complete, leaves it at the superficial inguinal ring. In other words, the hernial sac, formed by peritoneum and containing abdominal contents, takes the same course through the abdominal wall as the spermatic cord. Why is the term indirect applied to this type of inguinal hernia? An indirect inguinal hernia chooses an oblique and longer pathway through the abdominal wall than the direct type. The direct inguinal hernia enters the abdominal wall directly posterior to the superficial inguinal ring and therefore penetrates the inguinal canal through its posterior wall medial to the deep ring.

What is the cause of indirect inguinal hernia? The predisposing factor essential to the development of an indirect inguinal hernia is the persistence of the processus vaginalis. How is this structure defined? It is a diverticulum or outpouching of the peritoneum that, during embryonic development, precedes the testis in its migration into the scrotum, evaginating before it all layers of the abdominal wall it encounters in its descent. Whereas the lower portion of this peritoneal diverticulum remains patent as the tunica vaginalis testis, its upper part becomes obliterated. This obliteration normally takes place during the first postnatal year or even later.

Indirect inguinal hernia and inguinal canal

Can the presence of an open processus vaginalis be equated with an indirect inguinal hernia? A patent vaginal process, although predisposing to congenital inguinal hernia, is not at all identical to this clinical entity, as the latter requires the protrusion of a viscus or part of a viscus through the deep inguinal ring into this preformed sac. What is the deep inguinal ring, and at what point is it projected on the surface of the anterior abdominal wall? Simply defined, the deep ring is an opening in the transversalis fascia. Actually, it is the site where the transversalis fascia is continued as an attenuated out-pouching over the spermatic cord, forming its innermost sheath, the internal spermatic fascia. The deep ring is located about 0.5 inch above the midpoint of the inguinal ligament, the midinguinal point. Remember that the inguinal ligament does not extend to the midline but only as far as the pubic tubercle.

Because the normal inguinal canal represents a weakness of the anterior abdominal wall, what counteracts the formation of a hernia even in the presence of a partially or totally open processus vaginalis? The obliquity of the canal constitutes a natural obstacle to the formation of a hernia. An increase in intra-abdominal pressure, such as when coughing, straining, nose blowing, or crying, actually forces the walls of the canal closer together. If the cremaster muscle is well developed, a recoil-like action of its fibers pulls the cord like a plug toward the deep ring.

Herniation through the deep inguinal ring into the open processus vaginalis occurs only after the ring has become wide enough to permit some contents of the peritoneal cavity to extrude through the ring into the canal in conjunction with the spermatic cord. What is the relation of the hernial sac to the structures of the cord? The hernial sac lies within the substance of the cord, ensheathed by the internal spermatic fascia and cremaster muscle and fascia. These form the coverings of the cord within the inguinal canal. The ductus deferens lies immediately posterior to the sac (Fig. 25-2).

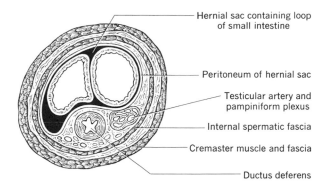

Hernial sac containing loop
of small intestine

Peritoneum of hernial sac

Testicular artery and
pampiniform plexus

Internal spermatic fascia

Cremaster muscle and fascia

Ductus deferens

Figure 25-2. Cross section through the spermatic cord and hernial sac containing a loop of small intestine. Notice that the hernia forms part of the contents of the cord and is surrounded by its coverings. Also notice the typical location of the sac in front of the ductus deferens.

What structure must be incised to open the anterior wall of the inguinal canal and make the spermatic cord and hernia visible? What forms the superficial inguinal ring, which is likewise cut by this incision, and where is it located? The aponeurosis of the external abdominal oblique muscle forms the anterior wall of the inguinal canal, reinforced laterally on its deep aspect by muscle fibers of the internal oblique arising from the lateral part inguinal ligament and the iliac fascia. The superficial inguinal ring is a triangular gap in the aponeurosis of the external oblique. To be specific, it is the site where the aponeurosis of the external oblique is attenuated to be continued over the cord as the external spermatic fascia, which forms the outermost sheath of a complete hernia. The superficial ring lies superolateral to the pubic crest. Its lateral (inferior) crus attaches to the pubic tubercle, and its medial (superior) crus inserts on the pubic crest.

In children with large hernias and in adults, a common additional step in the surgery of indirect inguinal hernia is suturing the conjoined tendon (falx inguinalis, conjoint tendon) to the inguinal ligament. This procedure strengthens the posterior wall of the inguinal canal. What is the conjoined tendon? It is a part of the lower arching aponeurosis of the internal oblique and transversus muscles that insert into the pubic bone. The conjoined tendon varies in composition and may be muscular, tendinous, or fascial in different individuals.

Anatomy of surgical complications

Endangered nerves.   During surgery in our case, as in every case of inguinal hernia, to what nerve is attention paid? The ilioinguinal nerve is particularly endangered because it lies in the operative field and passes through the superficial inguinal ring. It supplies the skin of the anterior portion of the scrotum and the adjacent region of the thigh with sensory fibers. If it is divided within the canal, numbness of the scrotum and inner aspect of the thigh results. If it is included in a suture or embedded in scar tissue, postoperative neuritic pain will ensue.

Do the ilioinguinal and the more superiorly located iliohypogastric nerves, both of which lie in the operative area, carry motor fibers? Both of these nerves have motor components that supply the lowermost portions of the internal oblique and transversus muscles. To section these nerves at this level would interfere with the nerve supply to the muscles and thus lead to weakness of the posterior wall of the inguinal canal, which might result in recurrence of the hernia.

Endangered blood vessels.   Postoperative hemorrhage is probably the most common complication of inguinal hernia. What blood vessels are encountered in this operation in the deep part of the subcutaneous tissue? Of what vessels are they branches? The superficial epigastric artery and vein, ascending in a medial direction across the midportion of the inguinal ligament, are divided and ligated in this operation. They are branches of the femoral artery and great saphenous vein, respectively. The superficial external pudendal artery and vein, which are branches of the same vessels, may also be encountered superficial to the spermatic cord.

What major vessel lies in close relation to the deep ring, the injury of which may cause serious hemorrhage? The inferior epigastric artery, one of the two main branches of the external iliac artery, may be inadvertently cut. If it is not ligated after such an accident, severe bleeding will result. What is the relation of the inferior epigastric artery to the deep ring, and therefore to the point of entrance, of an indirect inguinal hernia into the abdominal wall? It lies medial to the deep ring but forms the lateral boundary of the inguinal triangle, which is the site of entrance of a direct inguinal hernia. Review the boundaries of the inguinal triangle. The lateral boundary is the inferior epigastric artery, the medial leg of the triangle is the lateral border of the rectus abdominis, and the base is the inguinal ligament.

Injury to the ductus deferens and bladder. Another undesirable accident in herniorrhaphy is inadvertent cutting of the ductus deferens when the hernial sac is dissected free. In what relationship to the sac does the ductus deferens lie, and how can it be identified by palpation? It lies immediately posterior to the sac and can be recognized by its hard and cordlike feel when it is rolled between the thumb and index finger. Division of the ductus deferens will result in sterility on this side. An attempt at reuniting the divided ends should be made. Damage to the testicular artery and pampiniform plexus should likewise be avoided because it will cause hemorrhage and may also result in infertility on one side.

What organ situated in the lesser pelvis in the adult lies in a more abdominal location in the infant and may be in close proximity to the deep ring? In infants the bladder may overlap the deep ring and may be inadvertently incised in herniorrhaphy. This complication, although not harmless, can be taken care of by suture closure if it is recognized during surgery.

Incarceration and strangulation. Define the complications of incarceration and strangulation of a hernia. In incarceration the hernia is irreducible and there is obstruction to the passage of intestinal contents in the herniated portion of the intestine, but the blood supply to the viscus remains unaffected. In strangulated hernia the blood supply and lymph drainage of the herniated viscus are impaired or occluded. Depending on the degree of vascular occlusion, the intestinal loop will lose its viability within hours unless the hernia is attended to immediately.

26   **Biliary Colic and**
        Cholecystectomy

A 46 year-old woman is brought by ambulance to the hospital; she is in acute distress with symptoms of severe pain in the right upper abdominal region. In the past she had repeated attacks of severe pain in the right upper quadrant of the abdomen, frequently following a heavy meal. These attacks were accompanied by nausea and vomiting. She suffers from indigestion and "gas pain on her stomach," particularly after eating fatty foods.

EXAMINATION

The patient is a short, stocky, and rather obese woman, who has had five deliveries and two miscarriages. She complains of severe, sharp, constant pain that started in the epigastric and umbilical regions and then became localized in the right hypochondriac area. The pain radiates around the right chest to and below the inferior angle of the scapula. She is nauseated and vomits occasionally. There is marked tenderness and some rigidity in the right hypochondriac region. She has moderate fever. Her white blood cell count is elevated. Ultrasound examination without the use of contrast medium shows multiple stones in the gall bladder (Fig. 26-1).

DIAGNOSIS

Biliary colic and chronic calculus cholecystitis (inflammation of the gall bladder accompanied by gallstone formation) with acute exacerbation are diagnosed.

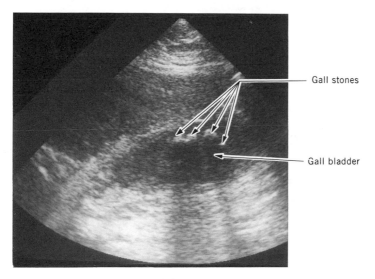

Figure 26-1. Ultrasound image of the gall bladder. The gall bladder is the dark, transversely oriented structure that contains several whitish gall-stones.

THERAPY AND FURTHER COURSE

The patient is given Demerol for her pain, prepared for surgery, and put under general anesthesia. The abdominal wall is opened by a subcostal incision that begins at the tip of the xiphoid process and is directed laterally and downward, paralleling the costal margin about two finger breadths inferior to it. After the anterior layer of the rectus sheath has been split, the rectus abdominis muscle is cut in a direction paralleling the skin incision. The incision is continued laterally through the external oblique, the internal oblique, and the transversus muscles in a direction paralleling the skin incision. The posterior layer of the rectus sheath is likewise divided, as is the transversalis fascia, the extraperitoneal fat, and the peritoneum. During this procedure an attempt is made to preserve intercostal nerves as they are seen within the rectus sheath deep to the rectus muscle by retracting them out of the way.

After the peritoneal cavity has been opened, it is explored with one hand with particular attention to the stomach, duodenum and transverse colon, and dome of the liver. The organs in question are found to be free from gross pathology in our case, except for numerous adhesions in the neighborhood of the gall bladder. The gall bladder is identified and on palpation is found to be thick-walled. It is contracted by scarring and seems to contain numerous hard stones. The operative field is walled off with gauze pads.

The surgeon then introduces a finger into the epiploic foramen and between this finger, and the thumb palpates the common bile duct within the hepatoduodenal ligament for evidence of stones, thickening, and dilatation. In this case the common bile duct (CBD) appears normal. With the gall bladder being retracted out of the way by its fundus, an incision is made into the hepatoduodenal ligament close to its free border. By blunt dissection, the cystic duct is exposed at its junction with the neck of the gall bladder and doubly clamped and divided. Next the cystic artery is identified, doubly ligated, and likewise divided between ligatures. Invariably, the cystic artery is located in the cystohepatic triangle (Calot), formed by the common hepatic duct on the left, the cystic duct on the right, and the liver above. The peritoneal attachment of the gall bladder to the liver is incised to free the gall bladder, and the gall bladder is separated from its bed by blunt and sharp dissection. After the gall bladder has been dissected free, it is turned upward and resected.

Venous bleeding from the gall bladder bed is controlled with electrocautery, and the gall bladder bed is covered by suturing the peritoneal flaps over it. The field is inspected for bleeding, and a small drain is placed into the subhepatic area. The incisions are closed in layers. The gall bladder, on being opened, shows fibrous thickening of its walls and an inflamed mucosa filled with numerous small multifaceted stones.

Postoperatively the patient is given intravenous glucose and saline solution. Gastric suction through a tube is applied for two days. In the absence of bile leakage, the drain is removed after three days. The patient is permitted out of bed for a few minutes on the first postoperative day, and this time is gradually increased each day, as is her diet after suction is discontinued. The further postoperative course is uneventful, and the patient is discharged from the hospital on the postoperative day 10.

Laparoscopic cholecystectomy

Laparoscopic biliary surgery, first performed in 1987, is rapidly becoming an alternative to the traditional operative procedure described above. Laparoscopic cholecystectomy reduces the amount of recovery time and pain associated with the traditional operation. According to some sources, 95% of patients can now be considered suitable for this procedure, and most patients are able to ambulate and return home the next day. It involves the use of endoscopic video equipment, which includes a tiny video camera attached to the laparoscope with cable connections to transmit images of the operative field to a monitor and specially designed surgical instruments, all of which are inserted into the abdominal cavity through small puncture sites.

The peritoneal cavity must be distended by creating a pneumoperitoneum with insufflation equipment to make room for lighting and the manipulation of the surgical instruments in the operative field. Carbon dioxide is the standard gas used for producing the pneumoperitoneum. Irrigation-aspiration devices are also used to keep the operative field clean and remove debris. Forceps and electrocautery devices are used to dissect the tissue and to achieve hemostasis of small blood vessels.

The procedure itself is performed under sterile conditions, and patients are prepared for both a laparoscopic procedure and an open cholecystectomy in the event complications develop during laparoscopic surgery. After anesthesia is established, the bladder is catheterized and a nasogastric tube is inserted in the stomach to empty it. The pneumoperitoneum is created and the patient is placed in the head-down position (reverse Trendelenburg). Four small abdominal wall incisions are made to act as passageways for the laparoscope and for three trocars and sheaths used for passing instruments.

A blunt forceps is placed on the fundus of the gall bladder to push the right lobe of the liver toward the diaphragm. Another is used to expose and dissect the gall bladder and porta hepatis. Dissection to free the gall bladder begins along its sides and proceeds toward the union of the cystic and common hepatic ducts. The cystic artery is located in the cystohepatic triangle and is dissected free from the surrounding tissues before the cystic duct is divided. It is important for the surgeon to locate both the anterior and posterior branches of the cystic artery. The arteries and cystic duct are ligated. After the gall bladder has been opened and the gallstones removed, the collapsed gall bladder is removed by using a grasping instrument.

DISCUSSION

By virtue of her sex, age, obesity, and numerous past pregnancies, this patient has the most common characteristics of a person prone to gall bladder disease. Although it is not quite clear whether gall-stones form as a result of infection or metabolic disturbances, the latter seems more likely. These metabolic deviations, in conjunction with stagnation of bile in the gall bladder through spasm or organic obstruction of the duct system, encourage the formation of gall-stones of various types. Later on, the accumulation of gallstones, combined with frequently superimposed secondary infection, re-sults in an acute or chronic inflammation of the gall bladder with the classic symptoms of epigastric pain, "gas on the stomach," indiges-tion, nausea, and vomiting, particularly after fatty meals. These symptoms are due to reflex spasms of the pylorus and probably the sphincter of the CBD which delay the emptying of stomach and gall bladder. The acute flare-up or biliary colic found in this case, as in many others, is caused by impaction of stones in the neck of the gall bladder.

Name the various parts of the gall bladder involved in this case. They are the fundus, body, and neck of the gall bladder, with the neck opening into the cystic duct (Fig. 26-2).

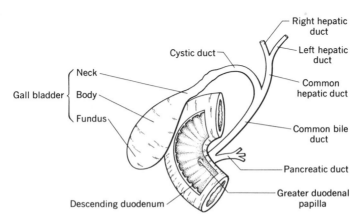

Figure 26-2. Extrahepatic biliary passages in the typical arrangement.

Anatomy of biliary pain and rigidity

Typical for biliary colic is the appearance of sudden, sharp, severe pain that starts in the epigastric and umbilical regions. It then becomes localized in the right hypochondriac area and radiates toward the inferior angle of the scapula and inferior to it.

How do you explain the location of pain in the right hypochondriac region and its typical radiation to the back, particularly to the scapular and infrascapular areas? The pain in the right hypochondriac area is caused by direct inflammatory stimulation of the sensory nerve endings in the parietal peritoneum contacted by the gall bladder. Innervation of the centrally located parietal peritoneum on the undersurface of the right dome of the diaphragm is provided by the right phrenic nerve. If this region is irritated by an inflamed gall bladder, pain is sometimes referred to the ipsilateral neck and shoulder region. The pain in the scapular region is referred pain, which is common in diseases involving the viscera. For physiologic reasons, pain arising in sensory nerve endings in the viscera, in this instance the gall bladder, is referred to areas of the body surface that send sensory impulses to the same segment of the spinal cord that receives sensory impulses from the affected organ.

Sensory fibers from the gall bladder run in plexuses along the biliary duct, closely intermingled with sympathetic efferent fibers. They pass through the celiac ganglion, the greater splanchnic nerve, sympathetic chain ganglia, and via white rami communicantes to spinal nerves and their dorsal roots and ganglia. Here their cell bodies are located. Central fibers from the dorsal root ganglia terminate in the seventh to ninth thoracic spinal cord segments. It is in the dermatomes innervated by these cord segments that the radiating pain to the scapular and infrascapular areas is localized.

Explain the muscular rigidity that is found over the diseased area. This rigidity is a state of involuntary contraction of the muscles of the anterior abdominal wall, particularly the rectus abdominis, which is a reflex response to stimulation of the nerve endings in the parietal peritoneum in the region of the gall bladder.

Topography of the abdomen

In this case history, two different topographic terminologies, both common in clinical descriptions, are used. The simpler one divides the abdomen into four quadrants by a midsagittal and a horizontal plane laid through the umbilicus. A second, more complex terminology introduces nine regions, outlined by two vertical and two horizontal planes. What is the location of these planes, and what are the names of the regions? The two vertical planes are erected from the midpoints of the inguinal ligaments. The upper horizontal plane is laid through the lowest point of the tenth costal cartilage. The lower horizontal plane passes through the level of the highest points of the iliac crest. The regions outlined are the right and left hypochondriac, the right and left lateral, the right and left inguinal, the epigastric, umbilical, and pubic.

Clinically important relations of the gall bladder

The abnormal findings in this case include the presence of dense adhesions to the organs in the neighborhood. Identify the organs that are in such intimate relationship to the gall bladder that not only adhesions may form between it and these viscera but also rupture and discharge of pus and stones may occur from the gall bladder into these organs through fistulas joining the two organs. They are the liver, the first part of the duodenum, the jejunum, and the transverse colon. Perforation may also occur into the peritoneal cavity or through the anterior abdominal wall. The greater omentum is frequently adherent to the gall bladder.

Is the gall bladder normally separated from the visceral surface of the liver by a layer of peritoneum? The gall bladder lodges in its own bed on the visceral surface of the liver, to the right of the quadrate lobe, with only connective tissue but no peritoneum intervening. This bed is often called the bare area for the gall bladder. In other words, the peritoneum that covers the visceral surface of the liver passes over the sides and inferior surface of the gall bladder only and does not cover the area in direct contact with the liver. Although operations on the biliary tract are as common as surgery for inguinal hernia and appendicitis, complications in gall bladder surgery are far more frequent than in the other two operations. These complications are due mainly to a lack of appreciation of anatomical variations that occur so frequently in the extrahepatic biliary system. A comprehensive knowledge of these anatomical deviations can prevent many complications. Cautious dissection will help in identifying the important structures and will protect them from injury.

The first surgical step in cholecystectomy is an incision into the hepatoduodenal ligament close to its free border. Define the lesser omentum, and name the structures encountered between its two layers near the free (right) edge. The lesser omentum is a double layer of peritoneum derived from the ventral mesogastrium that connects the lesser curvature of the stomach and first part of the duodenum with the liver. Consequently, its two continuous parts are named the hepatogastric and the hepatoduodenal ligaments. Between the two layers of the hepatoduodenal ligament and close to its free margin lie three important structures: the CBD farthest to the right, the proper hepatic artery to the left of the common bile duct, and the portal vein between and posterior to them. (A justified mnemonic is "ductus-dexter, portal vein-posterior.") Other structures surrounding this triad are autonomic nerve and lymph plexuses.

Anomalies of the cystic duct

It is the task of the surgeon first of all to identify the cystic duct and then doubly clamp, ligate, and divide it. With the liver and gall bladder retracted, the cystic duct, about 3 to 4 cm long, runs posteriorly, inferiorly, and to the left, and joins the common hepatic duct to form the CBD (choledochus). Most important to the surgeon are variations in the length and course of the cystic duct and the site of junction with the common hepatic duct (Fig. 26-3). If the cystic duct is unusually long, it may run alongside the common hepatic duct for a variable length of the latter's course, often attached to it by connective tissue. The cystic duct, instead of joining the common hepatic duct on its right side, may pass in front or behind the common hepatic duct, uniting with it on its left side (Fig. 26-3). If the anomalies mentioned are not recognized, the common hepatic duct may be mistaken for the cystic duct and may be clamped, ligated, or even partially resected. Blind clamping or ligation of bleeding blood vessels may also lead to injuries or occlusion of the common hepatic duct.

The result of complete occlusion of the common hepatic duct is severe jaundice, which is fatal unless the patient undergoes reoperation. Patency of the common duct must be reestablished or bile drainage otherwise instituted. Milder injuries to the CBD lead to drainage of bile into the hepatorenal recess and through a drain to

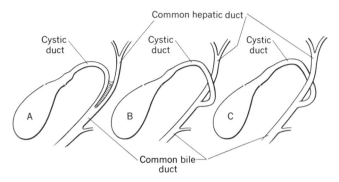

Figure 26-3. A. Unusually long cystic duct attached to the common hepatic duct by connective tissue. B. Cystic duct joining the common hepatic duct on its left side by passing in front of it. C. Cystic duct joining the common hepatic duct on its left side by passing behind it.

the outside, which may or may not require surgical intervention. If large amounts of bile enter the free peritoneal cavity, bile peritonitis and possibly death from shock result.

Anomalies of the cystic artery

Recognition of vascular anomalies, particularly of the cystic artery, is of equal clinical importance. The typical arrangement to be described occurs in only two thirds of all cases. Here the cystic artery arises from the right hepatic artery to the right of the common hepatic duct. After a course that varies in length, the cystic artery divides into a superficial and a deep branch, one going to the peritoneal, the other to the attached surface of the gall bladder. The cystic artery may also arise from the proper hepatic artery at the site of its bifurcation or before it divides into the right and left hepatic arteries. Other rarer origins of the cystic artery are from a hepatic artery that is a branch of the superior mesenteric artery. Finally, there may be accessory cystic branches from any of the previously mentioned arteries.

If the surgeon is unfamiliar with the possible multiplicity of the cystic artery or its abnormal course, profuse unexpected hemorrhage may result, which can be temporarily controlled by compressing (between index finger and thumb) the proper hepatic artery within the layers of the lesser omentum (Pringle maneuver). If the right hepatic artery is mistaken for the cystic artery, and if it is ligated instead of the cystic artery, necrosis of the liver occurs, with serious consequences and possibly death. Significant postoperative hemorrhage from injury to abnormal blood vessels is a grave complication that requires immediate reoperation. It is best avoided by carefully identifying all blood vessels at the time of cholecystectomy, being always aware of the possibility of aberrant blood vessels.

Stomach Distress

A 32-year-old schoolteacher is referred by her physician to the department of internal medicine with the diagnosis of dyspepsia. The patient complains of frequent nausea, heartburn, occasional vomiting, and a sense of fullness and abdominal discomfort soon after intake of food. The attacks of vomiting occur when she is upset in her work as a teacher.

In the last few months, after the death of her mother, with whom she lived, her symptoms have become increasingly severe. She now also complains of frequent headaches, fatigue upon slight exertion, insomnia, and loss of appetite.

EXAMINATION

The patient appears frail, underdeveloped, and undernourished. The epigastrium is slightly sensitive on palpation, but there are no other abnormalities. Radiologic examination of the gastrointestinal tract shows the stomach lacking in tonus. The stomach is quite long, sagging down into the lesser pelvis with the lowest point of the greater curvature three finger breadths above the symphysis pubis. The pylorus is at the level of the fifth lumbar vertebra to the left of the midline (Fig. 27-1). There are no signs of organic changes in the stomach or duodenum. The stomach empties fairly normally, being free of contrast medium after 4.5 h. On radiographic examination, the gall bladder appears elongated and low in position but otherwise

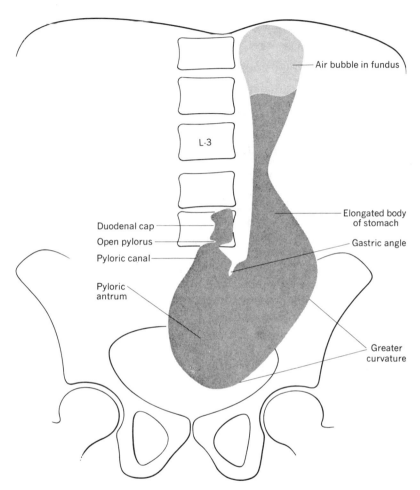

Figure 27-1. An x-ray of an elongated stomach after swallowing barium with the lowest point of the greater curvature three finger breadths above the symphysis pubis. The pylorus is at the level of the fifth lumbar vertebra to the left of the midline. This finding is consistent with normal function.

normal. There are therefore no signs of organic abnormalities in the upper gastrointestinal tract.

DIAGNOSIS

Stomach distress caused by emotional distress is diagnosed.

THERAPY AND FURTHER COURSE

During follow-up, the patient is seen on numerous occasions by a psychiatrist. In these interviews she reveals that she feels insufficient to accomplish her tasks, particularly since the death of her mother, on whom she relied heavily. She appears hypersensitive to frustrations and reacts to them emotionally and with the previously described gastric symptoms.

With the physician assuming a sympathetic and supportive attitude toward her problems, the patient's health gradually improves. She gains more confidence in herself, and her gastric symptoms are greatly alleviated. Under dietary supervision, mild sedation, symptomatic medical treatment, and with continuance of occasional psychotherapeutic interviews, the patient gains 15 pounds and finds her mild gastric discomfort quite tolerable.

DISCUSSION

The original clinical diagnosis by her local physician was gastroptosis, which refers to descent and sagging of the stomach, this condition supposedly being responsible for her clinical symptoms. The term implies a "standard" or "normal" position of the stomach, which in this patient's case deviated in an inferior direction.

Position of the stomach in the cadaver and in the living person

What is the "normal" position of the stomach? The formulation of the question in this manner, although frequently posed in the clinical and anatomical literature, is incorrect and unacceptable. The concept of a "standard" or "normal" gastric position is based on data collected at the turn of the century by the British anatomist Addison, who divided the abdominal region into small squares and allotted to the viscera fixed places in this scheme. The opinion prevailed that each organ, thoracic, abdominal, or pelvic, has its definite shape and position, a knowledge of which was necessary to recognize deviations. The corollary of this theory was the assumption that deviation from this standard position, particularly in an inferior direction, results in clinical symptoms. The descent or sagging of a viscus was called ptosis, and the literature of the past is replete with descriptions and case histories of gastroptosis, coloptosis, and generalized enteroptosis. Surgical procedures were devised that aimed at anchoring organs in their "allotted" location. As recently as 30 years ago, the surgical literature mentioned various techniques of surgical gastropexy, which meant the fixation of a "dropped" stomach in a higher position by suturing it to the abdominal wall or other structures.

Addison's work consisted of a statistical evaluation of variations in the topography of abdominal organs in the cadaver. What factors make the position of an organ in a cadaver an unreliable index of its location in the living? What is the state of the smooth and striated musculature in the dead body? What are the postmortem pressure conditions in the abdomen? The smooth and striated musculature, which includes the diaphragm, is either completely relaxed or abnormally rigid from rigor mortis. The thorax is in a state of maximal expiration with collapse of the lung and elevation of the diaphragm. Embalming and dissecting procedures change the pressure conditions in the thoracic and abdominal cavities and within the vasculature. The elasticity of connective tissue is lost and the fat is solidified.

Thus, the study of visceral topographic anatomy in the dissecting room in embalmed cadavers is of limited value in the assessment of visceral shape and position in living persons. Yet even the modern anatomical and clinical literature frequently ignores the available evidence of this discrepancy.

Returning to the living, list the physiologic variables that lead to alterations in the position of the stomach and other abdominal viscera. Body posture and respiratory phase are responsible for a wide range of shape and position of the abdominal viscera. The stomach descends in the upright position and with the descent of the diaphragm, that is, in inspiration. If you were to demonstrate on two consecutive x-ray films the extremes of variation in gastric position, how would you manipulate the variables of respiration and body position? One film would be taken in inspiration and in upright position, the other in expiration and in supine position.

What other striated muscles, in addition to the diaphragm, affect gastric position? The state of contraction of the muscles of the anterior abdominal wall has the greatest influence on the position of the stomach. This can easily be demonstrated under the fluoroscope by letting the subject retract his abdomen or by causing sudden contractions of the anterior abdominal wall by making the subject laugh. Needless to say, the degree of filling of the stomach will alter its position, although not to the extent that classic anatomists assumed, and so does the state of filling and size of organs in the neighborhood, such as the colon and spleen.

Tonus of the stomach

What is meant by the term "tone" or "tonus" of the stomach, and how does it affect gastric location? Tonus, in contrast to peristalsis, refers to the continuous state of contraction of the smooth musculature of the stomach. In this patient we find considerable loss of tone, in other words, a relaxation of the gastric wall, resulting in an inferiorly directed outpouching, especially of the greater curvature.

What nerve structures govern the tonus of the smooth musculature of the stomach? The latter is mainly under control of the intrinsic myenteric plexus in the wall of the organ, but it is also influenced by its extrinsic innervation, the vagus and the sympathetics. What are the results of vagal and sympathetic stimulation on the tonus of the stomach? In part, they depend on the degree of tonus at the time of stimulation as well as on the frequency and strength of the stimulus. In general, the vagus increases the tonus of the organ; the sympathetic innervation is inhibitory to the stomach wall. There is evidence of cortical and subcortical control of gastric tonus. Centers in the cortex most likely act on the hypothalamus, which in turn affects the vagal and sympathetic outflow. Acute emotional upsets result in increased activity of the thoracolumbar (sympathetic) division of the autonomic nervous system and of the adrenal medulla and are therefore generally accompanied by a decrease in tonus of the gastric wall and sagging of the stomach. Thus, we understand that the temporary emotional disturbance of the patient enhanced the descent of her stomach.

How do the autonomic components of the nervous system reach the stomach? The stomach is supplied from the celiac plexus via postganglionic sympathetic nerve fibers that follow the gastric arteries. Preganglionic vagal fibers reach the organ by direct gastric branches from the two vagal trunks or through the celiac plexus, which receives a parasympathetic contribution. Most of the preganglionic vagal fibers synapse in the intrinsic autonomic plexuses of the organ.

Stomach and constitutional type

If physiologic variables, such as body posture, respiratory phase, state of filling of the stomach, and adjacent viscera, are standardized, and emotional upsets are excluded, is there conformity in the site of the organ? Studies on groups of people, even of the same age, have shown that gastric position correlates to a certain extent with body build. Persons with a frail and slender physique, such as this patient, generally show a lower diaphragm and a lack of tonus of the skeletal musculature, with sagging of the anterior abdominal wall and to a certain extent of the pelvic support of the viscera. This, combined with the spaciousness of the pelvis and the scarcity of abdominal fat, results in a low position of the viscera, including the stomach. On the other band, in the heavy-set stocky individual with a high diaphragm and roomy upper abdomen, the viscera generally are in a more superior position.

Transpyloric plane and stomach bed

Two conventional anatomical terms referring to the stomach, the so-called transpyloric plane and the stomach bed, require further elucidation. What is your definition of the transpyloric plane that was introduced by Addison and which by its name seems to refer to the site of the pylorus? The transpyloric plane is a horizontal plane midway between the suprasternal notch and the pubic symphysis. It is supposed to pass through the disk between the first and the second lumbar vertebrae. What position in the living is the pylorus most apt to lie in or near this plane? In an x-ray anatomical study, it was shown that, with the subject supine, the pylorus of the empty stomach was in the transpyloric plane in about 20 percent of all cases; in another approximately 15 percent, it was superior to the transpyloric plane. Even in this position, however, when the stomach is most elevated, the pylorus was inferior to the transpyloric plane in more than 60 percent of all cases. For the standing male in no case did the pylorus lie in the transpyloric plane but was always inferior to it. Thus, for the living, particularly in the anatomical, that is, upright position, the term is a misnomer.

What is the definition of the stomach bed? It refers to the structures to which the posterior surface of the stomach is related in the supine position. What are these structures? From superior to inferior, they are the diaphragm, the left suprarenal gland, a small part of the left kidney, the splenic artery along the upper border of the pancreas, the body of the pancreas, the spleen to the left of kidney and pancreas, and the transverse mesocolon descending from the pancreas. All these structures are separated from the stomach by the omental bursa. The spleen lies at the left extremity of the bursa and is connected to the stomach by the gastrosplenic ligament. In the upright position, the relationships of the stomach change greatly. The organ descends and rests essentially on the transverse mesocolon and adjacent intestines, which in turn are supported by the anterior abdominal wall and the pelvic organs.

What is the most fixed part of the organ? The cardia changes least in position with physiologic alterations. By contrast, the pylorus is quite mobile, being suspended from the liver by the mesentery-like lesser omentum. The pylorus not only moves up and down, as has been pointed out, but also from right to left of the midline.

Where does the pylorus lie in this patient? In the upright position it is at the level of the fifth lumbar vertebra to the left of the midline (Fig. 27-1). The following well-worded quotation summarizes this discussion on the stomach bed: "The stomach bed, once given the rigidity of an ancient four-poster bed, now has become the malleable bed of a flowing river on which floats the visceral fleet" (O'Rahilly).

With one exception, the kidney, it should be stated that normal function of the abdominal viscera does not depend on their position because, for example, a stomach or transverse colon that has descended into the pelvis usually functions as well as one that lies higher in the abdomen. There is, therefore, no justification for the clinical diagnosis of gastroptosis or coloptosis, although low position of the kidney (nephroptosis) may cause clinical symptoms by kinking the ureter. In that particular situation, downward displacement of the kidney is a pathological condition.

28 Perforated Ulcer of the Stomach

A 36-year-old-high school teacher was well until two years ago, when he began to suffer periodic attacks of nausea, heartburn, and epigastric pain. During these periods the pain worsened when the stomach was empty and was relieved by food and antacids. The present illness became acute soon after a heavy lunch when suddenly, while reaching over a desk in his office, he experienced agonizing pain in his abdomen. A physician who was called immediately transferred the patient to a hospital by ambulance.

EXAMINATION

On arrival at the hospital, the pain is still excruciating, sharp and knifelike. The pain is located in the epigastrium and constant, but from time to time increases in intensity. The patient appears prostrate. His face has an anxious expression, and his forehead is covered with cold sweat. His breathing is rapid and shallow, and the abdominal wall does not seem to participate in respiratory movements. Temperature is normal, pulse rate only slightly elevated, and blood pressure normal. There is a boardlike rigidity of the abdomen, most marked in the epigastric area and left hypochondriac region and somewhat less pronounced in the umbilical region. Abdominal tenderness on palpation is most marked in the epigastrium.

DIAGNOSIS

On the basis of the past history, which made the presence of a gastric or duodenal ulcer likely, the diagnosis of acute perforation of the ulcer is made, and the patient is sent to the operating room.

THERAPY AND FURTHER COURSE

On opening of the abdomen with the patient under general anesthesia, the general peritoneal cavity shows the presence of moderate amounts of turbid fluid and some food particles, which are removed by suction. No sign of a ruptured ulcer on the duodenum or anterior wall of the stomach is demonstrable, however. In view of the clinical findings and the presence of fluid and food in the peritoneal cavity, perforation of an ulcer on the posterior wall into the omental bursa (lesser sac) is assumed and the omental bursa opened by an incision through the gastrocolic ligament, avoiding the blood vessels along the greater curvature of the stomach. In the bursa a considerable amount of gastric secretion and food is found, which is removed by suction. The stomach is turned upward for adequate exposure, and a perforated ulcer, 0.5 cm in diameter, is visualized 2 cm from the lesser curvature on the posterior aspect of the pyloric region of the stomach (Figs. 28-1 and 28-2). The ulcer is excised, and frozen sections of the ulcerous area show it to be nonmalignant. In the absence of cancer, the defect in the stomach is closed.

The patient has a fairly stormy convalescence with spiking temperatures. Postoperative care includes constant gastric suction through a nasogastric tube, intravenous fluids, and antibiotics. The patient gradually improves and is put on a strict ulcer diet. Three weeks after operation, greatly improved, he is discharged and continues on his diet. Three months after operation he is reported to be recovered and working.

DISCUSSION

The outstanding symptoms in this patient are abdominal tenderness, which is abnormal sensitiveness to touch, and excruciating pain. The latter made immediate intervention necessary. Recently it has been discovered that many ulcers of the stomach and duodenum are caused by the bacteria, *Helicobacter pylori* and are treated suc-

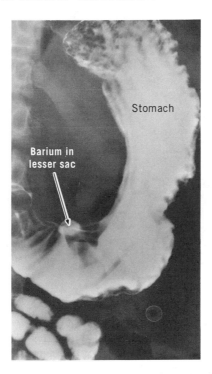

Figure 28-1. An x-ray of the stomach after swallowing barium showing the ulcer extending through the wall of the stomach. The small, white oval demonstrates barium in the omental bursa.

cessfully with antibiotics. Despite this advance in therapy, diagnosis must still be based on recognition of the signs and symptoms discussed in this case study; if perforation has occurred, surgery is required.

Anatomy of ulcer pain

In dealing with the anatomy of the various modalities of pain present in this case, we must separate the chronic ulcer pain that the patient complained of in his history, and which is often described as gnawing and ill-defined in location, from the sharp, stabbing pain after the perforation had taken place. The former, often identified as visceral, is mediated through afferent fibers that accompany the sympathetic efferent fibers from the wall of the stomach through the celiac ganglia, greater splanchnic nerves, sympathetic chain ganglia, white

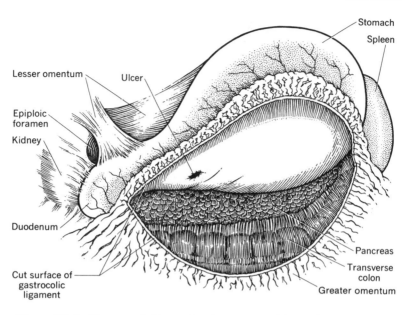

Figure 28-2. The omental bursa has been opened by an incision through
the gastrocolic ligament. The stomach has been turned up, and the perforated ulcer is shown on the posterior aspect of the body of the stomach,
fairly close to the lesser curvature.

rami communicantes, spinal nerves, and then by way of posterior
roots to spinal ganglia. Here their cell bodies are located. Central
fibers from these ganglion cells continue into the spinal cord. Pain of
this type, elicited in the stomach by the ulcer, is generally referred
to the epigastric region. By contrast, the sharp, knifelike pain after
perforation is due to peritoneal irritation by the gastric secretion and
contents and is mediated by somatic sensory fibers of the body wall
that supply the parietal peritoneum. Remember that the parietal
peritoneum, as well as the skin, in the area of the umbilicus is
supplied by the 10th intercostal nerve. Thus, the sharp pain, which
is fairly well localized in the epigastric region starting just below the
xiphoid process, would point to involvement of the sixth to the ninth
intercostal nerves. Does the vagus conduct sensory impulses, including pain, from the stomach? It seems to mediate mainly those
sensory impulses concerned with gastric reflexes, but it is generally
assumed not to transmit pain from the stomach.

What is the cause of the rigidity of the abdominal wall and the costal character of the patient's respiration? The rigidity is due to contraction of the muscular wall and is a reflex response of the abdominal muscles to abnormal stimuli arising from the involved area. The costal-type breathing with avoidance of abdominal respiratory excursions can be explained as a protective mechanism shielding the abdominal wall and parietal peritoneum from painful movements.

Surgical anatomy of the omental bursa (lesser sac)

The perforation in this case involves the omental bursa, into which the gastric secretions and food have spilled through the opening of the perforated ulcer (Fig. 28-3). How do you explain the presence of extraneous material in the greater peritoneal sac? Does the greater

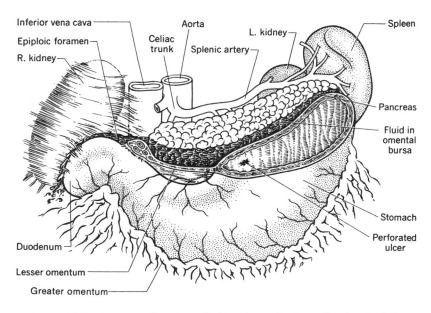

Figure 28-3. Cross section through the stomach above the level of the perforated ulcer. Notice the collection of fluid in the omental bursa and its communication with the general peritoneal cavity through the epiploic foramen. Also notice the relation of the pancreas and splenic artery to the posterior wall of the stomach, separated from it only by the omental bursa.

peritoneal sac communicate with the omental bursa? Locate the epiploic foramen, which is the opening of the omental bursa into the greater peritoneal sac, and give its boundaries. The foramen is bounded anteriorly by the free (right) border of the lesser omentum, more specifically, the hepatoduodenal ligament, containing the common bile duct, the proper hepatic artery, and the portal vein; posteriorly by the inferior vena cava; superiorly by the caudate lobe of the liver; and inferiorly by the first part of the duodenum (Fig. 28-3). What aspect of the stomach bounds the bursa anteriorly? Perforating lesions of what portion of the stomach would be most likely to involve the bursa? Into what space do ulcers of the anterior wall of the stomach perforate? Is the lesser omentum part of the anterior wall of the bursa? The lesser omentum and the posterior wall of the stomach form the important anterior boundaries of the main part of the omental bursa. Thus, whereas ulcers of the anterior wall of the stomach are apt to perforate into the greater sac (free peritoneal cavity), ulcers of the posterior wall may rupture into the omental bursa, as in this case.

Recesses of the omental bursa

What is meant by the terms "superior and inferior recesses" of the omental bursa? What lobe of the liver, covered by peritoneum, forms part of the boundary of the bursa? How do you explain the variations in the inferior extent of the inferior recess? If this recess extended into the greater omentum, between which layers of the omentum would it be located? Would this variable extension of the inferior recess be anterior or posterior to the transverse colon? The superior recess extends behind the liver, with the caudate lobe protruding into it from above. The inferior recess between the inner layers of the greater omentum extends below to a variable extent, depending on the degree of fusion of these layers. Usually it reaches only as far as the transverse colon but would extend anterior to it if the layers of the greater omentum remained unfused.

Pancreas and the omental bursa

Normally the space of the bursa is only potential; so the posterior wall of the stomach is in contact with the anterior aspect of the pancreas, separated only by two layers of peritoneum. What are these? They are the serosal covering of the posterior wall of the stomach (visceral peritoneum) and the parietal peritoneum lining the posterior wall of the bursa in front of the pancreas. Consequently, which organ is most apt to be invaded if an ulcer on the posterior wall of the stomach slowly perforates through the gastric wall? Actually, penetration into the pancreas from a posterior gastric ulcer, with fixation of the stomach to the anterior aspect of the pancreas and walling off of this perforation by peritoneal adhesions, is more common than the massive acute perforation described in this case. What major branch of the celiac trunk would be subject to erosion and possible fatal hemorrhage if this slow perforation and fixation were directed along the upper margin of the pancreas? The splenic artery would be involved.

Surgical access to the bursa

How was the omental bursa (lesser sac) opened in this case? Strictly speaking, the term gastrocolic ligament denotes that portion of the greater omentum that extends from the greater curvature of the stomach to the transverse colon and implies that the lower part of the omental bursa is obliterated. What vessels in the uppermost portion of this peritoneal duplicature are to be avoided in this surgical approach? The right and left gastroepiploic arteries form an anastomotic arch inferior to the greater curvature of the stomach. It is helpful to remember that the term epiploic in the name of these vessels refers to the greater omentum.

What further accesses to the lesser sac could be used in addition to the narrow pathway through the epiploic foramen and the inadvisable approach through the lesser omentum? Entrance could also be obtained by going from below, through the transverse mesocolon, although at the risk of injuring the artery to this part of the colon. Name and locate this artery and give its origin. The middle colic artery, a large branch of the superior mesenteric artery, runs between the layers of the transverse mesocolon. British surgeons have occasionally recommended access to the omental bursa through the gastrosplenic ligament. Locate it. What vessels would be endangered in this approach? The surgeon must guard against injury to the short gastric and left gastroepiploic vessels, which run within the gastrosplenic ligament.

29   Arteriomesenteric Occlusion of the Duodenum

A 33-year-old medical secretary comes to the physician's office complaining of nausea and vomiting of bile-stained food, with sensations of bloating, belching, discomfort, and pain in the upper abdomen. These symptoms come on about 1 to 2 after meals. After a respiratory infection, she suffered a marked weight loss amounting to 25 pounds during the last six months. Since then, her symptoms have gradually worsened.

On inquiry she states that since adolescence she has had alternating periods of well-being and abdominal discomfort accompanied by vomiting. Since the recent aggravation of her symptoms, she has felt extremely fatigued and has lost her appetite. She further states that when she has these attacks of pain and vomiting, she can obtain relief by lying on either side or in the knee chest position.

EXAMINATION

On physical examination, we find a rather apprehensive patient of asthenic habitus, particularly conspicuous because she shows evidence of recent marked weight loss. She has flaccid abdominal walls, and her liver, kidneys, and spleen can be palpated easily. As common in asthenic persons, she has a marked lumbar lordosis. The epigastrium is rather tender, but otherwise no signs of acute intestinal illness, such as rigidity of the abdominal wall or indications of intestinal obstruction, can be elicited. The patient is advised to seek admittance to the hospital for further studies.

In the hospital a full-blown attack is observed, which came on after a fairly large meal with a meat course and dessert. She was stricken with nausea and fairly severe cramping pain in the right upper abdominal quadrant. She vomited bile-stained food that she had eaten recently. The vomiting relieved her pain. Before the attack subsided, the examining physician noted that the patient displayed tenderness and visible peristalsis in the right upper abdominal region.

Radiographic study of the upright patient under the fluoroscope with a radiopaque meal shows rapid emptying of the stomach, which permits exclusion of pyloric stenosis. The first three portions of the duodenum fill rapidly and are considerably dilated. Under active peristalsis, the duodenum finally empties part of the barium into its fourth portion, but there is marked indentation of the barium filling at the site of transition of the third and fourth portions of the duodenum at the level of the third and fourth lumbar vertebrae, which corresponds to the cutoff point at the time of the beginning of filling of the duodenum. Radiographic examination 6 h after the barium meal shows a marked and abnormal residue of barium in the duodenum.

DIAGNOSIS

Chronic type of arteriomesenteric occlusion of the duodenum is diagnosed.

THERAPY AND FURTHER COURSE

The patient is put on a strict diet with small caloric liquid feedings every 2 h. She is advised to assume alternatingly the prone, right and left lateral, and knee-chest positions, the last particularly after meals. Because she prefers to sleep in the supine position during the night, the foot of the bed is elevated during this period. Gradually, her meals are increased in frequency and solids are added. She is allowed to get up intermittently, first for short periods. The time out of bed is increased gradually. She is also given exercises to strengthen her abdominal muscles. During the next two weeks, she gains 10 pounds, and her pain attacks become less frequent. She is discharged from the hospital with a recommendation to assume the supine or knee-chest position after each meal. She is also given an abdominal binder for support and told to exercise her abdominal muscles. She continues her weight gain and shows overall improvement in her general well-being, accompanied by decreased frequency of abdominal attacks. She is allowed, therefore, to return to work. Six months later she has regained her normal weight and feels comfortable. Her attacks occur quite infrequently, not more than once or twice a month. She is advised to be careful about her diet by avoiding coarse or stringy foods and to continue her muscle-strengthening exercises.

DISCUSSION

Obstruction of the third portion of the duodenum as a clinical entity is an interesting phenomenon. Enthusiasm for this diagnosis has waxed and waned since the disease was first defined in the middle of the nineteenth century. Some authors deny the occurrence of such an entity, but most clinicians are now convinced of its existence, particularly when confirmed by radiographic evidence. What are the underlying facts? Anatomists and pathologists have known for a long time that postmortem casts of the duodenum frequently show an imprint of the superior mesenteric vessels on the anterior wall of its third part. The equivalent of this imprint has been demonstrated in vivo by radiologic means as a filling defect in the same location.

Underlying anatomy of the condition

Define the third part of the duodenum. What is its relation to adjacent structures, particularly the parietal peritoneum, transverse colon, transverse mesocolon, pancreas, aorta, and superior mesenteric vessels? In the early part of training, the medical student in dissection, and the surgeon at the operating table frequently have difficulty identifying this portion of the duodenum because it lies entirely retroperitoneal and is crossed by the mesentery, from which the loops of the small intestine are suspended. It is also overlain by the transverse mesocolon and transverse colon. These latter structures must be lifted and the mesentery of the small intestine turned to the left to expose the parietal peritoneum of the posterior abdominal wall that covers the third part of the duodenum. It can then be palpated to the right of the mesenteric root. This part of the duodenum, which is also often called the inferior or horizontal portion, is about 3 inches long, begins at the inferior duodenal flexure as the continuation of the descending portion, and generally crosses the third lumbar vertebra. At its left extremity, it becomes the fourth or ascending portion that terminates as the duodenojejunal flexure (Figs. 29-1 and 29-2).

As stated, the third part of the duodenum is covered anteriorly by the parietal peritoneum except for a small area where the superior mesenteric vessels cross it at the site of its transition into the fourth part to enter the mesenteric root. It is separated from the vertebral column by the inferior vena cava to the right of the column and the abdominal aorta in front of the column. The transverse mesocolon, with the transverse colon suspended from it, crosses

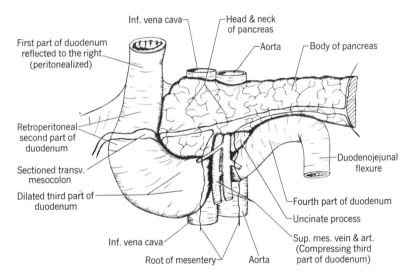

Figure 29-1. Front view of the duodenum in a case of arteriomesenteric occlusion of the third portion of the duodenum. Notice the prestenotic dilatation of the duodenum and compression of its third portion by root of mesentery and superior mesenteric vessels. Observe that the superior mesenteric artery arises from the aorta posterior to the neck of the pancreas but crosses in front of the uncinate process. The crossing of the root of the transverse mesocolon over the second portion of the duodenum and the anterior surface of the pancreas is also shown.

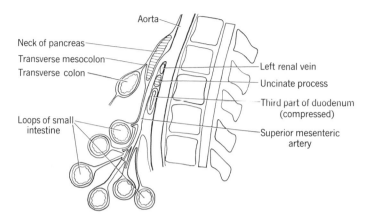

Figure 29-2. Midsagittal section showing the superior mesenteric artery stretched over the third portion of the duodenum and left renal vein by low-lying loops of small intestine in case of severe weight loss and depletion of mesenteric fat. Notice compression of the third portion of the duodenum. The normal relationship of the artery behind the neck, but in front of the uncinate process of the pancreas, is also shown.

superior to the third part of the duodenum by passing over the second or descending portion. The transverse mesocolon divides the duodenum into supracolic and infracolic portions. The pancreas is likewise located superior to the third part of the duodenum.

Superior mesenteric artery and vein

The superior mesenteric artery is given off the front of the aorta as the second of the unpaired visceral arteries (the celiac trunk being the first), generally at the level of the lower portion of the first lumbar vertebra and therefore superior to the third part of the duodenum. The artery is accompanied by its vein as it passes over the third part of the duodenum to enter the mesentery and to supply the small and large intestines from the distal duodenum to the left colic flexure. The superior mesenteric vein drains the same area of intestine and courses to the right of the artery (Figs. 29-1 and 29-2). Their relationship to each other is easy to remember by keeping in mind that the artery arises from the aorta in the midsagittal plane and the vein drains into the portal vein in its course toward the liver, which is essentially a right-sided organ.

What is the relation of the superior mesenteric artery to the pancreas? It arises from the aorta behind the neck of the pancreas but crosses in front of the uncinate process. In its course, the artery is surrounded by the superior mesenteric nerve plexus. Because the artery runs posterior to the neck of the pancreas, it is, of course, also posterior to the transverse mesocolon, which arises from the anterior surface of the pancreas. It is worthwhile to keep in mind that, while the origin of the superior mesenteric artery is superior to the third portion of the duodenum, the origin of the inferior mesenteric artery is inferior to this part of the duodenum. It is also easy to remember that the superior and inferior mesenteric veins, which accompany the two mesenteric arteries, both lie outside the arteries, that is, closer to the lateral abdominal wall than to the arteries.

Changing position of the duodenum

The duodenum, with the exception of its first portion, is a retroperitoneal structure; its position is therefore less variable than organs having a mesentery. Nevertheless, it is surprising that the duodenum is relatively mobile in vivo. Its location varies with body posture, being lowest in the upright, highest in the prone position. It also changes with the degree of its filling and the state of contraction of the anterior abdominal wall. It descends with age. Thus, the level of the third lumbar vertebra, or the disk inferior to it, represents only a mean as a landmark for locating the third portion of the duodenum, with the range extending from L2 to L5.

Embryological explanation of the retroperitoneal and retrovascular position of the third part of the duodenum. How do you explain, on an embryological basis, the retroperitoneal position of the major part of the duodenum and the retrovascular location of the third portion of this viscus in relation to the superior mesenteric vessels? During embryonic development, the intestinal tube forms an anteriorly convex loop in the midsagittal plane and is suspended from the posterior wall of the abdomen by a mesentery. The tube rapidly increases in length and, adjusting to the available space, undergoes a counterclockwise rotation by 270° as viewed from the front, with the superior mesenteric artery acting as the axis of rotation. As the distal part of the intestinal loop turns over the proximal portion, the superior mesenteric artery comes to lie in front of the third part of the duodenum but posterior to the transverse colon. At a later stage,

the duodenum, together with certain other portions of the intestinal
tract, loses its mesentery by peritoneal fusion and, except for its first
portion, becomes fixed to the posterior abdominal wall in a retroperitoneal position.

Pathogenesis of arteriomesenteric occlusion of the duodenum.   The
cardinal point of this discussion is, of course, the pathogenesis (i.e.,
mode of origin and development) of the clinical entity exemplified
by our patient. Whereas normally the superior mesenteric vessels
pass gently over the third part of the duodenum, in our case we have
to visualize the third part of the duodenum as being markedly compressed, as in a vise, between the aorta or lordotic vertebral column
posteriorly and the taut mesenteric vessels anteriorly. This happens
if, due to severe weight loss in an asthenic patient with insufficient
abdominal muscular support, the intestines drop inferiorly to an
undue degree. Thus, marked traction is exerted on the superior
mesenteric vessels at the site of the mesenteric root, which can lead
to acute or intermittent chronic obstruction of the duodenum at this
level.

Asthenic habitus

What is meant by the term asthenic habitus, so well demonstrated
by this patient? The asthenic habitus represents one extreme of a
continuous spectrum that extends from the short, stout, and stocky
person with well-developed musculature and heavy bony framework, to a body type characterized by tall, frail, and slender stature
with a delicate skeleton, weak and underdeveloped musculature,
and a low gastrointestinal tract reaching down into the pelvis. Other
terms besides asthenic used for this body type are ectomorphic and
linear. Such a body build is perfectly consistent with normal health
and body function.

Explanation of symptoms

How do you explain the patient's symptoms in the acute stages of her
illness? What is the reason for the intermittent occurrence of her
attacks with free intervals between? From her history we learn that
she has had acute periods of illness characterized by nausea, vomiting, belching, and pain in the right upper abdomen since adoles-

cence. This is consistent with intermittent compression of the third part of the duodenum as the cause of the described symptoms. Vomiting temporarily relieves the overloading of stomach and duodenum proximal to the site of the compression. The free intervals, which vary in length, can be explained by the force of peristalsis overcoming the obstruction and propelling the contents into the jejunum. The radiographic examination of the patient reveals, in addition to the dilatation of the duodenum proximal to the obstruction, increased peristalsis leading to emptying of the duodenum through the duodenojejunal flexure. Records of other cases also show hypertrophy of the duodenal musculature with dilatation proximal to the obstruction. It is understandable that incomplete constriction can become complete with exhaustion of the propelling muscular force. We then face an acute, life-threatening clinical picture that requires immediate surgery.

The recent aggravation of all symptoms in the patient is due to severe loss of weight and increased flaccidity of her abdominal musculature. The weight loss resulted in diminution of the fat cushion in the mesenteric root that so far had protected the duodenum from complete and lasting compression. The accompanying loss of fat in the pelvis, greater omentum, and retroperitoneal structures, and the weakening of her abdominal musculature, led to further sagging of the intestines into the pelvis and an increase of the drag on the vessels, which further decreases the acute angle between aorta and superior mesenteric artery, a process that has been compared with the action of a nutcracker clamping down on the third part of the duodenum.

Clinicians and radiologists have reported that manual pressure on the lower abdomen in a upward direction with the patient in the supine position will relieve the retention by lifting the intestine out of the true pelvis. Pathologists have obtained similar results at autopsy by raising the viscera after opening the peritoneal cavity and have observed the passage of liquid contents or air beyond the point of obstruction after this maneuver.

What other factors contribute to arteriomesenteric occlusion by tightening the vise on the inferior part of the duodenum? The patient's swayback or accentuated lumbar lordosis, which frequently accompanies the asthenic habitus, particularly in female patients, in combination with the defective abdominal musculature, increases the constriction.

Contributing developmental abnormalities

What faults in the development of the intestinal tract and its peritoneal relations can accentuate the tendency to obstruct the duodenum? A mobile cecum and an ascending colon suspended by a mesocolon will exert traction on their supply arteries, thus increasing the pull on the superior mesenteric artery and the degree of compression of the duodenum. Occasionally a rigid arteriosclerotic superior mesenteric artery is thought to be a contributing factor.

Duodenal arterial supply from the superior mesenteric artery

It has been mentioned previously that the superior mesenteric artery contributes to the blood supply of the duodenum. Which arteries does it use? At the level of the pancreatic notch, it gives off the inferior pancreaticoduodenal artery, which then divides into two branches, the anterior and posterior inferior pancreaticoduodenal arteries. These form arcades between the pancreas and the descending part of the duodenum by communicating with the superior pancreaticoduodenal artery from the gastroduodenal artery. They thus establish an important anastomosis between the celiac and superior mesenteric arteries.

Left renal vein exposed to compression

Is another important blood vessel located in the angle between the aorta and superior mesenteric artery that may likewise be compressed by the downward traction of the superior mesenteric vessels? The left renal vein, in its course toward the inferior vena cava, crosses the aorta deep to the origin of the superior mesenteric artery above the third part of the duodenum. It has been asserted that increased acuteness in the previously mentioned angle may cause compression of this renal vein and circulatory changes in the left kidney, sometimes resulting in albuminuria (Fig. 29-2). This may also explain the increased frequency of varicocele of the left testicle, as the left testicular vein drains into the left renal vein proximal to the site of compression, whereas the right testicular vein is a tributary of the inferior vena cava.

Surgery for treatment of arteriomesenteric occlusion of the duodenum

Fortunately for the patient, her complaints were relieved by conservative medical management, but a small percentage of cases will require surgery because of the severity and life-threatening character of the symptoms. The surgical treatment of duodenal obstruction consists of a bypass operation. The third part of the duodenum is exposed by an incision through the parietal peritoneum of the posterior abdominal wall after the transverse colon and its mesocolon have been turned upward. The posterior parietal peritoneum is reflected, and the retroperitoneal areolar tissue in front of the anterior aspect of the duodenum is dissected away. The prestenotic portion of the duodenum to the right of the superior mesenteric vessels is then connected in a side-to-side anastomosis with the proximal jejunum, thus bypassing the obstructed area.

30   Liver Abscess with Rupture into the Lung

A 37-year-old geologist spent the last 12 years in Central and South America working for an oil company. He is referred to the hospital by his physician for a diagnosis of chronic intestinal amebiasis. His symptoms started gradually several years ago and consisted of intermittent attacks of diarrhea with abdominal discomfort and 5 to 10 stools daily. Nonetheless, he had a good appetite and continued to work. Slowly, his symptoms worsened. He lost a great deal of weight and became disabled. A diagnosis of amebic dysentery was made, and he was sent back to the United States. He now complains of loss of appetite, frequent abdominal cramps, and numerous bloody stools. His pain is particularly noticeable in the right upper abdomen and lower chest with extension into the right shoulder and neck. The pain in the lower part of the right chest is quite severe and aggravated by deep inspiration. Recently he also developed a cough, leading to expectoration of large quantities of reddish brown, bloody sputum.

EXAMINATION

On examination we find a patient in poor nutritional state who appears listless and quite ill. He seems dehydrated, and his temperature reaches a peak of 101° F. On palpation, the whole abdomen is quite sore, but there is particular tenderness in the right hypochondriac region. The liver is enlarged and palpable 3 inches below the right costal margin. Pressure by the examining fingertips over the right anterior lower intercostal spaces indicates a particularly tender area that corresponds to the convexity of the right lobe of the liver. On percussion and auscultation of the lungs, there are signs of immobility of the right diaphragm and marked lung involvement with numerous rales and dullness on percussion. The white count is quite elevated. The dark reddish sputum contains the organism responsible for amebic dysentery, *Entamoeba histolytica*. Sigmoidoscopic examination reveals amebic ulcers with hyperemia and edema of the mucosa. Blood-stained mucus is recovered in which typical motile amebae can be demonstrated. Fluoroscopy and plain films of the abdomen show elevation and immobilization of the right diaphragm and consolidation of the lower medial portions of the right lung field. There is an abscess cavity demonstrable, which, on profile view, can be placed in the right middle lobe.

Using local anesthesia and careful aseptic conditions, fluoroscopically guided puncture of the right lobe of the liver is done and pus is aspirated by syringe. The material obtained consists of a paste-like, brownish substance; on microscopic examination, it is identified as necrotic liver tissue, red cells, some pus cells, and pathogenic amebae.

DIAGNOSIS

Amebic intestinal dysentery with an hepatic abscess, which has ruptured into the middle lobe of the right lung, is diagnosed.

THERAPY AND FURTHER COURSE

The puncture of the liver and aspiration of its abscess relieves the pain and greatly improves the patient's clinical condition. He is given narcotics, sedatives, and bed rest and receives frequent small feedings of a high-protein diet and adequate fluids. The patient is immediately started on specific chemotherapy. A broad-spectrum antibiotic is also given to prevent bacterial superinfection. Under this treatment, the patient improves rapidly, the enlargement of the liver gradually subsides, and his appetite increases. The pain disappears and his cough ceases. On the x-ray, only pleural scarring can now be demonstrated. After two weeks, three stool examinations for amebae are negative and the patient is discharged for home care. A reexamination six months later shows the patient well and without gastrointestinal symptoms. He has gained 25 pounds and has returned to work.

DISCUSSION

Mode of spread of amebic infection to the liver

This patient has a chronic ulcerative disease of the large intestine, which is caused by an ameba, the *E. histolytica*. He acquired this disease in the tropics, where it is found more frequently than in the United States. How does this lesion of the colon spread to the liver? It is known that amebae enter the capillaries and venules of the submucosa and muscularis of the colon, where they can be demonstrated. What is the venous drainage of the colon? The superior mesenteric vein drains (in addition to parts of the stomach, pancreas, and small intestine) the cecum, appendix, ascending colon, and transverse colon. The cecum, appendix, and ascending colon are favorite sites of amebic dysentery. The inferior mesenteric vein drains the rest of the large intestine. Here sigmoid colon and rectum are frequently involved in the disease. Both mesenteric veins, together with the splenic, form the portal vein, which then branches like an artery to terminate in the sinusoids of the liver. By this pathway, the amebae are brought to the liver, where they may cause hepatic necrosis and abscess cavities. Typically, these amebic abscesses are single and occur most frequently in the right lobe near the dome of the liver. This was also the location of the hepatic abscess in our patient.

Mode of spread of hepatic abscess to the lung

How do you explain the involvement of the lung in our case and the absence of peritoneal infection? The amebic infection of the lung is the result of direct extension of the liver abscess into the lung. How many layers of serous membranes must be traversed by rupture of the hepatic abscess into the lung? Two layers of peritoneum and two layers of pleura are eroded by the pus from the hepatic abscess. Identify these layers. They are the visceral peritoneal layer covering the dome of the liver, the parietal layer of the peritoneum lining the undersurface of the adjacent diaphragm, the diaphragmatic part of the parietal pleura, and the visceral pleura covering the base of the right lung (Fig. 30-1).

How can you explain the noninvolvement of the free peritoneal and pleural cavities in this case? As so often happens when the hepatic abscess enlarges, it approaches the diaphragm and causes formation of adhesions between the visceral peritoneum covering the abscess and the parietal peritoneal lining of the diaphragm. Slow development of the penetration of the diaphragm also allows pleural adhesions to form between its parietal and visceral layers. Thus, the general peritoneal and pleural cavities are sealed off at the site of the hepatic abscess, which then breaks through into the lung.

Site of lung abscess

What is the site of the secondary abscess in the lung? It is located in the right middle lobe. Later, breakthrough into a bronchus allows some of the pus from the lung abscess to be expectorated. How do

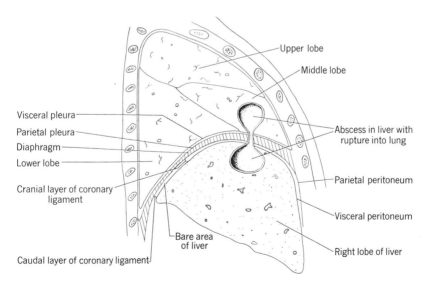

Figure 30-1. Profile view of the right lung and liver in a parasagittal plane shows abscess cavity in the convexity of the right lobe of the liver that has ruptured into the middle lobe of the right lung, causing a daughter abscess.

you explain the fact that the middle lobe, and not the lower lobe, is involved in this rupture into the base of the lung? The student is inclined to think of the lobes of the lung as vertically stacked tiers, the upper lobe being above the middle lobe, and the middle lobe above the lower lobe, with only the lower lobe forming the base of the lung. This is erroneous. The middle lobe forms the anterior part of the base of the lung, and both lower and middle lobes are in contact with the diaphragm with only pleurae intervening (Fig. 30-1).

What segments form the base of the lung?

Give the total number of bronchopulmonary segments that form the base of the right lung. Six segments participate in the base: the lateral and medial segments of the middle lobe, and the medial, anterior, lateral, and posterior basal segments of the lower lobe (Fig. 30-2).

Which segments of the left lung are in contact with the diaphragm? Often it is not realized that, in addition to the basal segments of the inferior lobe, the inferior segment of the lingular portion of the left upper lobe also reaches the diaphragm, although only in a small area. Theoretically, it is conceivable, but not very probable, that abscesses of the left lobe of the liver may extend directly into this segment of the left upper lobe (Fig. 30-2).

Homologies of right and left lungs

The oblique fissure divides the left lung into two lobes which, from their location and spatial relationship, might have been more appropriately identified as anterosuperior and posteroinferior lobes rather than as upper and lower lobes. Of what portion of the left lung is the right middle lobe a homologue? By bronchial similarities and location and by the occasional presence of a horizontal fissure on the left, the right middle lobe and the lower part of the left upper lobe are regarded as homologous. This portion of the left lung is called the lingula (little tongue), and its bronchus is the inferior (lingular) division of the upper lobe bronchus. What is the homologue of the left upper lobe on the right? The right upper and middle lobes together correspond to the left upper lobe.

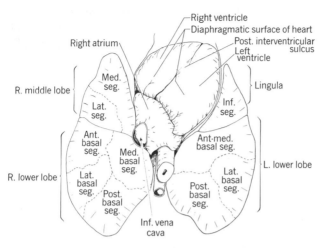

Figure 30-2. Basal view of the diaphragmatic surfaces of both lungs and the heart, showing the individual segments of middle and lower lobes on the right and upper and lower lobes on the left that are in contact with the diaphragm, with only pleurae intervening. Notice that both segments of the middle lobe and four basal segments of the right lower lobe have a diaphragmatic aspect. Observe particularly that the left upper lobe with its inferior segment of the lingula also borders on the diaphragm. In addition, three or four basal segments of the left lower lobe have a diaphragmatic surface.

Perforation of amebic abscess into serous cavities and adjacent organs and structures

If the destructive process in the liver is more acute, the abscess may rupture without adhesions having been formed to wall it off. In this case, the abscess may break through into the pleural or peritoneal cavities, causing dangerous infection in these spaces. On occasion, an amebic abscess of the liver ruptures into the pericardium, causing a suppurative (pus-producing) and generally fatal pericarditis. In which lobe of the liver is such an abscess most likely located? It is the left lobe of the liver, which underlies the pericardial sac and from which abscesses may perforate into this cavity.

Can you visualize a liver abscess rupturing into the abdominal cavity and causing a subphrenic abscess without involvement of the peritoneal cavity? Perforation through the bare area of the liver results in such an extraperitoneal subphrenic abscess. This complication is not infrequent. The literature lists rarer perforations of a liver abscess into the following organs and structures: stomach, duodenum, small and large intestines, spleen, inferior vena cava, right renal pelvis, and through the skin to the outside. All these structures are in close relation to the liver and may be anchored to the site of the abscess by previously formed adhesions.

Pain pathways involved in this case

Additional interest centers on the anatomical pathways responsible for the pain pattern in the patient. In the case history, we notice that the patient complains of pain in the right hypochondriac region and right lower chest. The pain increases in deep inspiration and radiates into the right neck and shoulder. Tenderness on digital pressure is quite marked in the thoracic and abdominal walls overlying the liver.

In defining the anatomical pain pathways involved, we must realize that visceral pleura and visceral peritoneum are insensitive to pain. There are, then, essentially three channels along which pain fibers travel. Visceral pain is due to stretching of the capsule of the liver. This pain is mediated through afferent fibers that accompany the efferent fibers.

The afferent fibers course by way of the hepatic plexus in the free margin of the lesser omentum and pass without synapse through the celiac ganglia, greater and lesser splanchnic nerves, thoracic sympathetic chain ganglia, white rami communicantes, spinal nerves and then by way of the posterior roots to spinal ganglia T6 to T10. Here their cell bodies are located, and the centrally directed fibers of the ganglia reach the spinal cord.

On the other hand, the pain in the thoracic and abdominal walls, including their serous linings, is somatic sensory in character and is mediated by the sensory component of the thoracoabdominal nerves that supply the body wall of this region. It is this pain that is increased by digital pressure. In contrast to their visceral portions, the parietal layers of peritoneum and pleura are quite sensitive to pain and irritated in this case by the underlying infection of liver and lung.

A third component of the patient's pain pattern is mediated

through the phrenic nerve, which, in addition to its well-known motor function, supplies the central portion of the diaphragmatic portion of the parietal peritoneum, diaphragm, and central part of the diaphragmatic pleura (also the pericardium and mediastinal pleura). This type of pain is frequently referred to the neck and shoulder. One explanation often given for the phenomenon of pain referral is that pain arising in the interior of the body, particularly in the viscera, is interpreted as coming from that area of the body surface that sends sensory impulses to the same segments of the spinal cord that receive visceral sensory impulses. The phrenic nerve arises from cervical segments three, four, and five, which also supply the periphery of neck and shoulder with sensory fibers by way of the great auricular and supraclavicular nerves. These nerves are the mediators of referred pain in our patient.

31   Appendicitis

A 22-year-old male university student and collegiate athlete who has been in excellent health was suddenly seized in the middle of the night by a severe attack of "indigestion" accompanied by cramplike pains above and around the umbilicus. He tried to move his bowels but did not succeed. Next morning, he felt hot and uncomfortable and decided to stay in bed. He had no appetite and some nausea and did not eat anything. By evening the pain had moved to the right lower abdominal region. He consulted a physician, who transferred him to a hospital.

EXAMINATION

On examination the patient lies on his back with his right thigh flexed. He has a slightly increased temperature of 99.6° F; his pulse rate is somewhat elevated. The patient now localizes his pain in the right lower abdominal region. On palpation of the abdomen, marked localized tenderness and some rigidity in the right iliac fossa are noted. Pressure with the fingertip shows that the area of greatest tenderness is located near McBurney's point (Fig. 31-1). Rectal examination reveals a definite difference in sensitivity in palpating the right and left sides of the rectovesical pouch: The right side is distinctly more tender.

DIAGNOSIS

The typical history of acute onset with loss of appetite, nausea, and constipation and the change in the site of pain from the epigastric and umbilical to the right iliac region, make the diagnosis of acute appendicitis most likely. This diagnosis is confirmed by the localized tenderness elicited on the abdomen and by rectal examination.

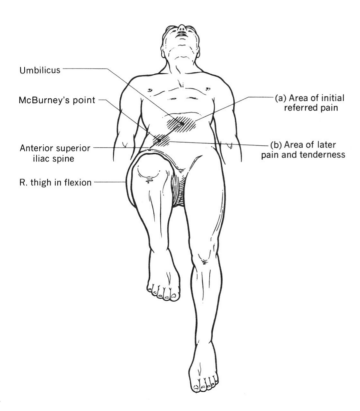

Figure 31-1. The two areas of pain: (a) initial referred pain in the unbilical and paraumbilical region; (b) later pain in the right iliac region caused by irritation of the parietal peritoneum. McBurney's point is at the site of greatest tenderness. Thigh is flexed to relieve tension.

THERAPY AND FURTHER COURSE

In view of the diagnosis of acute appendicitis, and to forestall complications such as perforation and peritonitis, immediate operation is
advised and performed. A right lower muscle-splitting (McBurney)
incision through the abdominal wall is chosen to obtain access to the
appendix. In this incision the external and internal abdominal
oblique muscles and the transverse abdominal muscle and their
aponeuroses are split in the direction of their fibers. Next the transversalis fascia, the extraperitoneal fat, and the parietal peritoneum
are incised, and the appendix is visualized. In our case the appendix
is greatly inflamed and distended, and its visceral peritoneal covering is quite red. The appendix crosses the psoas major muscle and
reaches into the true pelvis with its tip hanging over the pelvic brim.
It is raised and manipulated into view.

The mesoappendix or mesentery of the appendix is clamped
and divided, and the appendicular vessels and their branches are
ligated. Next the base (root) of the appendix is clamped, crushed,
and ligated, and the appendix is amputated distal to the ligature.
The stump of the appendix is cauterized, inverted, and buried by
sutures within the wall of the cecum. The peritoneum and the other
components of the abdominal wall are closed in layers.

Under administration of intravenous fluids and antibiotics, the
patient progresses satisfactorily and is discharged from the hospital
six days after operation.

DISCUSSION

Appendicitis is generally brought about by occlusion of the lumen of
the appendix vermiformis by a fecal stone or by some food particle,
with subsequent distension of the blind sac distal to the obstruction.
Infection and inflammation develop in the distended portion, which
may lead to tissue death, perforation, and abscess formation. The
appendix has often been called the "tonsil of the abdomen," which
refers to the accumulation of lymphatic tissue within its wall and its
proneness to infection.

Anatomy of pain transmission in appendicitis

How can the changing pattern of pain, shifting from the region of the
umbilicus to the right iliac area, be explained? The initial pain in the

epigastric and umbilical regions originates in visceral sensory fibers in the wall of the inflamed appendix. What is the course of these sensory fibers? Where are their cell bodies located?

The sensory impulses from the appendix travel in visceral sensory fibers, which are closely intermingled with sympathetic efferent fibers, through the superior and inferior plexuses and ganglia, greater and lesser and lumbar splanchnic nerves, the sympathetic chain ganglia, and via white rami communicantes to spinal nerves and their dorsal roots and dorsal root ganglia. Their cell bodies are located in the dorsal root ganglia. Central fibers from these ganglion cells continue into the spinal cord. For physiologic reasons, the pain arising in the appendiceal wall is referred to areas of the body surface that send sensory impulses to the same segments of the cord that receive pain impulses from the appendix, that is, the ninth thoracic to first lumbar nerves. What segment of the spinal cord is mainly responsible for the innervation of the skin area around the umbilicus? The tenth thoracic cord segment supplies the area around the umbilicus with overlap from the 9th and 11th segments.

The later pain in the right iliac region seems to be caused by stimulation of somatic sensory fibers supplying the parietal peritoneum of the abdominal wall. What spinal nerves carrying somatic sensory fibers from the abdominal wall are involved in transmission of this type of pain? The 11th intercostal, the subcostal, and the first lumbar nerves (iliolumbar and ilioinguinal) carry somatic sensory (pain) fibers from this area. Tenderness on palpation and the protective muscle contraction, which expresses itself as rigidity of the right lateral abdominal wall, are likewise the result of irritation of the parietal peritoneum.

McBurney's point

What is the location of McBurney's point? It is classically defined as a point one third of the way to the umbilicus on a line joining the right anterior superior iliac spine to the umbilicus (Fig. 31-1). Experienced surgeons recognize that this "spinoumbilical line" marks the myoaponeurotic transition of the external abdominal oblique muscle into its contractile element and its aponeurosis. The external oblique layer, while maintaining its downward and medial directionality, commonly appears thin, white, and glistening rather than red and fleshy under McBurney's point.

As originally conceived by McBurney, this point is supposed to correspond to the site of origin of the appendix, but variability in the position of the umbilicus, in the degree of descent of the cecum, and in the location of the origin of the appendix makes this point a somewhat questionable landmark.

Positive psoas test and rectal findings

How do you explain the preference of the patient for flexion of the right thigh? What muscle is a posterior relation of the appendix and also a flexor of the thigh? In this case the appendix crosses the psoas major muscle, and the patient prefers flexion of the thigh to relieve tension of the inflamed area (Fig. 31-1). The opposite movement, hyperextension of the thigh, puts the psoas muscle and its inflamed fascia on the stretch and is painful and resisted by the patient (psoas test in appendicitis).

What is the explanation for the difference in sensitivity on rectal examination in palpating the right and left sides of the rectovesical pouch? Define the latter pouch. It is the outpouching of the inferiormost extent of the peritoneal cavity between the bladder and rectum in the male. The increased tenderness on the right side of this pouch indicates irritation or inflammation of the parietal peritoneum in this area.

Anatomy of the right lower abdominal muscle-splitting incision

The approach to the appendix in this case was a right lower abdominal muscle-splitting incision through the abdominal wall. What is the direction of the fibers of the three lateral abdominal muscles in this area? The fibers of the external abdominal oblique muscle run from lateral above to medial below ("as if you put your hand in your front pocket"). What is the direction of the fibers of the internal abdominal oblique and transversus abdominis muscles in the right iliac region? The fibers of both muscles generally run transversely in this area. Why is the direction of the fibers of the internal oblique muscle at a somewhat higher level? They run at right angles to the external oblique fibers ("as if you put your band in your back pocket"). Care must be taken not to injure what important nerves that lie deep to the internal oblique muscle in the operative field? The iliohypogastric and ilioinguinal nerves may be damaged by this incision. Keep in mind that the deep circumflex iliac artery, a branch of the inferior epigastric, is found between the internal oblique and the transversus muscles and will cause unnecessary bleeding if accidently cut.

Should this incision be done in females who are in their childbearing years? Disease of the female internal genitalia, for example, infections of the uterine tube or other parts of the female adnexa, may produce signs and symptoms very similar to those of appendicitis that cannot be ruled out by physical examination. If disease of the female pelvic organs is a diagnostic possibility, the McBurney incision should not be done. By its design, the McBurney is a small incision that cannot be extended sufficiently to give adequate surgical exposure of the female pelvic organs. Surgical exploration of these organs generally requires a longer incision such as that allowed by a midline incision. If a McBurney incision is used when the diagnosis of appendicitis is incorrect, a needless second incision might have to be made.

Location of appendix and its blood supply

What arrangement in the longitudinal musculature of the cecum assists in locating the origin of the appendix (Fig. 31-2)? The anterior

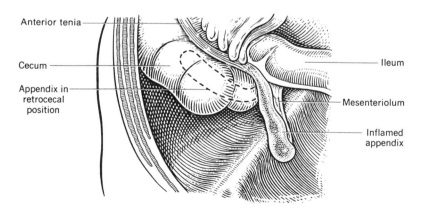

Figure 31-2. Appendix vermiformis is inflamed and distended in its distal portion with its tip hanging over the pelvic brim. Notice how the anterior tenia acts as a guide to the orgin of the appendix. Notice also how a retrocecal appendix might be difficult to approach surgically.

tenia coli forms the best guide to this point. In our case, the position of the appendix facilitated its removal. What common location of the appendix would be apt to cause technical difficulties at surgery? Retrocecal position of the appendix could make the operation more difficult.

What blood vessels are ligated in the mesentery of the appendix? The blood vessels that are ligated are the appendicular artery and vein and their branches and tributaries. Of what artery is the appendicular artery usually a branch, and how does it run in relation to the last part of the ileum? The appendicular artery generally is a branch of the ileocolic artery from the superior mesenteric artery and passes posterior to the terminal portion of the ileum to enter the mesentery of the appendix.

The appendicular artery and its branches are end arteries, that is, arteries that do not anastomose with other arteries. Therefore, if it or one of its branches is blocked by pressure from a fecal stone or by thrombosis, local necrosis occurs, leading to abscess formation and perforation and at worst to generalized peritonitis and death.

Identify the named veins through which an ascending infection in the appendicular vein would have to pass to reach the liver and cause liver abscesses. The infection would travel by way of the appendicular, ileocolic, superior mesenteric, and portal veins to the liver.

32   Hydronephrosis due to an Aberrant Renal Vessel

A five-year-old girl with a history of periodic febrile attacks and complaints of intermittent sharp pain in the left loin is brought to a physician's office. The mother states that the attacks occurred every few months and lasted one or two days. They were accompanied by nausea and vomiting. She also complains that the child eats poorly and has not gained any weight during the last eight months. The patient is admitted to Children's Hospital for further study.

EXAMINATION

The physical examination shows a rather poorly nourished but normally developed child with a slightly enlarged and tender left kidney. Urine examination reveals numerous pus cells. Her temperature is 99.6° F and her white count is elevated.

A plain x-ray film of the abdomen and an intravenous pyelogram (IVP), a radiographic study of the kidneys made while an opaque dye is excreted by the kidney, are obtained. The IVP of the kidneys, with opacified pelves and calyces, shows a moderate enlargement of the left pelvis and calyces. The right kidney appears normal. Under local anesthesia, the girl undergoes cystoscopy, and catheters are inserted into both ureters. The urine flowing from the right ureter is clear, but the urine from the left is cloudy and contains pus. The catheter on the left is then inserted into the pelvis of the kidney and 10 ml of an x-ray opaque medium are injected to visualize the pelvis and calyces (retrograde pyelography). After withdrawal of the catheter into the lower portion of the left ureter, further injection of contrast medium demonstrates the ureter. The films of the left urinary tract taken at various stages of the procedure show a dilated renal pelvis and calyces and a distinct indentation and narrowing at the ureteropelvic junction (Fig. 32-1A).

DIAGNOSIS

Moderate hydronephrosis (dilatation of pelvis and calyces) of the left kidney with obstruction at the ureteropelvic junction, possibly due to an aberrant blood vessel, is diagnosed.

THERAPY AND FURTHER COURSE

The patient is operated on. At operation the left kidney appears enlarged and the pelvis bulging. An accessory artery passes from the aorta in front of the left ureter to the lower pole of the left kidney. This artery compresses the ureter (Fig. 32-1B). On easing the artery away from the ureter, the distended pelvis empties promptly.

The artery is temporarily compressed, and the area of the lower portion of the kidney supplied by the artery is inspected. Only a slight discoloration is noticed, which lasts only a few minutes. The aberrant artery is then ligated and divided.

Postoperatively, antibiotics are given, and convalescence is uneventful. Periodic urinalysis shows continuous improvement of the kidney infection. Serial x-ray studies with intravenous application of dye at six-month intervals reveal that the kidney and calyces gradually return to a more normal size and capacity. Two years later the mother reports that the child is well and without complaints.

DISCUSSION

Aberrant renal vessels to the inferior pole of the kidney occur in 4 to 6 percent of all kidneys and may be a cause of obstruction of the upper urinary tract. How do you explain, from an embryological point of view, the appearance of supernumerary renal arteries at levels different from the main renal artery? During fetal development, where are the kidneys located, and how do they reach their definitive location in the lumbar region? The kidneys develop origi-

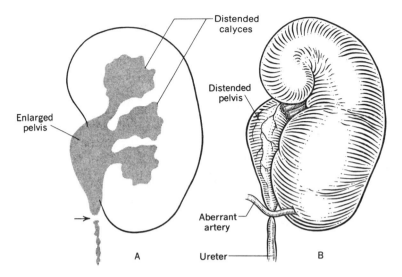

Figure 32-1. A.—Radiograph of the left kidney shows dilated renal pelvis and calyces and an indentation of the ureter at the ureteropelvic junction (see arrow). B.—Diagram shows the enlarged kidney with an accessory (aberrant) artery going to the lower pole and indenting and compressing the left ureter.

nally in the pelvis and migrate from there superiorly by gradual retroperitoneal ascent. Although located in the pelvis, they are supplied by blood vessels in the neighborhood originating from the common, external, or internal iliac arteries, the inferior mesenteric artery, or aorta. Most of these regional vessels disappear as the kidneys ascend, but some persist as supernumerary or aberrant arteries supplying portions of the kidney, particularly the lower pole.

Clinical significance of aberrant arteries

What is the clinical importance of this anomaly? In crossing the ureter, more commonly anteriorly than posteriorly, these aberrant vessels may cause an intermittent or continuous obstruction to urinary drainage from the renal pelvis. How do you explain the progressive enlargement of the renal pelvis and calyces (hydronephrosis) and the eventual destruction of the renal cortex in these cases? Pressure of the backed-up urine may gradually distend and enlarge the pelvis and calyces of the kidney and destroy the cortex. An important factor in this progressive destruction of the kidney is interference with the intrarenal blood supply by increased intrarenal pressure. What is the cause for the frequently superimposed infection of the kidney? The insufficiently nourished and diseased kidney with its stagnating urine may readily become the site of blood-borne infection originating in the upper respiratory tract or elsewhere.

What is the clinical significance of the accessory arteries to the upper pole of the kidney, and from what arteries are they derived? They may be inadvertently torn in renal surgery, leading to severe or sometimes fatal hemorrhage. They are most commonly derived from inferior phrenic or suprarenal arteries. In the x-ray findings, what in our case pointed to the diagnosis of an aberrant vessel as the cause of hydronephrosis? The indentation and narrowing of the ureter just inferior to the enlarged pelvis were certainly significant.

To what extent would ligation of an accessory polar renal artery interfere with the blood supply to the kidney? This is a serious problem in the design of surgery for the condition under discussion because severance of a major artery to the kidney would entail loss of function of that portion of the kidney supplied by the artery and may result in renal necrosis and infection. If the amount of renal parenchyma involved is more than a fourth of the organ, the artery should be left intact and circumvented by microsurgery to establish a junction of the ureter and pelvis unencumbered by the aberrant artery. Temporary compression of the artery at the time of surgery and observation of resulting color changes in the area of the kidney supplied by the artery will furnish a clue to the importance of the artery.

Other causes of ureteral obstruction

Is it possible that the crossing of the ureter by the aberrant artery is not the primary cause of the obstruction but coincides with some internal stenosis of the ureter at the same site and acts only as a contributing factor on an already enlarged pelvis that is sagging over the accessory vessel? This hypothesis has been put forth in the literature by a number of authors who ascribe the primary intraureteral stenosis to congenital mucosal valves or inherent narrowing of the ureter. Such malformations certainly do occur as a cause of hydronephrosis, and not all supernumerary lower polar vessels cause obstruction of the ureter. Consequently, the ureter must be opened at the time of surgery if there is a suspicion of an internal stenosis, in which case microsurgery of the ureter is indicated.

33   Psoas Abscess

A 30-year-old homeless man was transferred to the University Hospital from a tertiary care center known for its treatment of tuberculosis patients, where he has been for a year with a diagnosis of pulmonary tuberculosis. Several years earlier, his grandmother died of tuberculosis of the lung. For the preceding six months, he has complained of backache, which has become more severe during the last few weeks. He also has lost weight and suffers from cough and night sweats.

EXAMINATION

On physical examination the patient appears poorly nourished and shows evidence of tuberculous involvement of the upper right pulmonary lobe, which is confirmed by radiographic examination. There is marked pain in the area of the lower thoracic and upper lumbar vertebral column and tenderness over the spinous processes of the last thoracic and first lumbar vertebrae. The left hip is flexed and externally rotated. Forceful extension of the left thigh is painful and resisted by the patient. A reducible, painless, fist-sized swelling is present in the femoral triangle. There also is some fullness in the left iliac fossa. Radiographic examination of the vertebral column shows an area of destruction on the left side of the anterior portions of the 12th thoracic and first lumbar vertebrae, with narrowing of the intervertebral disk space between these two vertebrae. There is a slight left and posteriorly convex angulation of the vertebral column corresponding to the area of destruction. In the anteroposterior view, a left-sided bulging of the lateral contour of the psoas shadow is noted.

DIAGNOSIS

Tuberculosis of the 12th thoracic intervertebral disc with involvement of the adjacent vertebrae and left-sided psoas abscess (compartment syndrome) becoming superficial in the femoral triangle were diagnosed.

THERAPY AND FURTHER COURSE

During the next eight weeks, the patient is put on specific chemotherapy, including isoniazid for his lung and bone tuberculosis. A nutritious diet and bed rest on a hard mattress are also prescribed. Under this treatment, the patient improves, he gains some weight, and his cough subsides.

Under general anesthesia an operation is performed. The retroperitoneal area is entered through a large oblique incision parallel to and one finger breadth above the iliac crest. The three anterolateral muscles of the abdominal wall and the transversalis fascia are divided without opening the peritoneal cavity or entering the kidney bed. The fascial covering of the psoas is brought into view by blunt dissection, and the psoas fascia is divided to expose the tuberculous abscess within the psoas compartment. The inguinal ligament is divided where the pathway of the abscess is dissected on its way downward beneath it. A second incision is made over the femoral triangle to expose the extension of the psoas abscess to the area of the lesser trochanter. The whole extent of the fascial sac, with the abscess and surrounding scar tissue, is excised. The area of destruction in the 12th thoracic intervertebral disc and the adjacent two vertebrae is now approached and curetted (scraped), and the infected material and debris are cleaned out. During this procedure, care is taken not to injure the left ureter or the sympathetic trunk. With this in mind, a catheter has been inserted into the ureter previously. The inferior vena cava, the testicular vessels, and the exposed branches of the lumbar plexus lying within the psoas are also identified and protected. Antibiotic solution is injected into the large wound, and soft rubber drains are placed into the upper and lower margins of the incision. The divided transversalis fascia and the three abdominal muscles, the subcutaneous tissue, and skin are sutured. The patient is put in a body cast, and strict bed rest is prescribed. Chemotherapy, including antibiotics, is continued for another eight months. Four months after the excisional surgery just described, a fusion operation is done that unites the spinous processes and laminae of the diseased vertebrae with a bone graft taken from the tibia of the patient; the purpose of this surgery is permanent immobilization of the involved vertebrae. The cast and bed rest are continued for another six months after the fusion operation. The patient is then gradually allowed to get up and walk using a brace.

Examinations, one year and two years after operation, show the patient to be fully active and employed. He has gained 25 pounds, his general status is improved, and his tuberculosis in the lung and vertebral column seems arrested.

DISCUSSION

We are dealing here with tuberculosis involving a circumscribed area of the vertebral column that has led secondarily to an involvement of portions of the posterior abdominal wall (posterior to the peritoneal cavity) and posteromedial to the kidney and its fascia.

Not long ago it was hoped that tuberculosis would be eliminated from the United States early in the twenty-first century; instead, the incidence of tuberculosis is rising, especially among the homeless and acquired immunodeficiency syndrome (AIDS) patients. From 1953 to 1984, however, the number of reported cases decreased by about 5.6% each year. From 1985 to 1993, however, the overall number of cases increased by 14%; 25,313 cases were reported in 1993 in the United States. Moreover, an increase in the number of drug-resistant strains of *Mycobacterium tuberculosis* has made it more difficult to treat some cases of tuberculosis.

Psoas muscle, fascia, and compartment

The affected area can be designated the psoas compartment because it comprises the psoas major muscle and its fascia and extends downward to the insertion of the iliopsoas muscle (Figs. 33-1 and 33-2). Where is the psoas major located? Where does it arise and insert?

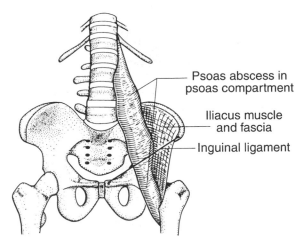

Figure 33-1. A psoas abscess that originated in the spinal column and broke into the psoas compartment. Notice the bulging of this compartment and the extent of the abscess that reaches under the inguinal ligament into the femoral triangle in front of the trochanter minor.

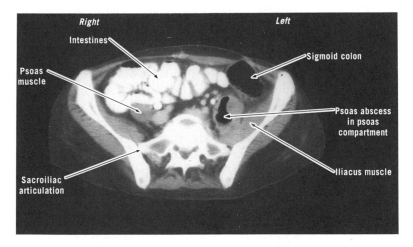

Figure 33-2. CT at the level of the sacroiliac articulation with constrast in the intestines and vessels making them appear white. The sigmoid colon is black because it is distended with gas. The left-sided psoas abscess (dark) has expanded the psoas compartment considerably.

What is its nerve supply and main action? The psoas major is a thick, fleshy muscle (the filet mignon cut of beef) that lies in a trough between the bodies and transverse processes of the lumbar vertebrae. The muscle has a continuous origin from the 12th thoracic to the upper half of the fifth lumbar vertebra, where is arises from the lateral surface of the vertebral bodies, the transverse processes, and the intervening intervertebral disks. It also takes origin from four fibrous arches that bridge the waist of the vertebral bodies and transmit the four lumbar arteries and veins and rami communicantes to the lumbar nerves. The muscle courses downward, forward, and laterally, and passes into the thigh beneath the inguinal ligament just lateral to the iliopectineal eminence (identify this on the skeleton). It fuses with the iliacus muscle before passing deep to the inguinal ligament to become the iliopsoas muscle and inserts into the anterior surface of the lesser trochanter of the femur. The muscle is innervated by direct branches of the lumbar plexus. It is the most powerful flexor of the thigh, wherein it plays a prominent role in kicking and doing sit-ups. When acting from its insertion, it flexes the lumbar vertebral column and bends it toward the same side.

What is meant by the term psoas fascia? What is the extent of this fascia and its clinical importance? The anterior surface of the psoas major is invested by a well-defined, thin, but fairly strong deep fascia, the psoas fascia. With the inclusion of the fascia of the quadratus lumborum laterally, the inferior fascia of the diaphragm above, the fascia of the iliacus muscle below, the psoas fascia may be considered part of the transversalis fascia, the inner deep fascial lining of the abdominal wall. A superior thickening of the psoas fascia, which extends from the body of the second lumbar vertebra medially to the transverse process of the first lumbar vertebra laterally, forms the medial lumbocostal arch from which part of the diaphragm arises. The psoas fascia forms a funnel-shaped sheath that envelops the muscle and also serves as a container for pus originating from diseased thoracic vertebrae. Under the influence of a bacterial infection, which is most often tuberculous, the fascia becomes inflamed and thickens and thus retains the accumulated pus under the clinical picture of a psoas abscess. Gradually destroying the psoas muscle itself and following gravity, assisted by the milking action of the psoas, the abscess descends within the psoas compartment and frequently becomes superficial in the femoral triangle in front of the insertion of the psoas into the lesser trochanter beneath the fascia lata (Figs. 33-1 and 33-2). The medial boundary of the psoas compartment in the abdomen corresponds to the attachment of the psoas muscle and fascia to the vertebral column. In the greater pelvis, the psoas fascia is continuous anterolaterally with the denser iliac fascia.

Anatomy of a typical psoas abscess

How do you visualize the pathological pathway of the disease in our case? As the tuberculous infection leads to destruction of the 12th thoracic intervertebral disc and the adjacent vertebrae, these structures are no longer able to sustain the weight of the overlying column, and they partially collapse at the site of the disease. This explains the radiographic appearance of narrowing of the disc and partial destruction of the adjacent vertebrae, with distortion of the axis of the vertebral column at this point. The partial collapse of the vertebrae squeezes bony debris and pus into the region of least resistance, that is, into the adjacent psoas compartment.

Why does the abscess not invade the spinal canal posteriorly or the region immediately anterior to the vertebral column? The anterior and posterior longitudinal ligaments offer resistance to the spread of the tuberculous process.

Do we have radiographic findings in our case to indicate that the tuberculous abscess has invaded the psoas compartment? Normally, the lateral margin of the psoas is demonstrable on the x-ray film as a straight (noncurving) and laterally descending line that extends from the level of the first lumbar vertebra to the pelvis. In our case, the left psoas margin is characterized by a curving contour corresponding to the bulge of the psoas abscess.

How do you explain the flexed and laterally rotated position of the left thigh, a position the patient naturally assumes and tries to maintain by external support? This position relaxes the muscle and is an attempt to relieve the muscular tension and to prevent pressure on the lumbar nerves in the psoas compartment.

Lumbar plexus

What are the nerves in the psoas compartment? They are branches of the lumbar plexus that are also exposed to injury during surgery for psoas abscess. Which are the most important nerves, and what is their location in relation to the psoas muscle? The femoral and obturator nerves are the principal structures that may be paralyzed in this disease or that may be injured during surgery. The femoral nerve (ventral rami, L2, 3, and 4) forms within the psoas muscle and courses in the groove between psoas major and iliacus; it must be closely guarded during surgical exposure. The obturator nerve (also L2, 3, and 4) branches from the lumbar plexus just anterior to the origin of the femoral nerve. It then leaves the field of surgery by traveling medially into the lesser pelvis to enter the medial compartment of the thigh, where it supplies the adductor muscles of the thigh. Other branches of the lumbar plexus likely to be exposed in radical surgery for psoas abscess are the iliohypogastric and ilioinguinal nerves, which pass under the medial lumbocostal arch, and the lateral femoral cutaneous nerve. These three nerves lie lateral to the psoas major muscle. A fifth nerve, the genitofemoral nerve, pierces the anterior surface of the psoas muscle as well as its fascia and may be damaged by disease or surgery, but this is not of serious consequence.

Other pathways of psoas abscess

Can you conceive of any other pathway that a psoas abscess may follow besides the one that has been described? In general, it can be stated that the pus collections follow the lines of least resistance. Their position and extent, therefore, are greatly affected by fascial planes and fascial attachments. An example of the latter is the rarity with which a psoas abscess breaks into the lesser pelvis. The firm attachment of the iliopsoas fascia to the pelvic brim precludes the entrance of the abscess into the lesser pelvis. The resistance of the peritoneum makes perforation into the peritoneal cavity and involvement of the intraperitoneal organs an exceptional event.

On the other hand, the patient's body position, such as the upright posture or lateral decubitus (lying on one side) will facilitate extension of the abscess in the corresponding direction. Thus, it may spread laterally under the fascia of the quadratus lumborum and come to the surface in the lumbar triangle, leading to an outpouching of the thin floor of this triangle. What muscle forms the floor, and what structures form the boundaries of this triangle? The internal abdominal oblique muscle forms the floor, and the latissimus dorsi, the external oblique, and the crest of the ilium form the boundaries of this triangle. A psoas abscess may also extend laterally under the iliacus fascia to appear just medial to the anterior superior iliac spine. Following the usual course into the femoral triangle, the abscess may enter and involve the femur at the lesser trochanter. It may also track along the medial femoral circumflex vessels and present itself along the posterior aspect of the thigh or perforate there; or the abscess may follow the femoral vessels through the adductor canal and appear in the popliteal fossa.

What are the boundaries, floor, and contents of the femoral triangle, which is so important in this case history? It is bounded laterally by the medial border of the sartorius, medially by the medial border of the adductor longus, and superiorly by the inguinal ligament. The iliopsoas and pectineus muscles form its floor, the fascia lata its roof. Important contents of the triangle are the femoral nerve and femoral vessels, which must be protected in surgery draining a psoas abscess. After the femoral vessels leave the apex of the femoral triangle, they enter the adductor canal, which extends from the apex of the femoral triangle to the opening in the adductor magnus by which the femoral vessels appear in the popliteal fossa.

What are the boundaries of the adductor canal? The vastus medialis bounds it anterolaterally, the adductor longus and magnus posteromedially, and the fascial bridge uniting these boundaries forms the roof of the canal, covered by the sartorius. This is the pathway that an occasional psoas abscess takes on its way to the popliteal fossa.

In rare cases the vertebral abscess may break through the posterior longitudinal ligament into the vertebral canal, with consequent involvement of the spinal cord. It may also penetrate through the anterior longitudinal ligament in front of the vertebral column and following gravity track down with the aorta and its terminal branches to reach the gluteal region, either cranial or caudal to the piriformis muscle. It arrives there with the branches of the internal iliac artery, that is, the superior and inferior gluteal arteries.

One final pathway should be mentioned because it has important anatomical and clinical implications, that is, the involvement of the iliopsoas bursa by a psoas abscess. This bursa is one of the largest and most important in the human body. Where is it located? It lies in front of the capsule of the hip joint where the iliopsoas tendon passes adjacent to the iliopectineal eminence. Does this bursa communicate with the hip joint? In 10 to 15 percent of cases, it opens into the joint. If a psoas abscess breaks into the bursa, it may involve the hip joint and lead to the serious complication of tuberculosis of the hip joint.

This case serves as an instructive example of the clinically well-known fact that the spread of abscesses is frequently determined by fascial attachments and that knowledge of fascial anatomy allows us to predict the various pathways that abscesses may take. This also holds true for the fascial compartments in the neck, where the anatomy of the different layers of cervical fascia affects the direction of the spread of infections, including the entrance of pus into the mediastinum.

V PELVIS AND PERINEUM

34   Prolapse of the Uterus

A farm wife, aged 42 years, comes to the outpatient department with the following complaints. She has a "bearing down" sensation in her womb; "something seems to come down," she says. This discomfort increases when she strains or lifts heavy loads. She often has backaches, particularly if she is on her feet all day. She also complains of urinary symptoms, such as frequency of and burning on urination. She fatigues easily. The patient has had four children. Her menstrual flow is increased, and her periods are somewhat irregular.

EXAMINATION

On general examination, the patient appears nervous and anxious. She is underweight and rather frail. Otherwise, the general examination does not show any abnormalities.

Gynecological examination reveals a moderate downward bulging of the anterior vaginal wall that increases on straining. On examination in the erect position, the cervix of the uterus is found in the vagina close to the vestibule. It recedes somewhat when the patient is supine but does not assume its normal position. The cervix is elongated (Fig. 34-1).

DIAGNOSIS

Prolapse (descensus or downward displacement) of the uterus into the vagina and cystocele (bulging of the bladder into the anterior vaginal wall) are diagnosed.

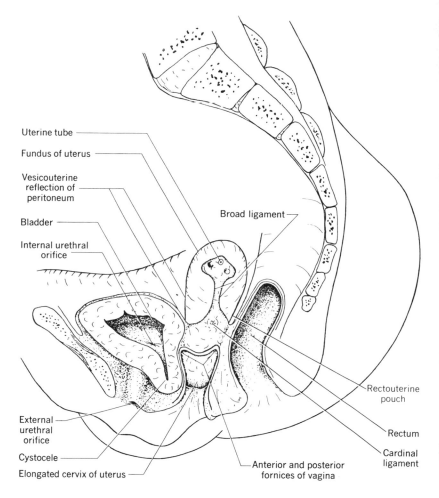

Uterine tube

Fundus of uterus

Vesicouterine
reflection of
peritoneum

Broad ligament

Bladder

Internal urethral
orifice

Rectouterine
pouch

External
urethral
orifice

Rectum

Cystocele

Cardinal
ligament

Elongated cervix of uterus

Anterior and posterior
fornices of vagina

Figure 34-1. Prolapse of the uterus and cystocele. Notice the retroverted
position of the partially descended uterus and the elongation of the cervix.
Observe the bulging of the bladder into the anterior vaginal wall.

THERAPY AND FURTHER COURSE

Because the patient is otherwise in good health and relatively
young, reconstructive surgery is recommended and agreed on. Under general anesthesia, the patient is placed in the lithotomy posi-

tion (that is, she is on her back, legs are flexed on the thighs, and thighs flexed on the abdomen and abducted).

Examination under anesthesia reveals that with traction, the cervix descends to the level of the hymenal ring. Associated with the uterine prolapse is the cystocele, which also descends to this level. There is marked loss of the urethrovesical angle, clinically referred to as rotational urethral descent. The posterior vaginal wall in this patient has not collapsed, and there is no rectocele. The perineal body and vaginal axis are normal.

The surgery, done vaginally, consists mainly of vaginal hysterectomy and shortening of the uterosacral and cardinal ligament complexes, which will form the mainstays of support for the apex of the vagina after hysterectomy. After the uterus is removed, redundant peritoneum of the rectouterine pouch (of Douglas) is excised. After the hysterectomy, the anterior vaginal mucosa is incised in the midline to the urethral meatus. The anterior wall is dissected free from the posterior aspect of the bladder. The fascia of the bladder is imbricated (folded) in the midline to reduce the cystocele anteriorly. The urethrovesical angle is corrected, and resupport of the urethra is achieved by shortening the pubovesical ligaments.

The following are the actual steps of these procedures: An elliptical incision is made through the anterior fornix, extending into the lateral fornices. Using sharp dissection, a plane between the bladder and the cervix is developed within the intervening fascia. The peritoneal cavity is entered by cutting through the peritoneum forming the vesicouterine fold. The rectouterine pouch is entered similarly by sharp dissection through the posterior fornix. The uterosacral and cardinal ligament complexes and the uterine artery are clamped, divided, and ligated with sutures. The ends of the uterosacral ligaments and cardinal ligaments are held separately for later use in the repair.

The uterus, round ligaments, the ovarian ligaments, and the uterine (fallopian) tubes are extracted through the vagina. The ovaries may also be removed (oophorectomy). Now the rectouterine pouch is reentered to remove any excess peritoneum from the rectum to prevent collapse of the rectum anteriorly (rectocele). The sutured uterosacral ligaments are brought across the rectum and attached to each other in the midline, which effectively shortens them and obliterates the rectouterine pouch.

Resuspension of the vaginal cuff is done by suturing the reconstructed uterosacral ligaments to the posterior wall of the vagina. Likewise, the ends of the cardinal ligaments are sewn into the lateral vaginal walls for additional support. A pursestring suture, laced through peritoneum, is placed high in the peritoneal cavity to gather peritoneum to eliminate the communication between the peritoneal cavity and the vagina. The vaginal wall and mucosa are then closed. The vagina should now be of normal length and within normal limits of caliber. With the patient in the supine position, the vaginal axis should be angled slightly posteriorly. A normal urethrovesicle angle should have been achieved.

Postoperatively, an indwelling transurethral catheter is used for 48 h, and the patient is taught to perform self-catheterization. Only rarely is the patient able to void normally for the first few days after this type of repair. After two weeks, however, the great majority of patients are voiding normally and their preoperative urinary symptoms have resolved. The patient would be discharged from the hospital on the third day after surgery. Reexamination after three and six months shows no recurrence of the prolapse.

DISCUSSION

How do you explain the patient's discomfort, including a feeling of heaviness in the lower abdomen and backache? Although this discomfort remains poorly understood, most gynecologists believe it is related to venous congestion and traction on the nerves and support structures of the pelvic floor by the pull of the prolapsed organ. How do you explain the urinary symptoms, such as frequency and burning in the cystocele? Because of the dislodgment of the bladder and change in the urethrovesical angle, residual urine remains in the bladder after urination, resulting in periodic infection of the stagnating urine and cystitis. Frequency and burning are typical signs of this disorder that result from urinary retention.

Flexion and version of the uterus

What is the normal position of the uterus? What angles do the terms "anteversion" and "anteflexion" indicate in relation to the uterus? The uterus is a very mobile organ, subject to constant changes in position depending on the state of filling of the organs in its neighborhood, mainly the bladder and rectum. With these organs empty or nearly empty, the most common position of the uterus is that of anteversion, denoting an anteriorly open angle of somewhat more than 90 degrees between the long axes of the cervix and vagina. In addition, the uterus is generally also anteflexed, which denotes an anteriorly open angle between uterine body and cervix. When the bladder fills, the uterus is readily elevated or even retroverted by the upper surface of the bladder, whereas filling of the rectum may increase its anteversion and anteflexion (Fig. 34-2). In what direction does the ostium of the cervix face if the uterus is in its typical anteverted position? It opens posteriorly into the vagina. On the other hand, the cervical opening faces anteriorly if the uterus is retroverted.

In contrast to former teaching, retroversion and retroflexion by themselves are of questionable clinical significance. Only if uterine

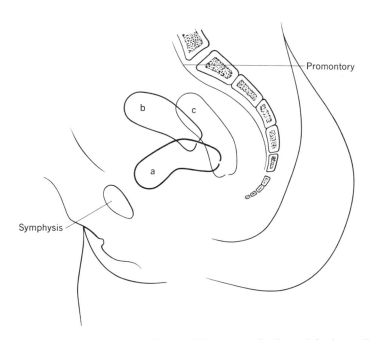

Figure 34-2. Variable positions of the uterus in the pelvis depending on the state of filling of the rectum and bladder. Position of the uterus (a) with bladder and rectum empty, (b) with bladder and rectum filled, and (c) with full bladder and empty rectum (after Merkel).

supports are weakened does a retroverted and retroflexed position of
the uterus tend to promote descent of the uterus because it then lies
in the extension of the longitudinal axis of the vagina (Fig. 34-1).
Intraabdominal pressure further accentuates the downward displacement of the cervix. Congestion and swelling gradually result in
elongation of the cervix as in our patient.

Uterine support

Uterine prolapse, often combined with a cystocele, as in this patient, is one of the most frequently encountered gynecological disorders. What is the cause of the uterine prolapse and the cystocele?
Advancing age brings increased relaxation and loss of tonus of the
pelvic diaphragm and the ligaments that constitute the support of
the pelvic viscera. This fact is mainly responsible for the disorder.
Do multiple childbirths contribute to the occurrence of uterine prolapse? Tearing and overstretching of the supporting tissues during
childbirth greatly enhance the chances for prolapse.

The pelvic diaphragm is a thin, conical muscle that is composed
of the paired levator ani and coccygeus muscles and covered on both
surfaces by deep fascia. Its muscular part is often partly replaced by
connective tissue after having been stretched during childbirth. Its
two halves are separated in front by a narrow gap through which the
vagina, urethra, and anal canal pass to the perineum. What is the
name of the gap? It is called the urogenital hiatus. The importance of
the pelvic diaphragm for the support of the uterus is exemplified by
cases where, because of its congenital paralysis in malformations of
the spinal cord, there is already a prolapse of the uterus in the early
years of childhood. Support of the uterus by the pelvic diaphragm
and the urogenital diaphragm is mainly indirect, however, in that
the uterus rests on organs that on their part are sustained in position
by the intact pelvic and urogenital diaphragms. These organs are the
bladder, on which the normally anteverted and anteflexed uterus
rests, and the ampulla of the rectum, which supports the cervix of
the uterus and the vagina inferiorly and posteriorly.

Particularly controversial is the role of the cardinal (lateral or
transverse cervical) ligaments. Define these ligaments. They are
condensations of parametrial connective tissue in the base of the
broad ligaments, surrounding the uterine vessels and its autonomic
nerves. The cardinal ligaments extend from the lateral pelvic wall to

the cervix and upper part of the vagina. The utcrosacral ligaments are continuous with the cardinal ligaments but extend posteriorly toward the sacrum, where they fan out into condensations of pararectal tissue inserting into the connective tissue anterior to the sacrum. Although they do not directly attach to the sacrum, they contain some of the sensory nerves of the uterus and are shortened in most vaginal repairs for prolapse.

Finally, the fibrous connective tissue between the vagina and bladder and vagina and urethra should be mentioned as providing support. Clinicians have given them the names of vesicovaginal and urethrovaginal septa or fasciae. They are a part of the pelvic visceral fascia and cover the walls of the bladder, vagina, and rectum.

Applied anatomy of prolapse surgery

What important structures are endangered when the cardinal ligaments are shortened? What is the position of these structures in relation to the uterus and the uterine artery? The ureters are usually somewhat displaced from their normal position next to the lateral vaginal fornices. Great care must be exercised during division of the cardinal ligaments to prevent damage to the ureters. The ureters pass by the sides of the lateral fornices of the vagina at a distance of only 1 to 2 cm. Here they are located in the base of the broad ligaments. The uterine artery crosses superiorly and in front of the ureter (water runs under the bridge) giving a small branch to it. The ureter may be mistaken for the uterine artery and erroneously ligated in surgical removal of the uterus.

35 Vasectomy

A 32-year-old geologist had a vasectomy, or excision of a segment of the ductus deferens (vas deferens, vas) five years earlier for the purpose of sterilization after his first wife died. He has remarried and his second wife desires children. He consults a urologist to find out whether reunion of the deferent ducts could be done. The urologist recommends the operation but does not promise success.

THERAPY AND FURTHER COURSE

With the patient under local anesthesia, an incision into the scrotum is made at the site of the former operation. Biopsy of the epididymis verifies the presence of active spermatozoa. Both ends of the previously ligated ductus deferens are freed for 2 cm and brought to the surface. They are trimmed back to the point where patency can be observed. Then an end-to-end anastomosis is established with all layers of the duct being properly approximated. The duct of the opposite side is repaired in the same manner. The incisions are closed and a support is prescribed to immobilize the scrotal contents. Laboratory studies on two occasions within the next months prove the presence of live spermatozoa in the semen. Six months later the patient reports that his wife is pregnant.

DISCUSSION

Applied anatomy of vasectomy

How is this operation performed? Under local anesthesia a skin incision is made on the front of the scrotum just above the level of the head of the epididymis, and the ductus deferens is identified among the other constituents of the spermatic cord. What are the constituents of the spermatic cord, and what are the characteristic features of the ductus deferens? The essential components of the spermatic cord are the ductus deferens with its artery, vein, and some fine nerves that pass to the epididymis; the testicular artery, which is accompanied by testicular nerves; the pampiniform plexus of veins, lymph vessels, and the strandlike remnants of the processus vaginalis in the anterior part of the cord. All these structures are embedded in areolar connective tissue that is in continuity with the extraperitoneal connective tissue (Figs. 35-1 and 35-2).

The ductus deferens lies in the posterior part of the spermatic cord and is identified by its hard and whipcord-like feel when it is rolled between the thumb and index fingers. How do you explain the firm consistency of the duct? This firmness is due to the thick muscular wall surrounding a narrow lumen. The muscular coat consists of outer and inner longitudinal fibers and a heavy circular middle layer, and it delivers by its peristaltic action the semen into the prostatic urethra during ejaculation. Is the ductus deferens the most posterior structure of the spermatic cord at the level of the incision? At this level the pampiniform (tendril-like) plexus consists of 8 to 10 veins, most of which lie in front of the ductus deferens. This larger anterior group surrounds the testicular artery. A smaller group, comprising two or three veins, is located posterior to the duct (Figs. 35-1 and 35-2).

To pick the duct for ligation, the coverings of the spermatic cord are separated. What are these coverings? Although not easily identified individually, they consist of three layers: (1) the thin internal spermatic fascia derived from the transversalis fascia, (2) the cremasteric muscle and fascia derived from the internal oblique muscle, and (3) the external spermatic fascia, representing the continuation of the fascia of the external abdominal oblique muscle over the cord.

After the duct has been stripped free of the areolar tissue in its

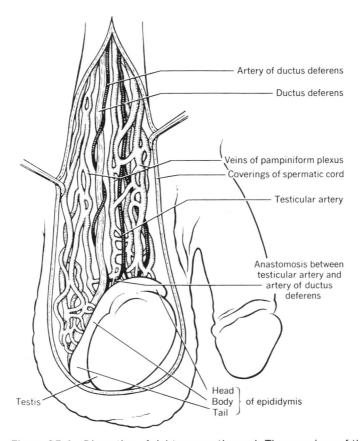

Figure 35-1. Dissection of right spermatic cord. The coverings of the cord have been incised and the contents separated. Notice the veins of the pampiniform plexus in front and behind the ductus deferens.

neighborhood, it is grasped with forceps. The small artery of the ductus deferens is either pushed aside or ligated. Of what artery is it a branch? It is derived from one of the vesical arteries, which are branches of the internal iliac artery, and generally accompanies the deferent duct from the pelvis through the inguinal canal as far as the testis. A small segment of the duct, 1.5 to 2 cm long, is removed and both ends are ligated. The two ends are separated and cauterized to reduce the possibility of recanalization of the duct. Then the wound is closed with sutures and the operation repeated on the other side.

Does ligation of the ductus deferens lead to atrophy and non-functioning of the testes? Clinical and experimental evidence has shown that after ligation of the duct neither the seminiferous epithelium nor the interstitial cells degenerate. In most cases, potential for spermatogenesis is preserved after ligation. Only the ejection of spermatozoa from the testes is prevented.

What is the rationale of reunion and recanalization of the ductus deferens after previous surgical vasectomy? Can it occur spontaneously? The preservation of spermatogenesis after ligation of the duct makes it feasible to reanastomose the ligated ends to restore the anatomical and functional integrity of the ducts. In that case, fertility may be reestablished in 95 percent of patients when modern microsurgical techniques are used.

Three arteries travel within the spermatic cord and provide the blood supply of the testis. They usually form an efficient anastomotic system, establishing testicular circulation. Therefore, one of these arteries is damaged in the performance of the vasectomy; neither the contents of the cord nor the testis are under major risk of infarction. Identify them and give their origin. They are, in descending order of their importance for the survival of a functioning testis, the testicular artery which descends directly from the abdominal aorta; the artery of the ductus deferens, which anastomoses with the testicular artery at the tail of the epididymis; and the cremasteric artery, a branch of

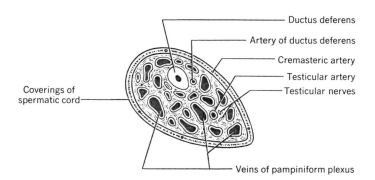

Figure 35-2. Cross section of the spermatic cord at the scrotal level showing ductus deferens, veins of pampiniform plexus, testicular artery, artery of ductus deferens, and cremasteric artery.

the inferior epigastric artery. The cremasteric artery supplies the coverings of the spermatic cord and the scrotal sac and enters into functioning anastomotic connections with the testicular artery and the artery of the ductus deferens in two thirds of men.

Failure of vasectomy

Spontaneous reunion may take place, partly depending on the surgical technique, thus defeating the purpose of the procedure. The regenerated adventitia of the two ends of the duct apparently serves as a splint guiding the separated fragments to reanastomosis. What other reasons, in addition to spontaneous recanalization, could explain failure of vasectomy to result in sterility? Sperm apparently stay alive in the ductus deferens for as long as six weeks or more. During this period after ligation the patient remains, of course, potentially fertile. Other reasons for failure of vasectomy are the presence of accessory ducts that bypass the ligated site and the surgeon's failure to identify correctly and remove a segment of the ductus deferens.

Is the old concept that the seminal vesicles are the main storehouse for semen still tenable? The answer is no. It is the function of the seminal vesicles to add bulk and nutritive material to the semen through their secretory activity. Live spermatozoa are stored mainly in the ductuli efferentes, which connect the testes with the head of the epididymis, and in the duct of the epididymis. Nevertheless, the fact that fertile spermatozoa can be delivered for several weeks after bilateral ligation of the ductus deferens makes their storage in parts of the efferent portions of the reproductive system above the site of ligation (superior to the epididymis) a certainty. Therefore, patients are advised that they will normally remain fertile until residual sperm are flushed away by several ejaculations.

Other consequences of duct ligation

Is potency affected by ligation of the ducts? Potency, the ability of the male to have intercourse, is based on hormonal production, mainly by the testis. What cells in the testes are the source of testosterone, the testicular hormone? Does ligation interfere with secretion of these cells? The interstitial cells of the testes, which produce this hormone, remain unaffected by ligation. How does this hormone leave the testis? It is secreted into the blood stream, and thus potency does not suffer. Is there any justification for the opposite theory, that ligation of the duct through suppression of spermatogenesis results in an increase in hormone production and therefore in improved potency? Ligation of the ductus deferens for purposes of rejuvenation and increase in masculinity was quite popular some years ago, but it is based on false claims.

Does exclusion of spermatozoa from the ejaculate after ligation make a noticeable difference in the amount of the semen? What other glands participate in the production of the ejaculate? The bulk of the semen is composed of secretions from the deferent ducts, the seminal vesicles, mainly the prostate, and the mucus glands of the urethra, including the bulbourethral (Cowper's) glands. The amount is not altered much by the absence of spermatozoa.

In general, how many spermatozoa per ejaculation are necessary for fertility? Normally, about 200 to 500 million spermatozoa are present in the ejaculate. When the total number of sperm cells in the ejaculate falls below 50 million, sterility usually results.

A 22-year-old student comes to the clinic with a history of having had sexual relations with a casual acquaintance about three weeks ago. Five days after this exposure, he complained of tingling and itching at the tip of his penis and in the anterior portions of the urethra. He also noticed a discharge, which was at first thin and watery, but soon became purulent. There was pain and burning on urination. The discharge gradually increased and became greenish yellow. A physician in the student health service gave him an intramuscular injection that he was told was penicillin. After this injection the urethral discharge decreased in amount and became more serous. But within a week it returned to its previous color and consistency. The patient now suffers from fever, discomfort in the perineum, a feeling of fullness in the rectum, urinary frequency and urgency, and severe pain on urination. His main complaint, however, is a very painful swelling of about fist-size in the upper portion of the scrotal sac.

EXAMINATION

On examination, the penis is slightly edematous, particularly around the urethral meatus, which is everted and red. It is tender on slight pressure, especially the corpus spongiosum. The right epididymis is greatly swollen and hard, and it is quite painful on palpation. The swelling continues upward into the inguinal canal. Rectal examination reveals a somewhat enlarged and soft prostate, which is exquisitely tender to touch. The seminal vesicles are swollen and painful and can be palpated superior to the prostate. On slight massage of the prostate by rectum, pus exudes from the urethral orifice. A smear is taken for microscopic examination.

On general examination, there are no abnormal findings concerning the vital organs. The patient's temperature is 101° F degrees. The urine is turbid and blood-streaked and contains threads of desquamated cells. After a sample of urine is taken, a sterile platinum loop is inserted slightly into the urethra. With the loop pressed against the urethral wall, a smear is obtained for staining. This, as well as the pus expressed from the prostate, demonstrates gram-negative diplococci, typical for *Neisseria gonorrheae*. Special cultures confirm this identification of the organism.

DIAGNOSIS

Gonorrheal anterior and posterior urethritis, prostatitis, funiculitis, and epididymitis are diagnosed.

THERAPY AND FURTHER COURSE

A total of 4.8 million units of aqueous procaine penicillin is given by intramuscular injection into the buttocks, along with 1 g of oral probenecid. In view of the extensive spread of the infection, the patient also receives an oral broad-spectrum antibiotic for the next five days. For the symptomatic treatment of his complications, the patient is hospitalized and put on bed rest. Ice packs are applied over the scrotum, which is also immobilized by a well-fitted suspensory. He receives analgesics and sedatives and is told to drink plenty of fluids. Under this treatment, the patient becomes afebrile and his symptoms subside. The swelling of the spermatic cord and epididymis decreases. The patient is discharged on the sixth day and told to abstain from heavy work and sexual activities for another two weeks. Repeated laboratory studies of the urinary tract, including prostatic secretions, are negative and the patient is regarded as cured.

DISCUSSION

Urethra and its glands

Clinicians identify anterior and posterior portions of the urethra, whereas anatomists divide the tube, anteriorly to posteriorly, into the spongy or cavernous, membranous, and prostatic urethra. The spongy urethra to the anatomist is the anterior urethra to the clinician; the other two anatomical subdivisions make up the posterior urethra. The slitlike external meatus is variable in size and caliber, but any instrument that will pass through this opening usually should not encounter any difficulty in traversing the remainder of the urethra. The fossa navicularis (Fig. 36-1) is a fusiform dilatation of the spongy urethra extending inwards from the meatus for about 2.5 cm to the level of the corona of the glans penis. The distal end of the fossa navicularis near the external opening is lined by stratified squamous epithelium, and the remainder of the spongy portion is lined by epithelium of the stratified columnar type. The bulbous urethra of the clinician represents another fusiform dilation of the spongy urethra. It is that part of the urethra that enters the bulb of the penis just below its passage through the urogenital diaphragm.

Blind pockets or crypts (lacunae of Morgagni) are found throughout the spongy urethra (Fig. 36-1). In addition, numerous, mucus-secreting glands (Littre's glands) are located in and beneath the mucosa. Their ducts frequently terminate in the crypts.

Preputial glands (Tyson's glands) are bilateral sebaceous glands located outside the urethra on both sides of the frenulum of the prepuce. The secretion of these glands in the uncircumcised lubricates the prepuce.

The bulbourethral (Cowper's) glands are two small glands posterior and to the right and left of the membranous urethra. They are embraced by the deep transverse perineal muscle on the superior surface of the bulb. Each gland is drained by a duct that pierces the tunica albuginea of the bulb of the penis and terminates in the bulbous portion of the spongy urethra (Fig. 36-1). Normally, the bulbourethral glands have a mucoid secretion that is a component of the seminal fluid.

The membranous urethra, with its coat of external striated muscle, is the most fixed part of the male urethra. It extends from the apex of the prostate to the bulb of the penis and is only

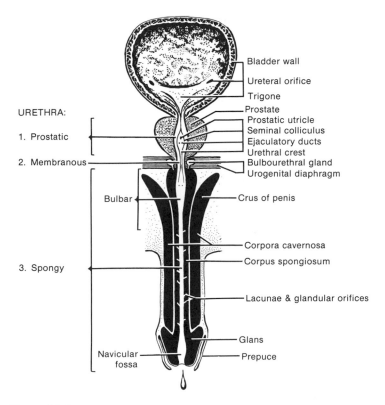

URETHRA:

1. Prostatic

2. Membranous

3. Spongy

Bladder wall
Ureteral orifice
Trigone
Prostate
Prostatic utricle
Seminal colliculus
Ejaculatory ducts
Urethral crest
Bulbourethral gland
Urogenital diaphragm

Bulbar

Crus of penis

Corpora cavernosa
Corpus spongiosum

Lacunae & glandular orifices

Glans

Navicular
fossa

Prepuce

Figure 36-1. Frontal section of the bladder, prostate, and urethra with the anterior wall of the bladder, prostate, and dorsum of the penis removed.

1.5 cm long. It is thin-walled and devoid of glands, in contrast to the prostatic portion, which offers numerous openings of ducts and crypts.

The prostatic portion of the urethra has a longitudinal ridge or crest along its posterior wall. By its protrusion into the urethral lumen, this crest makes the latter cresent-shaped on cross section. An eminence at the height of the crest is called the colliculus semi-nalis or verumontanum (Fig. 36-1), which literally means the ridge the mountain. It is a clinical term that has been in use for almost 300 years. The colliculus seminalis houses a blind pouch, the prostatic utricle. The prostatic sinuses, grooves on either side of the urethral crest, represent the sites where about 20 ducts drain the prostatic glandular tissue. The ejaculatory ducts open into the urethra on each side of the seminal colliculus.

Gonorrheal anterior urethritis

Usually gonorrhea starts as an urethritis; clinicians speak of gonorrheal anterior and posterior urethritis. In gonorrheal anterior urethritis, the gonococci seem confined to the anterior portions of the fossa navicularis the first few hours after intercourse. The crypts or lacunae of Morgagni and the glands of Littre are easily infected, as indicated by the purulent discharge. It is difficult to rid them of infection, however, because inflammation and edema of the mucosa and submucosa obstruct some of the crypts and ducts of the glands. Likewise, preputial glands of Tyson may be involved. When infected they appear as sensitive swellings on the under surface of the glans penis. The bulbourethral glands are also likely to be involved in gonorrheal infection, but usually one-sided. Here we find a painful swelling of bean to plum size on one side of the midline of the perineum. Cowperitis, as it has been called, may be mild and catarrhal in character, or it may lead to abscess formation or chronicity.

Phimosis, paraphimosis, and balanitis

In the uncircumcised male, phimosis, paraphimosis, and balanitis may accompany acute gonorrhea. Phimosis is a tightness of the prepuce or foreskin that makes its retraction over the glans penis impossible. In gonorrhea this is due to edema and inflammation of the foreskin. In paraphimosis the foreskin bas been retracted, but the patient is unable to bring it forward again to its normal position. The narrow preputial rim or edge acts like a rubber band constricting and producing edema of the glans. This is an emergency that can lead to gangrene of the glans. Balanitis is an inflammation of the surface of the glans penis that may occur in cases of infection and inflammation of the prepuce (posthitis), the inner layer of which is moist and has the character of a mucous membrane. Smegma, gonorrheal pus, and the products of secondary infection accumulate on the surface of the glans, which is continually bathed in the urethral discharge. Our patient, who has not been circumcised, has a wide opening into the preputial sac and does not suffer from any of these three complications.

Gonorrheal posterior urethritis

When our patient was seen at the clinic, he had all indications of gonorrhea of the posterior urethra with complications involving the internal sex organs. In other words, because of the resistance of the causative organisms to treatment or because of undertreatment, the infection had spread internally and represented a more serious illness, as evidenced by fever and malaise.

What parts of the genitourinary tract were involved in this later phase of the gonorrheal infection? Without doubt, the disease had spread from the spongy urethra through the membranous portion into the prostatic portion. It had probably also passed through the bladder neck to the interior of the bladder, as indicated by the urinary frequency, urgency, and pain (Fig. 36-1).

Normal variations in intravesical pressure as well as the increase in abdominal pressure caused by straining in coughing, lifting, voiding, and defecation had forced the infected secretions through the prostatic ducts into the prostate and through the ejaculatory ducts into the seminal vesicles, the right ductus deferens, and the right epididymis. The genital tract and its adnexae represent favorite sites of gonorrheal spread and complications, but the upper urinary tract, such as the kidneys and their pelves, the ureters, and most of the bladder (with the exception of the trigone) generally escape the infection.

Prostatitis

In our case, all signs of prostatic involvement were present. The patient complained of perineal pain and a feeling of fullness in the rectum. The prostate was softly enlarged and extremely tender on rectal examination. On light massage, pus containing gonococci was discharged from the external urethral meatus. Because prostatitis represents one of the outstanding complications of posterior urethritis, a brief look at the anatomy of the gland is indicated. The prostrate consists of smooth muscle (stroma) and glandular tissue (parenchyma). Except for the base, where it joins the bladder, and the apex, where it joins the sphincter urethrae, the prostate is surrounded by a fibrous capsule from which septae extend into the gland, dividing it into about 50 lobules. From these lobules, about 20 ducts empty into the prostatic urethra. During sexual activity the secretion of the prostate is expelled through the prostatic ducts by contraction of the prostatic musculature and is added to the ejaculate. In our patient, the posterior urethritis has spread via the various ducts into the gland itself, causing an acute gonorrheal prostatitis, an uncommon sequela.

Seminal vesiculitis

Acute seminal vesiculitis was one of the complications of the posterior urethritis in our patient. On rectal examination, the seminal vesicles felt doughy and swollen and painful on pressure. The infection of the seminal vesicle may be mild and overshadowed by the accompanying prostatitis or may, in undertreated cases, lead to a rather grave clinical picture that imitates acute peritonitis. This event is easily understood if one realizes that the seminal vesicle is capped by the cul-de-sac of peritoneal cavity; so adjacent infection may lead to peritoneal irritation. The seminal vesicle, because of its tortuosity and multiple outpouchings (Fig. 36-2), forms an excellent nidus for bacterial organisms to lodge and multiply. Rupture of abscesses of the seminal vesicle into the peritoneal cavity, rectum, and posterior urethra has been reported.

Ampullitis and funiculitis

The duct of the seminal vesicle unites with the terminal portion of the ductus deferens (that is, its ampulla) to form the ejaculatory duct (Fig. 36-2). It is not surprising that gonorrheal infection of the prostatic urethra leads to ampullitis and infection of the ductus deferens. Our patient had a painful swelling on the right side with inflammation of the surrounding spermatic cord (funiculitis), which extended from the diseased epididymis to the superficial inguinal ring. Generally, pain radiates downward into the scrotum. In other cases, pain may be localized at the deep inguinal ring, where contraction of the abdominal muscles may compress the swollen and inflamed ductus deferens.

Swelling of the terminal portion of the ductus deferens where it runs adjacent to the ureter, close to the bladder wall (Fig. 36-2), may obstruct the ureter, causing symptoms of ureteral block with severe renal pain as a result of the backing up of urine. In general, this

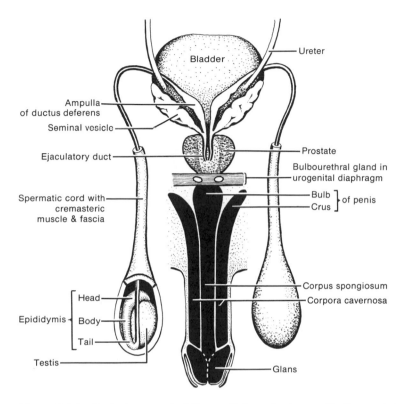

Figure 36-2. Posterior aspect of the genitals and adnexa with the prostate and left scrotal sac opened. The contents of the left scrotal sac have been rotated to give a profile view of the testis and epididymis.

ureteral blockage lasts only a short while, and the symptoms of urinary obstruction subside with treatment.

Right-sided funiculitis and seminal vesiculitis are frequently mistaken for appendicitis. Severe pain on digital examination of the right inguinal canal and on palpation of the deferent duct within the canal should, in most cases, allow a differential diagnosis.

Epididymitis

At one time gonorrheal epididymitis was the most common complication of posterior urethritis (affecting 5–10% of untreated patients).

It then became relatively rare compared with the number of cases of simple urethritis. The usual mode of infection is direct intracanalicular spread from gonorrheal involvement of the ductus deferens (Fig. 36-2).

The epididymis is composed of countless convolutions of a single tube that at its head receives efferents from the testis and continues at its tail into the ductus deferens. Between head and tail of the epididymis lies its body, where the number of coils is somewhat reduced. Topographically, the epididymis may be said to ride "piggyback" on the testis.

In this case, we found a marked enlargement and exquisitely painful swelling of the whole epididymis on the right side. On palpation, the organ is an indurated, tender mass on the posterior aspect of the testis. Occasionally, only the inferior end (tail), is involved. As a usual finding, there is accompanying edema of the surroundings of the epididymis. The skin of the scrotum is inflamed over the diseased organ.

Clinically, the pain and tender swelling in the acute stage of epididymitis gradually subside, even if untreated, but with certainty and considerably faster if sufficient antibiotics are given. Even today, there is one serious complication of bilateral involvement: fibrosis of the duct of the epididymis. This condition may lead to permanent localized obstruction of its lumen, resulting in lasting sterility. Another complication of no great clinical significance is an accompanying hydrocele, a collection of fluid within the cavity of the tunica vaginalis testis. It generally disappears with clearing of the infection.

The indurated inflammation of the epididymis or the accompanying hydrocele may be mistaken for inflammation of the testis (orchitis). Some pathologists, however, exclude intracanalicular spread from the epididymis as a cause of orchitis and assume that most gonorrheal cases of orchitis are due to transmission via the lymphatics or the bloodstream. The common spread to the testis in infectious orchitis (mumps or tuberculosis) is hematogenous in origin.

Proctitis

Another site of primary gonorrheal infection is the rectum. In contrast to the female, where the interfemoral crease channels the infected discharge from the urethra and vagina to the anal canal, in the male gonorrheal proctitis is nearly always due to genitorectal coitus, and rarely to the use of infected instruments or gloves. Although gonorrheal proctitis may be quite mild, it can also be a serious illness accompanied by tenesmus (straining) and pain with fever and the general symptoms of infection. In the case of purulent discharge from the rectum, we find dermatitis around the anal opening with occasional bleeding.

The stratified squamous epithelium of the lower part of the anal canal, in combination with the usually tightly contracted external anal sphincter, offers a limited impediment to the spread of gonorrheal infection to the rectal mucosa. Chronicity of the infection, accompanied by residual bacterial accumulations in rectal glands and anal sinuses, may lead to periproctitis, abscesses, and fistula formation as well as strictures.

Lymphadenitis

Inguinal lymphadenitis, an outstanding feature in most venereal diseases, is inconspicuous in gonorrhea. Inguinal nodes may be moderately enlarged and only slightly tender.

Gonorrheal eye infection

Direct involvement of the eye of the patient is a well-known danger caused by manual transfer of the gonorrheal organisms in careless handling of secretions from the genital organs. This spread to the eye results in conjunctivitis, blepharitis, and keratitis. These must be rigorously treated to avoid further complications.

Hematogenous spread

Invasion of the lymphatic system with rather benign involvement of the regional lymph nodes has been mentioned, but the metastatic spread of the organisms via the bloodstream is of much greater importance. This spread presupposes invasion of veins, and we can assume that in the male the penile and the prostatic veins are the main portals of entrance of the gonococci. Gonorrheal thrombophlebitis has been reported in both locations.

The veins of the penis drain in the following fashion: (1) the dorsal vein of the penis drains into the great saphenous, which empties into the femoral, which, in turn, is a tributary of the external iliac vein; (2) the deep dorsal vein of the penis, which receives numerous tributaries from the deep veins of the penis, terminates in the prostatic and vesical plexuses, which drain into the internal iliac vein; and (3) small veins from the penis connect with the internal pudendal vein, which is a tributary of the internal iliac vein. Of the veins listed, the prostatic plexus is the main recipient of venous blood from the penis. It is formed by large, thin-walled veins that are embedded in the prostatic sheath and is probably the main channel for hematogenous gonorrheal spread. The pathway goes from the internal iliac vein via the common iliac, the inferior vena cava, the right heart, the lungs, the left heart, and finally via the aorta into the general circulation.

Gonorrheal arthritis, tenosynovitis, and bursitis

Among the systemic manifestations of gonorrhea, arthritis is most prevalent. The incidence of this complication is 0.5 percent. Although the disease may start soon after the initial urethral infection, it generally takes several weeks for it to develop. Involved are joints such as the wrist, knee, ankle, shoulder and elbow. Smaller joints (e.g., the metatarsophalangeal and interphalangeal) may also become infected, although more rarely. The joints are red, hot, painful, swollen, and often contain an exudate. There is general malaise with fever. The primary site of the infectious metastasis within the joint is the synovial membrane. The synovial exudate is seropurulent, and cultures of the effusion may or may not show gonococci. The infection responds well to antibiotics in the proper dosage. If suppuration occurs because of delayed or insufficient treatment, permanent ankylosis (fusion of the articulating surfaces) may result. According to the older literature, involvement of more than one joint and recurrence in the same joint were observed quite frequently.

Closely related to metastatic gonorrheal arthritis are gonorrheal tenosynovitis and bursitis. Favorite locations for tenosynovitis to occur are the tendon sheaths of the extensor tendons of hand and foot. When involved, they appear tender and swollen. Gonorrheal bursitis most frequently affects the bursa between the Achilles tendon and the calcaneus.

More serious and fortunately rather rare manifestations of gonococcemia are endocarditis, myocarditis, and pericarditis, iritis, chorioretinitis, and meningitis. Gonorrheal endocarditis commonly involves the aortic valves and may lead to their destruction. Gonorrheal meningitis is often accompanied by other manifestations of hematogenous spread, such as skin lesions and multiple joint involvement. In these cases, much higher doses of antibiotics over a longer period are required.

Urethral stricture

Historically, the final sequela of gonorrheal urethritis is urethral stricture. A famous physician facetiously remarked: "The lieutenant has the gonorrhea, but the colonel has the stricture." The interval between acute urethral infection and clinically significant urethral stricture extends over years. A figure mentioned in the literature is 20 years. Present-day urethral strictures are still seen and are generally the consequence of preantibiotic infections. The most common sites of gonorrheal stricture are the bulbous urethra and the posterior region of the fossa navicularis. A stricture is the result of the acute inflammatory process of the urethral mucosa with periurethral invasion by the gonococcus resulting in scarring and a circumferential narrowing of the urethral lumen. Once formed, the stricture can be permanent. The signs and symptoms of a chronic urethral stricture are those of obstruction to the urinary outflow with urinary retention. Further complications of untreated strictures are secondary infection of the dilated prestenotic urinary passages, periurethral abscesses, and finally upper urinary tract dilatation with hydroureter and hydronephrosis, pyelonephritis, and uremia. The treatment of uncomplicated strictures consists of repeated urethral dilatations with bougies or sounds. If this method leads to complications or is unsuccessful, surgery is required. It was common for physicians to pass a urethral sound (a surgical probe) during the acute stages of gonococcal urethritis, and the traumatic role of the sound in the genesis of stricture has never been excluded.

Anatomy of Female Gonorrhea

An unmarried 24-year-old woman comes into the clinic requesting treatment for a gynecologic problem. She complains of chronic backache, increased menses, and chronic vaginal discharge.

This patient's history reveals that she has been sexually active since age 16. At age 18 she had an external genital infection on the inside of the right labium majus, which led to an abscess that was surgically drained. At the time, she also had urinary symptoms, particularly frequency and burning pain on urination. Later, she complained of low backache and a white-to-yellow discharge from the vagina. As a result of the symptoms of infection, she was treated with antibiotics. A few weeks later she had cramplike attacks of lower abdominal pain with loss of appetite, occasional vomiting, and fever. These attacks reappeared at approximately monthly intervals. Menstrual periods became more painful, lasted longer, and bleeding was considerably increased.

At the age of 20, an abscess that was apparently located in the rectouterine pouch (of Douglas) was drained by a transvaginal approach (culdocentesis). She was told by her physician that she had a gonorrheal infection and was treated again with antibiotics. Over the next few years, the pelvic symptoms decreased in intensity, although the lower abdomen was often sore and she had occasional attacks of mild fever and malaise.

EXAMINATION

The patient is seen in the clinic, and smears are taken from the urethra, cervix, rectum, and pharynx. On inspection, the external genitalia appear essentially normal except for a scar on the right side of the vestibule. During examination of the vagina with a speculum, a mucopurulent substance is observed at the os of the cervix. After removal of the substance, some erosions of the cervix are visible. On bimanual examination of the uterus and adnexa, there is lower abdominal pain and some resistance of the abdominal wall, particularly on the right. The uterus seems fixed in a retroverted position; the cervix is likewise fixed and pulled to the right side by adhesions; and the right uterine tube seems enlarged and transformed into irregular, hardened masses. On internal inspection, the rectum appears normal. Other vital organs are essentially normal. Laboratory studies and fluorescent antibody procedures confirm the clinical diagnosis of gonorrhea and demonstrate the presence of gonococci in cervix and rectum.

DIAGNOSIS

Chronic gonorrhea of the cervix uteri with right-sided salpingitis and local peritoneal involvement, with adhesions, and gonorrhea of the rectum are diagnosed.

THERAPY AND FURTHER COURSE

Treatment is started immediately. The patient is given 4.8 million units of aqueous penicillin intramuscularly in divided dosages, together with 1 g of oral probenecid. Both drugs are repeated the next day. A total dosage of 10 g of tetracycline hydrochloride is given orally over a period of five days (500 mg is given four times each day).

The patient is checked at weekly intervals for four weeks, and pelvic examinations are repeated twice over the next few months, each right after the menstrual period. On each of these occasions, there are no urinary symptoms, the discharge was decreased, and no gonococci could be demonstrated at any portal of the body; however, the uterine displacement and immobility persist as well as the palpatory findings concerning the adnexa.

DISCUSSION

The patient is fairly typical of the chronic, almost asymptomatic female patient who may serve as a carrier of the disease. In light of its complexity, it seems worthwhile to discuss the anatomy of the various forms and locations of female gonorrhea.

Urethritis

The common urogenital sites of acute gonorrheal infection in the female are the urethra and the cervix of the uterus. Older sources identify the urethra as the most common location of primary infection (up to 90 percent). In contrast to the male urethra, whose gross and microscopic structure is much more complicated, the female urethra is only about 4 cm long. It is directed downward and forward with a slight curvature; lies immediately in front of the lower, anterior part of the vagina, in which it seems embedded; and can be palpated through the anterior vaginal wall. Exudates can be expressed from the urethra by the gloved finger in the vagina. The external urethral orifice is located immediately anterior to the opening of the vagina, which explains the common occurrence of infection in sexual intercourse. Occasionally, the acute gonorrheal infection may be recognized at the external meatus of the urethra, which may be red, swollen, and everted (Fig. 37-1).

The mucous membrane of the urethra is thrown into longitudinal folds with the epithelium stratified or pseudostratified columnar in character, types for which the gonococci seem to have a preference. The epithelium forms little glandlike outpouchings that contain mucous cells, an arrangement resembling the urethral glands in the male. In addition, true glands also open through thin-walled ducts into the lumen of the urethra.

Infection of paraurethral glands

Paraurethral glands (Skene's) are located at both sides of the distal end of the urethra and drain through two ducts that open on the sides of or into the external urethral meatus (Fig. 37-1). The gonococci cause inflammation and a mucopurulent exudate containing desquamated epithelial cells. Ascent of the infection to the bladder is rare, but abscesses may develop in the paraurethral glands or

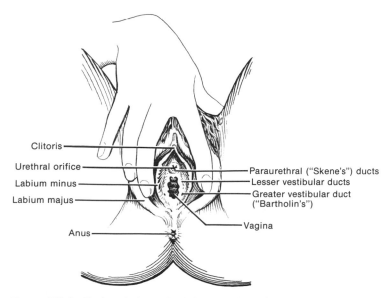

Clitoris

Urethral orifice

Labium minus

Labium majus

Anus

Paraurethral ("Skene's") ducts

Lesser vestibular ducts

Greater vestibular duct ("Bartholin's")

Vagina

Figure 37-1. Perineal sites of adult gonorrheal involvement: the urethra and its external meatus, the paraurethral glands (Skene's) and ducts, the greater and lesser vestibular glands and ducts, and the anus and rectum.

in the periurethral tissues. In contrast to the male, strictures resulting from past infections are rare.

Infection of the vestibule and the greater and lesser vestibular glands

The labia minora enclose the vestibule of the vagina. The stratified squamous epithelium of the vestibule protects them from gonorrheal infection in most adult females.

Specific gonorrheal infections in this region occur mostly in the greater vestibular (Bartholin's) glands. These two mucus-secreting, pea-sized bodies are situated beneath the posterior portion of the labia majora. Their ducts open into the grooves between the hymen or its remnant and the labia minora (Fig. 37-1). Frequently, they harbor the bacteria for longer periods than other areas. Their orifices may appear red and swollen. Glands commonly abscess, as in our patient, and must be drained, either from the inside near the openings of the ducts or from the labia majora. Mixed infection is a more common cause of Bartholin's abscess. Lesser vestibular glands, which are numerous and located around the vaginal orifice, may also become infected due to the character of their susceptible epithelium.

Vaginitis

To the surprise of most patients (and medical students), the vagina of the adult is uninvolved in gonorrheal disease. The epithelial lining is resistant to the infection. The vagina itself does not contain any glands in which the organism can live. Fluid in the vagina is an exudate derived from the blood of its tunica propria and may contain numerous sloughed cells of the superficial layers of the mucosa as well as nonpathogenic bacteria intermingled with normal mucus from the cervical glands. These substances are usually present in combination with infections caused by *Trichomonas vaginalis* and *Candida albicans*. It is debated whether true gonorrheal vaginitis occurs in the fornices. The presence of infected excretions at this site may also be due to discharge originating in the cervix.

In contrast to the absence of infection of the vagina in the adult, gonorrheal vulvovaginitis in infants and young girls up to the age of six years does occur, caused by either sexual molestation or poor hygiene, particularly where adults and children live in crowded conditions or in institutions, such as infant nursing homes and daytime nurseries. The explanation for the susceptibility of young girls to gonorrheal infection in the lower genital tract can be found in the aplastic condition of the vulva and vagina, which are lined by a transitional, loosely interconnected epithelium, which readily permits the entrance and spread of the organisms. The symptoms of the disease include a profuse purulent discharge and redness and edema in the affected area.

Cervical involvement in acute gonorrhea of the infant has been observed frequently and may in part be the cause of recurrence of vaginitis. As a corollary of the underdevelopment of internal genitalia in children, there is generally no ascent of the infection beyond the cervix, and the well-known complications in the internal genital organs are absent.

In the adolescent, estrogen, produced by the ovary, causes an increase in thickness of the vaginal wall, typical pubertal changes in vaginal pH and flora, and concomitant adult development of the external genitalia with growth of paraurethral and vestibular glands.

Cervicitis

In acute cases of gonorrheal infection, the cervix, next to the urethra, is the most common site of involvement. In chronic cases, the relationship seems reversed. The branching longitudinal folds of the cervix (*plicae palmatae*), the columnar epithelial lining, and the presence of numerous large and extensively branching and secreting glands form an excellent soil for the multiplication and spread of the infection (Fig. 37-2).

Whereas uncomplicated gonorrheal cervicitis may also be symptomless except for *leukorrhea* (white viscid discharge from cervix), patients may also complain of low backache and some suprapubic discomfort. Later, the discharge may become more purulent and profuse, and the external orifice of the cervix may appear inflamed and show some erosion. Our patient displays, in addition to the positive laboratory findings, all these signs of chronic gonorrhea.

Other patients display retention cysts (Nabothian follicles) of

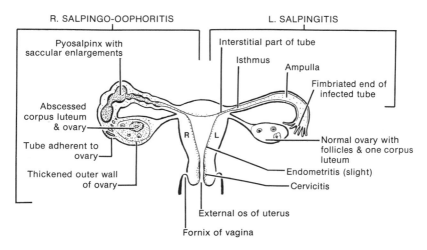

Figure 37-2. Sites of gonorrheal involvement of the internal genitalia. These are the cervix, the endometrium (?), the uterine tubes, and the ovaries with accompanying peritoneum.

the glands around the cervical os. These were first described by the German anatomist, Naboth, in 1707, who, interestingly enough, mistook them for ova, which explains their original name, ovula nabothi. A similar mistake was made in naming the disease gonorrhea meaning flow of seed. Physicians of this period believed that the discharge in the male was an involuntary loss or flow of semen instead of a discharge or pus.

Endometritis

The most dreaded and common ascending gonorrheal infection in the female involves the uterine tubes; however, the intervening uterine body is rarely involved. Evidence of gonorrheal endometritis is rather tenuous. Experts in this field have assumed that the main culprits that facilitate passage of gonorrheal organisms across the uterine mucosa to the uterine tubes are menstrual contractions and uterine blood. Followers of the theory of continuous spread via the endometrium and endometritis (Fig. 37-2) assume a self-healing course of the endometritis and confirm this by the absence of acute endometrial inflammation in cases where, due to severe complications, the uterus and its adnexa have to be removed.

Salpingitis

Gonorrheal salpingitis and its pelvic sequelae appear to occur most commonly if the infection takes place during or right after menstruation, when the epithelial structures of the uterus are sparse and desquamating tissues and blood are profuse. Other factors may include high-pressure vaginal douches, abortion, instrumentation, and labor contractions. Once the organisms have entered the uterine tubes, they invade the columnar epithelial lining and the luminal spaces from which they penetrate the subepithelial connective tissue and muscular layers. The mucous membrane of the widest portion of the tube, the ampulla, forms numerous profusely branching folds that leave only narrow luminal spaces between them.

The originally serous gonorrheal exudate inside the tube becomes purulent and sometimes, before the fimbriated peritoneal opening closes as a result of adhesions and scarring, pus exudes from the opening, causing pelvic peritonitis and oophoritis (Fig. 37-2). Closure of the peritoneal end and other portions of one or both tubes takes place, often resulting in permanent sterility. After total closure at the fimbriated end, further production of exudate inside the tube may cause pus pockets and outpouchings in the tubes, leading to what may be called tubal pseudoabscesses or pyosalpinx (Fig. 37-2). True abscesses and scarring and hardening of the tubal wall in combination with circumscribed outpouchings may give the palpatory and clinical picture that this patient shows.

The ascending type of infectious spread is typical for gonorrhea, whereas lymphatic or vascular channels may be used by septic and tuberculous infections for propagation to the tubes and ovaries.

Clinically, characteristic for the acute stage, bilateral lower abdominal pain, tenderness and rigidity with distention of the intestine, often accompanied by vomiting, fever, and leucocytosis, are usually prevalent. Backache accompanying ascending gonorrhea can be explained by referred pain to the back. The inflammatory edema in the connective tissue of the uterus and uterine tubes stimulates pain fibers that originate in the lower thoracic and upper lumbar segments.

Oophoritis

The most common source of gonorrheal infection of the ovary is the pus that exudes through the abdominal opening of the uterine tube (Fig. 37-2). After closure of the tubal opening, the organisms may migrate through the diseased wall of the tube to the adherent ovary, or the accompanying peritoneal infection may secondarily involve the germinal epithelium and penetrate into the interior of the organ. Because of inflammation, the ovary may seem quite enlarged on palpation. Ruptured ovarian follicles may also be a portal of entrance of the infection if the ovary is adherent to an infected tube. Thus, tubo-ovarian abscesses may occur in these cases (Fig. 37-2).

Oophoritis is generally one-sided and less common than salpingitis. In the further chronic course of salpingo-oophoritis, the purulent exudate gradually becomes more serous, and the gonococci may disappear. Acute recurring symptoms of fever and pain likewise disappear or appear only at intervals. Slight backache and minor menstrual irregularities may be the only residue of the disease.

Pelvic peritonitis

Peritoneal spread may comprise all stages of infection, from slight pelvic irritation to the circumscribed serous, fibrous, or purulent peritonitis. The last of these occasionally leads to abscesses in the rectouterine pouch that, as in this case, can be drained through the posterior fornix of the vagina or may rarely lead to breakthrough into adjacent organs, such as the rectum and bladder. Localized right-sided peritoneal involvement may result in the rather common erroneous diagnosis of appendicitis.

The most common after effects of gonorrheal peritonitis are adhesions with fibrous bands. The uterus is generally fixed, immobile, and often retroflexed and retroverted with the cervix displaced, as in this patient. These adhesions are often confirmed by surgery or autopsy. They are widespread and massive and frequently involve, in addition to the internal genital organs, the small intestine, sigmoid colon, rectum, and bladder. Partial and complete intestinal obstructions are occasional complications. Chronic invalidism, together with recurring infections, may make total hysterectomy, including adnexa, necessary.

Proctitis

About 10 to 40 percent of all women with gonorrhea harbor the gonococcus in the anal canal, as this patient did. Many rectal infections are locally asymptomatic; nevertheless, gonorrheal proctitis may lead to bacteremia with distant metastatic manifestations. As in the male, symptoms may be mild and consist essentially of only slight itching and burning in the anal region and some pain on defecation. On the other hand, the infection may represent a serious illness with tenesmus (straining), severe pain, particularly on defecation, occasional hemorrhage, fever, and general malaise. Chronic disease with residual bacterial accumulations in the rectal glands and anal sinuses may lead to mixed infection with periproctitis, abscesses, and fistula formation.

Pharyngitis

Another primary site of infection is the pharynx, where the infection is transmitted by oral-genital intercourse. The disease appears with signs and symptoms of streptococci pharyngitis, and only suspicion and awareness of the possibility of gonorrheal infection will lead to proper culturing and correct diagnosis.

Ophthalmia neonatorum

A primary site of gonorrhea in the newborn is the eye, where the infection is acquired during passage through the infected birth canal during delivery. It is the most dangerous organism in regard to potential harm to the eye. In addition to the conventional care of the newborn, preventive diagnosis and treatment of the mother during pregnancy is the most effective approach. Manual transfer of the organisms through careless transmission of genital by-products to the eyes of children or to the patient's own eyes is a danger resulting in conjunctivitis, blepharitis, keratitis, and panophthalmitis, which may eventually lead to blindness.

Metastatic spread of gonorrhea

Tenosynovitis and arthritis are the most common results of gonorrheal bacteremia. Papulopustular lesions of the skin may also appear. Much rarer are meningitis, endocarditis, pancarditis, uveitis (inner eye), and panophthalmitis. Because these metastatic infections are infrequent, they often are not diagnosed and consequently improperly treated, for example, with steroid therapy. They should be suspected, particularly in sexually active teenagers and young adults.

Lymphatic invasion can occur at any site where the organisms penetrate the loosened columnar epithelium and infiltrate the connective tissue and with it the lymph vessels. In contrast to other venereal diseases, this involvement of lymph vessels and nodes is relatively benign and hardly ever leads to lymph node abscesses. However benign, inguinal lymphadenitis, although more frequent in the male, has often been observed in female gonorrhea, particularly in infection of the greater vestibular glands.

Although lymphatic spread via the thoracic duct to the general venous circulation cannot be excluded, it is more likely that venous propagation occurs by gonococcal invasion of the peripheral thin-walled veins and capillaries that drain into the plexuses of the bladder, vagina, uterus, ovary, and rectum. The pathway then extends into the internal iliac vein and from there via the common iliac, the inferior vena cava, the right heart, the lungs, the left heart, and finally the aorta into the general circulation. Increase in the incidence of hematogenous spread accompanying the general increase in incidence of gonorrheal infection has recently been reported by several sources.

VI   UPPER LIMB

38   Fracture of the Clavicle

A 13-year-old boy scout fell on his left shoulder while running down a steep incline and immediately complained of severe pain in the area of his collarbone. All movements of his left arm are painful. He tries to avoid painful motion by holding his left arm close to his body and by supporting the left elbow with his right hand.

EXAMINATION AND DIAGNOSIS

The boy is brought to a physician, who diagnoses a fracture of the clavicle. The fracture is located at the middle of the bone. There is marked tenderness and some swelling at the fracture site. Upon passing the fingers along the border of the clavicle, the examiner can discern the projecting ends of the fragments. The sternal fragment is angulated upward (Fig. 38-1). Passive movement of the left shoulder is quite painful. A radiograph confirms the diagnosis of clavicular fracture at the expected site and shows depression of the outer fragment.

THERAPY AND FURTHER COURSE

The fracture is reduced by pulling the shoulder upward and backward, and correct alignment of the fragments is retained by application of a figure-8 bandage. This bandage allows the patient to use his left elbow, wrist, and finger joints, which are exercised at regular

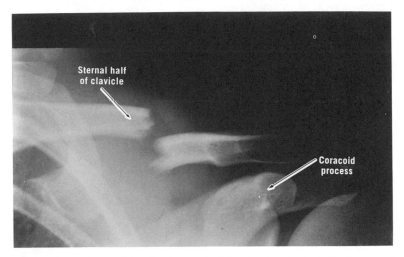

Figure 38-1. X-ray of the fractured clavicle showing typical displacement of the fragments. Notice that the sternal end is displaced upwards, whereas the distal end sags because of gravity.

intervals to avoid stiffening. The bandage is removed after five weeks, when clinical examination shows evidence of bony union.

DISCUSSION

Clavicular fracture is one of the most common fractures in the body. How do you explain this? The clavicle is the only skeletal connection of the shoulder girdle to the trunk, and it serves as a strut to maintain the shoulder and arm at the proper distance from the chest. As such, it is exposed to any force that tends to thrust the arm medially against the chest, as exemplified in our case, in which the patient fell on his shoulder. If unbroken, the clavicle maintains a constant distance between the acromion and the middle of the body; a decrease in this distance, compared with the normal side, is a rough indication of the amount of overriding of the fragments.

Ligaments anchoring the clavicle

What keeps the clavicle from dislocating at the sternoclavicular joint when an inward thrust is exerted on the shoulder? Inspect a skeleton and see whether there is secure adaptation of the articulating parts of this joint. As far as the bony contours are concerned, the joint seems quite unstable and vulnerable to dislocation. Why, then, is dislocation at this joint infrequent? Identify the ligamentous structures that protect the integrity of the sternoclavicular joint (Fig. 38-2). They are the strong costoclavicular ligament, the anterior and posterior reinforcements of the articular capsule, the anterior and posterior sternoclavicular ligaments, and the articular disk attached to the clavicle above and the first costal cartilage below. Is there an equally strong ligament at the lateral end of the clavicle that binds the clavicle to the scapula? The coracoclavicular ligament with its two parts, the conoid and trapezoid ligaments, protects the integrity of the acromioclavicular joint and prevents the acromion from being driven under the clavicle. Can you correlate the most common site of fractures of the clavicle in the middle third with the location of the major ligaments? These fractures occur between the attachments of the costoclavicular and the coracoclavicular ligaments that anchor the clavicle at either end.

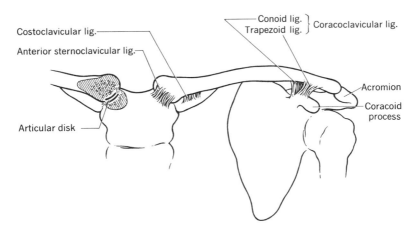

Figure 38-2. Ligaments of the clavicle. The disk, the sternoclavicular ligaments, and the costoclavicular ligament protect the integrity of the sternoclavicular joint and prevent dislocation. Notice that the disk is attached to the clavicle above and the first rib below. Also notice that fractures most commonly occur between the costoclavicular and the coracoclavicular ligaments.

Clavicular fracture at birth

Do fractures of the clavicle occur as birth injuries? Fractures of the clavicle are particularly common in the newborn. In fact, they are more frequent than all other birth fractures combined. The clavicle may be fractured by the hand of the obstetrician in breech (buttocks) presentation, or it may break on its own during passage of the child through the birth canal by being pressed against the maternal symphysis pubis. Can you give a reason why the clavicle at the time of birth would be rather rigid and unyielding? The clavicle starts ossification earlier than any other bone: during the fifth week of fetal life.

Muscles involved in clavicular fracture

Displacement of the fragments is rather characteristic and depends on the action of the muscles attached to the shoulder girdle and on the weight of the arm. The pull of what muscle displaces the medial fragment upward? The clavicular portion of the sternocleidomastoid muscle is responsible for the upward tilt of this fragment (Fig. 38-1).

On the other hand, the weight of the arm and the pull of what muscle would displace the lateral fragment downward? The deltoid arises from the lateral third of the clavicle and, combined with the weight of the limb, is responsible for this displacement. These factors cause the left arm to hang lower than the right. What large muscle connecting the thorax with the arm would adduct (pull) the arm toward the thorax, causing a decrease in the distance between acromion and midline and therefore an overlapping of the fragments? The pectoralis major, supported by the latissimus dorsi and smaller muscles, is responsible for this displacement. Because the medial rotators of the arm are stronger than the lateral rotators, and the bracing action of the clavicle is nullified by the fracture, the arm is also medially rotated. What muscles are responsible for this action? The pectoralis major, subscapularis, teres major, the latissimus dorsi are the medial rotators of the arm. This medial rotation of the arm also explains why the medial end of the lateral fragment commonly points posteriorly.

Despite the superficial location of the clavicle and the frequent presence of bony fragments at the site of fracture, piercing of the skin by osseous spicules is rather rare. Why? The subcutaneous location of the platysma, which allows the skin to move freely over the clavicle, protects the skin and usually prevents fragments from piercing it, thus preventing the occurrence of a compound (open) fracture with its dangers of secondary infection at the fracture site.

More important is the protective action of another muscle that lies deep to the clavicle, between it and the first rib. It guards important underlying structures against injuries from bony fragments. Name this muscle and the underlying structures. The subclavius, surrounded by its fascial sheath, derived from the clavipectoral fascia, runs from the first rib to the undersurface of the clavicle. It shields the subclavian vessels and the brachial plexus from damage in the clavicular fracture. Remember that these important structures pass over the first rib but under the clavicle on their way into the axilla. Do the curvatures of the clavicle allow for the course of these neurovascular structures? The medial half of the clavicle has its convexity anteriorly, increasing the space between it and the first rib. In visualizing the crowding of the subclavian vessels in the costoclavicular space, it might help to know that in many people the radial pulse becomes demonstrably weaker if the arm is pulled forcibly in a posterior and downward direction.

Injuries to blood vessels and nerves in clavicular fracture

Watson-Jones, in his textbook, Fractures and Joint Injuries, tells us that the founder of the London police force, Sir Robert Peel (from whom the members of this force derive their nickname "bobby") died of a fractured clavicle, with splinters from the fractured bone causing a fatal hemorrhage from the subclavian vein. Other cases are on record in which nonunion of the clavicular fracture or excessive callus formation was responsible for thrombosis of either the subclavian vein or artery, causing pulmonary embolism in the former and embolism in the brachial or basilar artery in the latter. Describe the course that a blood clot takes to reach the lung in the case of venous thrombosis and to lodge in the brachial artery in thrombosis of the subclavian artery. Right brachiocephalic vein, superior vena cava, right atrium, right ventricle, and pulmonary artery would be the pathway that a blood clot formed in the subclavian vein would take on its way to the lung. A blood clot formed in the subclavian artery would travel with the arterial bloodstream to the periphery of the upper extremity, where it would be arrested in one of the major arteries of the extremity, depending on the size of the clot. It also could go to the brain via the vertebral branch of the subclavian artery and lodge in the basilar artery at the base of the brain.

Injuries to the brachial plexus have likewise been described as early or late complications of clavicular fracture. The neurologic symptoms consist of paresthesias (sensations of tingling, burning, and numbness) in the area of distribution of spinal cord segments C8 and TI. Which trunk of the brachial plexus is involved? The lower trunk, particularly its first thoracic component, lies behind the subclavian artery on the first rib and is exposed to pressure against the rigid bone.

39   Cervical Rib Syndrome

A 39-year-old woman has suffered for many years from "rheumatic" pains in her right arm. Recently, after the patient took on additional work, the pain worsened and now radiates down the medial side of the arm and forearm into the hand. Her pain increases toward the end of the day and at night. Sometimes the fingers on the ulnar side of the hand tingle and feel numb. The right arm seems weaker than the left.

EXAMINATION

Examination shows some tenderness and resistance in the right supraclavicular area, but nothing definite can be palpated. Downward pulling on the arm increases the pain. There is obvious wasting of the right thenar eminence. On testing, the opponens pollicis and abductor pollicis brevis seem to be particularly involved.

DIAGNOSIS

The diagnosis of cervical rib in this case is based on the resistance in the right supraclavicular fossa and on the presence of subjective and objective neurologic signs pointing to involvement of the lower trunk of the brachial plexus; both sensory and motor fibers are affected. Radiography confirms the diagnosis and shows an accessory rib on the right side articulating with the seventh cervical vertebra, pointing forward and downward and ending bluntly.

THERAPY AND FURTHER COURSE

At operation the cervical rib is found to be continued anteriorly as a fibrous band attached to the first rib. The brachial plexus is elevated, as is the subclavian artery, both of which pass over the cervical rib. The inferior trunk of the plexus appears rather taut and stretched over the accessory rib (Fig. 39-1). The cervical rib is excised.

After removal of the cervical rib, the symptoms gradually disappear during the next few months. Strength seems to return to the hand and the wasting of the thenar eminence also gradually diminishes.

DISCUSSION

The sensory disturbances in this case do not correspond to the cutaneous distribution of any one peripheral nerve but involve an area that is supplied by at least three named nerves. Which are these? The medial brachial and antebrachial cutaneous nerves and the ulnar nerve supply the involved area with sensory fibers. In addition, the motor deficit in the thenar eminence concerns two muscles supplied by a fourth nerve (name it). The two affected muscles of the thenar compartment are supplied by the median nerve. The involvement of fibers distributed through four peripheral nerves makes a peripheral nerve lesion highly improbable.

Localization of neural lesion

A lesion involving sensory and motor nerve fibers, proximal to the level at which the nerves of distribution of the brachial plexus are formed, would explain all the sensory and motor defects in this case.

Using a dermatome chart (Fig. 39-2), state which neural segments are involved on the sensory side. The C8 and TI segments are affected on the sensory side. The opponens pollicis and the abductor pollicis brevis most commonly receive their main motor supply via the median nerve from segments C8 and Tl. These are the same segments that display the sensory defects.

It is most likely that the lesion is located outside the spinal cord distal to the point where sensory and motor fibers combine to form the mixed spinal nerve, as both types of fibers are involved. The lesion actually must be beyond the point of division of the mixed

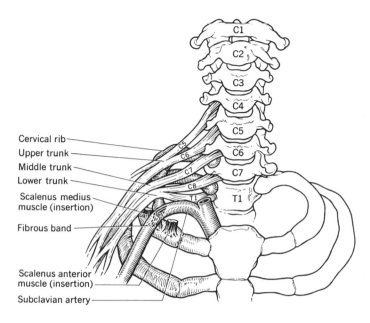

Figure 39-1. The cervical rib on the right side is continued as a fibrous band that attaches to the first rib. The brachial plexus and subclavian artery are elevated, and the lowest trunk of brachial plexus seems particularly taut and stretched by the cervical rib.

spinal nerve into ventral and dorsal rami because there is no sign of neurological deficiency in the dorsal rami of C8 and T1 spinal nerves.

Where in the course of the nerve fibers of spinal nerves C8 and T1 did the lesion most likely occur? The pathological picture as displayed at operation reveals that it is the inferior trunk of the brachial plexus that is exposed to the stretching effect of the accessory rib. All clinical signs also point to the inferior trunk of the brachial plexus as the site of the lesion, which would explain all the subjective and objective neurologic disturbances, including the motor deficits.

Clinical examination shows that in our case the opponens pollicis and the abductor pollicis brevis are particularly involved. How would the action of these muscles be tested? Keep in mind that it is the function of the abductor pollicis brevis to pull the thumb away

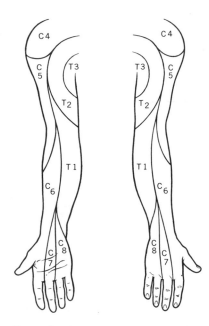

Figure 39-2. Dermatome chart of anterior and posterior aspects of upper extremity (after Foerster). Note particularly the representation of segments C8 and T1 on the medial side of the arm, forearm, and hand.

from the palm in a plane at right angles to the palm. It is the function of the opponens pollicis to advance the thumb across the palm in an arc, rotating it simultaneously, so that at the end of the motion, the palmar surfaces of the thumb and little finger are in opposition to each other. Consequently, these muscles are tested for integrity of function by letting them execute these motions against resistance.

Further clinical study reveals that certainly not all motor fibers coming from C8 and T1 are affected. The muscles of the hypothenar eminence seem to have escaped, a common occurrence in nerve lesions, that is probably explained on the basis of the location of nerve fibers within the trunk.

Why do the symptoms of the patient become noticeable later in life, although the underlying condition is congenital? With progressing age, the tone and strength of the muscles suspending the shoulder decrease, and there is less muscular resistance to the downward pull of the arm. A conservative alternative to the radical surgical removal of the cervical rib includes physical therapy to strengthen the muscles suspending the shoulder, therefore decreasing the stretching of the compressed neurovascular bundle and enlarging the space behind the scalenus anterior (interscalene triangle). Surgical section of the scalenus anterior (scalene myotomy) where it inserts into the scalene tubercle of the first rib has the same effect.

40 Subclavian Steal Syndrome

A 59-year-old postal worker is seen in the outpatient department and later admitted to the hospital. He reports that for the last three years he has experienced transitory periods of dizziness with vertigo, nausea, and occasional fainting spells. These episodes are accompanied by blurring of vision and generally last from only a few seconds to a few minutes. Now, however, they are occurring more often and interfering with his occupation. He also has noticed occasional pain and numbness in the left arm that increase on exercise. In addition, his arm fatigues easily.

EXAMINATION

On examination of this well-nourished, not acutely ill patient, a marked difference in blood pressure between right and left arm is noted. The pressure is 180/95 in the right, 93/70 in the left. The carotid pulsations are normal, but there is diminished pulsation in the left supraclavicular fossa, accompanied by a systolic bruit, that is, an auscultatory murmur. The brachial and radial pulses are diminished on the left compared to the right. On exercise of the left upper extremity, the patient complains of numbness and tingling in the arm, lightheadedness, and vertigo. Radiographic examination of the aortic arch and its branches by injection of a contrast medium via the left brachial artery (retrograde aortography) demonstrates severe narrowing of the left subclavian artery proximal to the origin of its vertebral branch (Fig. 40-1). Cineangiographic studies reveal retrograde flow in the left vertebral artery, with the flow directed toward the subclavian artery.

DIAGNOSIS

The diagnosis is subclavian steal syndrome on the left side, probably due to atherosclerotic plaques in the subclavian artery proximal to the origin of the vertebral artery.

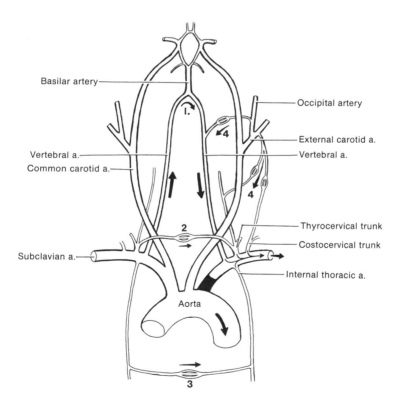

Figure 40-1. Various arterial pathways involved in proximal occlusion of the left subclavian artery. Collateral routes include branches of the two subclavian arteries such as the vertebrals (1), inferior thyroids (2), internal thoracics (3), and branches of the ipsilateral external carotid and subclavian arteries (4) distal to the occlusion.

THERAPY AND FURTHER COURSE

Because spontaneous relief cannot be expected, surgery is proposed. The surgeon's choices are (1) excision of the plaques from the intima of the subclavian artery at the involved site (endarterectomy), (2) replacement of the affected portion of the artery by an artificial patch-graft, or (3) bypass of the pathological area by means of a Teflon graft that will connect the portions of the artery proximal and distal to the stenosis. None of these operations requires intrathoracic or mediastinal approaches, which have been found to be more hazardous to the patient. The third alternative will have the same effect as the other procedures. In addition, it will replace the stenosed arterial portion completely. For this reason, it is chosen for this patient.

The operative findings confirm the preoperative diagnosis. There is almost complete occlusion of the left subclavian artery secondary to atherosclerotic lesions. The lesions are located not far from the origin of the artery from the aorta and extend 1.5 cm along its course. One year after the operation, the patient is asymptomatic with normal blood pressure and pulses in both arms.

DISCUSSION

Since the first reports of subclavian steal in 1960 and 1961, which identified an adaptive effort of the organism that has gone astray, more than 200 cases have been reported. In 80 percent of patients, associated lesions are present in other extracranial vessels. Familiarity with the anatomical course, distribution, and anastomoses of the subclavian and vertebral arteries is necessary for the understanding of the subclavian steal syndrome (Fig. 40-1).

Mechanics of subclavian steal

The term subclavian steal is of recent origin and rather colorful. To stay within the metaphor, what is "stolen" and who is the victim? There is a great decrease in pressure between the prestenotic portion of the left subclavian artery and its distal patent part. Therefore, there is "larceny" of blood from the vertebral artery of the right side. This blood would normally pass into the basilar artery on the inferior surface of the pons. Instead, the "stolen" blood courses down the vertebral artery on the left side in retrograde direction to supply the patent poststenotic portion of the subclavian artery. In functional terms, blood is siphoned from the left vertebral artery, which supplies important areas of the brain, to the distal portion of the right subclavian artery to ensure a supply to the upper extremity. This certainly does not exemplify the so-called "wisdom of the human body" or the saying that "nature always knows best," as deprivation of arterial blood from the brain is of far greater consequence than withdrawal of blood from an upper extremity. In our case, the flow of blood in the left subclavian artery is assured by withdrawing it from the right vertebral artery and its basilar termination inside the skull.

Anatomy of the subclavian artery

The term subclavian artery refers to the artery's location deep to the clavicle. The subclavian artery, one of the most important vessels in the body, supplies blood via its branches to areas as far cranially as the cerebral hemispheres. It also supplies blood as far inferiorly as the anterior portion of the thorax, including the breast and the anterior abdominal wall. Its blood courses as far distally as the fingers and as far medially to structures such as the vertebral column and thyroid gland. Students and physicians alike often think of the artery as being responsible for the blood supply to the upper extremity only.

Subclavian steal resulting from atherosclerotic plaques occurs much more commonly on the left side (more than 70 percent), which can be partially explained by the difference in origin and length of the right and left arteries. What is the difference? The right subclavian artery arises from the brachiocephalic trunk of the aorta behind the right sternoclavicular joint and arches upward and laterally often above the level of the clavicle. By contrast, the left subclavian artery arises considerably lower directly from the arch of the aorta and ascends through the superior mediastinum into the supraclavicular fossa. This difference in origin between the right and left subclavian arteries makes the left 3 to 4 cm longer than the right.

Factors that contribute to the formation of vascular lesions include changing viscosity of the blood, turbulent flow, cardiac thrust, and varying distensibility of blood vessels. Damage from these causes may stimulate fibrin production and the release of lipids that form the typical atherosclerotic lesion.

Anatomy of the vertebral artery

The main function of the vertebral artery, which is the first, largest, and most important branch of the subclavian, is to supply the brain and spinal cord. It has been estimated that the vertebrals supply the brain with about 25 to 30 percent of its arterial blood. After it courses through the transverse foramina of the upper six cervical vertebrae and the dura of the spinal canal, the vertebral artery passes through the foramen magnum to join its counterpart of the opposite side to form the basilar artery. Just before the formation of the basilar artery, it gives off its largest branch, the posterior inferior cerebellar artery; in addition, the vertebral artery sends off the anterior and posterior spinal arteries to the spinal cord.

The vertebral artery, together with the ascending cervical and deep cervical arteries, supplies the vertebrae in the cervical region only. Other arteries that supply the vertebral column as a whole include branches of posterior intercostals, subcostal, lumbars, iliolumbar, and lateral and median sacral arteries.

Arterial anastomoses

Stenosis (narrowing) or occlusion (blockage) of the first part of the subclavian artery results in blood being carried by various alternative pathways. The retrograde flow in the ipsilateral vertebral artery may be supplemented by extracranial anastomoses from the (1) contralateral vertebral artery and (2) ipsilateral occipital artery (Fig. 40-1). Anastomoses also occur between other branches of the ipsilateral external carotid artery and the thyrocervical and costocervical trunks of the subclavian artery. The ipsilateral internal thoracic artery also assists in supplying blood to the poststenotic left subclavian. These occurrences thus diminish the need for surgical interference with the cerebral blood flow. On the other hand, participation of the basilar artery in the arterial circle (circle of Willis) may add to the depletion of cerebral blood supply in this syndrome by withdrawing additional blood from the internal carotids of both sides.

Although not pertinent to this discussion, it is interesting to note that the arteries to the upper and lower extremities (i.e., branches of the subclavian and external iliac arteries) anastomose with each other by way of the superior and inferior epigastric arteries.

Explanation of objective signs and subjective symptoms

How do we explain the patient's objective signs and subjective symptoms in terms of his anatomy and physiology? A number of his disturbances, such as the episodes of fainting, dizziness, vertigo, nausea, and blurred vision, can be explained by ischemia (deprivation of blood due to mechanical obstruction) of the central nervous system (CNS). In our case, the combination of eye symptoms and general signs, such as fainting and vertigo, is due to temporary depletion of blood from the posterior cerebral cortex and the brain stem.

In this discussion, one must keep in mind that the classic distribution of blood vessels in the CNS does not always hold true; variations are fairly common. One variation that would preclude the left vertebral artery as a conduit for additional blood supply to the left arm would be its origin directly from the aorta, which occurs in 5 percent of cases.

How are the findings in the patient's left upper extremity explained? The differences in blood pressure between right and left extremities, the auscultatory phenomena over the left supraclavicular fossa, the decrease in the pulse volume on the left, and the subjective symptoms of tingling and numbness in the left arm are due to the narrowing of the first part of the subclavian artery. The extent of the blood pressure differential between right and left is an indication of the amount of narrowing present. The minimum degree of stenosis necessary to produce symptoms does not appear to be a fixed amount, however. The diagnosis of subclavian steal is confirmed in our patient by the simultaneous appearance of neurological signs of cerebral ischemia and vascular insufficiency of the extremity when the left arm is exercised.

Other steal phenomena

It is not surprising that recognition of the subclavian steal calls attention to similar vascular "thievery" in other locations. Thus, an aortoiliac "steal" was reported in a patient who underwent iliofemoral bypass for the relief of bilateral common iliac artery occlusion, but who also had atherosclerotic narrowing of the mesenteric arteries. The surgical intervention that shunted blood from the aorta and its mesenteric branches to the femoral arteries of the legs led to ischemia of the intestine and subsequent fatal necrosis of the bowel.

Steal phenomena have also been reported in other major vessels, such as the carotid, pulmonary, and coronary arteries. In the coronary circulation, vasodilating drugs can undesirably siphon arterial blood from the atherosclerotically narrowed vessels of the ischemic myocardium to portions of the heart with a normal blood supply, leading to maldistribution of coronary blood and causing angina pectoris with concomitant changes in the electrocardiograph.

Although redistribution of blood flow by way of anastomoses is a common adaptive phenomenon in the body, the last mentioned cases demonstrate that some of these adjustments can be harmful to the organism and illustrate cases in which the physician, to repeat the bioforensic jargon of the title, has become an "accomplice to the crime" of the steal phenomenon.

41   Embolism of the Brachial Artery

The patient, aged 51 years, is admitted to the hospital for generalized arteriosclerosis, lesions of the aortic valves, and cardiac failure. During his stay in the hospital, he suddenly complains of sharp pain and partial paralysis of the right forearm of about an hour's duration.

EXAMINATION

On examination the forearm is cold and pale, with the hand and fingers drawn up in a contracted position. There is loss of movement and sensation below the elbow. Radial and ulnar pulsations are absent.

DIAGNOSIS

Embolism of the brachial artery, that is, occlusion of the artery by a blood clot originating elsewhere in the bloodstream, is diagnosed.

THERAPY AND FURTHER COURSE

The patient is taken to surgery, where a long incision is made over the brachial artery in the groove along the medial aspect of the distal part of the biceps brachii muscle. The median nerve is dissected free and retracted out of the way. The incision is extended into the cubital fossa, and the bicipital aponeurosis (lacertus fibrosus) is cut, exposing the bifurcation of the brachial artery.

On exposing the brachial artery, the clot within the vessel is easily seen. The clot completely fills the brachial artery and extends about an inch into both the radial and ulnar arteries. The entire brachial artery is occluded as well as the deep brachial and all of the collateral branches, including the radial and ulnar collateral and recurrent vessels. Tourniquets are placed above and below the embolus. A small incision 1-inch-long is made into the brachial artery just above its bifurcation, and the extensions of the clot into the radial and ulnar arteries are removed with forceps. The remainder of the clot in the brachial artery is removed by a combination of suction and milking. A small, soft rubber catheter is introduced into the artery as a means of suction, and the milking action is carried out manually. The small arterial incision is then closed with sutures. The clot at operation measures 8 inches long and completely occludes the collateral arterial vessels. Amputation would certainly have been required if the patient had not undergone surgery.

Immediately postoperatively, the radial pulse at the wrist is easily felt. Motor power and sensation in the forearm and hand gradually return to normal, and four days later the patient is seen using his right hand to feed himself. He is discharged from the hospital.

Anticoagulants were administered.

DISCUSSION

The diagnosis of occlusion of the brachial artery by a blood clot originating elsewhere in the bloodstream was based on the appearance of sudden sharp pain, the loss of motor power and sensory function, the coolness and paleness of the extremity, and the absence of pulsations. All this took place in a man suffering from chronic heart and aortic disease, which is conducive to the formation of thrombi in the heart and aorta. The signs listed are typical of arterial embolism, that is, the spread of a blood clot, which in this case was formed in a diseased heart or aorta. Give the course of such a clot from the left ventricle to the right brachial artery. The clot traveled from the left ventricle to the ascending aorta, where, at the beginning of the aortic arch, it passed into the brachiocephalic trunk, from there into the right subclavian and axillary arteries, and then into the brachial artery, where it was arrested.

Location of pulse in ulnar and radial arteries

Both ulnar and radial pulsations were absent. Where would one try to find the pulse of either artery? Remember, the pulse is best felt in areas where the artery is superficial and resting on a firm structure such as a bone or a ligament. This is the case for both arteries at the wrist, where the ulnar artery lies superficial to the flexor retinaculum on the radial side of the pisiform bone and ulnar nerve. The pulse of the radial artery is felt on the lateral side of the wrist a little more proximally, lateral to the tendon of the flexor carpi radialis.

What is the cause of the partial motor paralysis and the loss of sensation? Remember that nerves and muscles can function only in the presence of sufficient blood supply, which was interrupted in our case by the arterial embolus (clot).

Surgically important relations of the brachial artery

During surgery the median nerve had to be identified and retracted. What is its changing relationship to the brachial artery? The median nerve in the arm usually crosses in front of, rarely behind, the brachial artery from lateral above to medial below. In the cubital fossa the median nerve is medial to the brachial artery (Fig. 41-1). Beginners often mistake the basilic vein and the medial cutaneous nerve of the forearm for the brachial artery and the median nerve. What separates the brachial artery from the basilic vein in the lower part of the arm? The deep brachial fascia and the bicipital aponeurosis separate the brachial artery from the more superficially located vein (Fig. 41-1). Remember also, the brachial artery usually is accompanied by two veins (venae comitantes).

What is the surgical landmark for the level of the bifurcation of the brachial artery? The neck of the radius is generally given as the usual level, but the bifurcation may be located more proximally.

Collateral circulation in blockage of the brachial artery

At surgery, the size of the clot was surprisingly large. It not only occluded the brachial artery but also its most important branches,

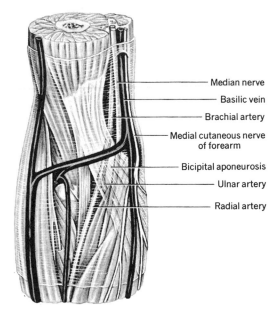

Median nerve

Basilic vein

Brachial artery

Medial cutaneous nerve
of forearm

Bicipital aponeurosis

Ulnar artery

Radial artery

Figure 41-1. Structures along the medial aspect of the cubital fossa.

the deep brachial and the two terminal branches, the radial and
ulnar arteries. The collateral branches around the elbow were likewise occluded. Undoubtedly, the large extent of the clot was due to
secondary thrombosis above and below the embolus. There was,
therefore, in this case no chance for the development of a collateral
circulation, but in milder cases the limb may survive without specific treatment because of the anastomosing channels around the site
of the obstruction. In case of nonintervention, survival of the limb
depends on the presence of anastomosing channels that bypass the
site of blockage to transport blood around the occlusion. What are
the anastomosing channels if the block in the brachial artery is above
the origin of the deep brachial artery? This is a most unfavorable
site, and the circulation relies essentially on the anastomosis between the descending branch of the posterior humeral circumflex
artery from the axillary artery and an ascending branch of the deep
brachial artery.

A block below the origin of the deep brachial artery is more
favorable. Here numerous anastomosing vessels are available both

above and below the block to reestablish the circulation. It is probably not necessary to familiarize oneself with the names of all these vessels if one realizes that the deep brachial divides into anterior and posterior descending branches and the brachial artery itself sends the superior and inferior ulnar collateral arteries distally. These descending vessels, which have "collateral" in their name, anastomose with "recurrent" branches from the radial, ulnar, and posterior interosseous artery in front of and behind the elbow. Cross-anastomoses from the radial to the ulnar side likewise exist. In addition, many unnamed vascular channels are available, particularly those present in the musculature.

As stated before, in this case the blockage was so extensive that a collateral circulation could not be established. Without the operation, it would have been necessary to amputate the limb.

REFERENCE

Duncan, R. D., and Myers, M. E. Peripheral arterial embolism. Brachial embolism successfully treated. *Am J Surg* 62:34, 1943.

42   **Peripheral Venous Access**

A 42-year-old homemaker arrives at the hospital with a history of heart disease following repeated attacks of rheumatic fever. At present the patient complains of cough, severe shortness of breath, and swelling of her legs.

EXAMINATION

On examination the patient appears to be in acute distress from shortness of breath. The heart is considerably enlarged, there is fluid in the pleural cavity, and the liver is increased in size. There is marked edema of the legs, particularly in the region of the ankles. The radiograph shows signs of pulmonary congestion with fluid in the pleural cavity.

DIAGNOSIS

The diagnosis is heart failure resulting from a rheumatic heart lesion.

THERAPY AND FURTHER COURSE

The patient is immediately given sedatives, cardiac medication, and diuretics. For the first few days of treatment, the intravenous route (i.v.) is chosen to accelerate the diuretic effect. The first three injections into the cubital veins are painless and well tolerated, but on the fourth injection the patient complains immediately of burning pain at the site of injection in a vein in the lateral portion of the cubital fossa. The pain increases during the day and radiates over the palmar aspect of the forearm. In the evening, the patient complains of numbness and prickling over the radial aspect of the forearm, and i.v. medication is continued in the other arm.

Under prescribed treatment the patient improves gradually and is discharged for ambulatory treatment. The numbness over the lateral part of the forearm persisted, however, and palpation of the cubital fossa showed an indurated area at the previous site of the painful injection. There is no muscular atrophy and motion of the forearm and hand is normal, but for all modalities there is complete loss of sensation over most of the area of the lateral antebrachial cutaneous nerve.

DISCUSSION

What is the rationale for i.v. medication? The i.v. route is chosen when a rapid effect is needed, and application directly into the bloodstream appears indicated. What is the favorite site for i.v. injections, and why is this location chosen?

Applied anatomy of the cubital and antebrachial veins

The median cubital vein is most frequently used for venipuncture taking of a blood sample, i.v. injection of drugs, and blood transfusions because the vein is large, superficially located, and therefore easily seen and felt. It is also unaccompanied by nerves and arteries. Which two superficial veins does the median cubital vein connect? In the most common type of arrangement, the cephalic and basilic veins on the lateral and medial sides of the forearm are joined by the median cubital vein, which crosses the roof of the cubital fossa in a medially ascending direction (Fig. 42-1). The vein that is present in about three fourths of all cases terminates in the basilic vein by ascending along the medial margin of the biceps brachii muscle.

Do other superficial veins likewise connect with the median cubital vein? It frequently also receives blood from the median antebrachial vein, which ascends on the palmar aspect of the forearm about halfway between the cephalic and basilic veins. Quite fre-

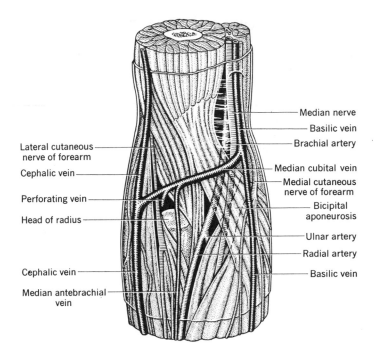

Median nerve
Basilic vein
Brachial artery
Median cubital vein
Medial cutaneous nerve of forearm
Bicipital aponeurosis
Ulnar artery
Radial artery
Basilic vein

Lateral cutaneous nerve of forearm
Cephalic vein
Perforating vein
Head of radius
Cephalic vein
Median antebrachial vein

Figure 42-1. Superficial veins of the elbow and forearm accompanied mostly by cutaneous nerves. Note the relationship of the basilic vein to the median nerve and brachial artery. Notice that the median cubital vein is unaccompanied by nerves. Notice also, its deep connection by a perforating vein.

quently, the median antebrachial vein bifurcates at the elbow into two veins, with one of these joining the cephalic vein and the other the basilic (Fig. 42-2). Thus, an M-shaped arrangement results. The two central limbs of the M are then frequently spoken of as the median cephalic and median basilic veins, the latter corresponding to the previously mentioned median cubital vein. Does this vein drain exclusively into the cephalic and basilic veins? There exists in addition a communication with the deep veins of the forearm which passes through an opening in the deep fascia (Fig. 42-1).

How is the state of distention of the superficial veins increased for the purpose of venipuncture? The following means are customarily employed: (1) keeping the arm in a dependent position for some time to slow the venous return, (2) compressing the veins by a tourniquet 1.5 to 2 inches above the site of the puncture, (3) applying heat by means of hot, moist towels or by immersing the hand and forearm into a basin of hot water, and (4) alternating opening and closing the hand. What is the effect of the last procedure, and what is the result if the tourniquet is applied too tightly? Muscular activity will increase the amount of arterial blood flow to the distal portion of the extremity. It is also possible that the opening and closing the hand will enhance the blood flow from the deep to the superficial veins by means of the perforating veins. On the other hand, maximum tightening of the tourniquet may obstruct the arterial flow to the forearm.

Thrombosis formation with occlusion of the injected vein is a possible consequence of i.v. injection. This obliteration of the vein may be asymptomatic, or it may transform the vein through the

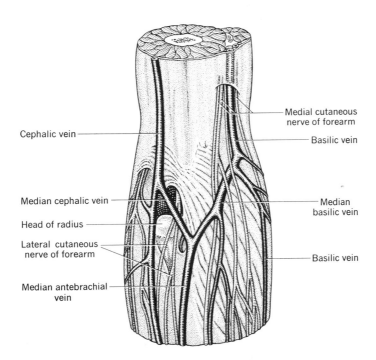

Figure 42-2. The M-shaped arrangement of cubital veins.

accompanying inflammatory process into a knotty cord, which may remain painful and tender for many months. Obliteration of the vein can be caused by the simple trauma of venipuncture or, more frequently, as a direct result of the irritating effect of the injected drug. It then becomes necessary, as in our case, to inject other veins in the cubital region or in the forearm. The cephalic, basilic, and median antebrachial veins are available. What are the risks of using any of these veins? Unlike the median cubital vein, these veins are accompanied by cutaneous nerves that may be injured (Fig. 42-1).

Nerve injuries by intravenous injection

In case of leakage of the injected drug from the vein after withdrawal of the needle or through faulty extravenous injection of part of the drug, some nerves may be damaged. Identify them. They are the lateral antebrachial cutaneous nerve, whose branches course with the cephalic and median antebrachial veins, and the medial antebrachial cutaneous nerve, which accompanies the basilic vein. What is the origin of these two nerves, and what cutaneous area do they supply? The lateral antebrachial cutaneous nerve is the terminal cutaneous branch of the musculocutaneous nerve. It pierces the deep fascia lateral to the biceps tendon above the elbow joint and divides into anterior and posterior branches to supply the front and back of the radial side of the forearm. It may also supply a variable area of skin on the dorsum of the hand. By contrast, the medial antebrachial cutaneous nerve is a direct branch of the medial cord of the brachial plexus. It pierces the deep fascia medial to the biceps at the middle of the arm and, dividing into anterior and ulnar branches, supplies the skin on the front and back of the ulnar side of the forearm. What nerve was involved in our case? The injection injured the anterior branch of the lateral antebrachial cutaneous nerve.

What precautions should be taken to prevent extravenous injection of medication? The gauge of the needle should be as small as possible, the needle should be sharp, the skin over the site of the injection tightened, and the piston of the syringe withdrawn and blood aspirated to verify the location of the needle in the vein. Finally, the injection should be done slowly to prevent leakage during injection and after withdrawal of the needle. Which is the important motor nerve that is exposed to damage by i.v. injection in this area (Fig. 42-1)? Injury to the median nerve, often in combination with impairment of the medial antebrachial cutaneous nerve, has been described. The result is severe loss of motor function in the muscles supplied by the median nerve and sensory deficits in the territory of the median and medial antebrachial cutaneous nerves. For this reason, it is recommended not to give any injections in the basilic vein above the bend of the elbow.

Inadvertent intra-arterial injection

Another complication, likewise quite serious, is accidental intra-arterial injection. What artery may be involved, and what separates this artery from the basilic vein (Fig. 42-1)? Realizing that only the deep fascia and the bicipital aponeurosis separate the basilic vein from the brachial artery enables one to understand that such accidents occur not too infrequently. What is a clue that the needle is in the brachial artery instead of in a vein? The aspirated blood would be bright red, not dark red. In the case of irritating drugs, the clinical picture of arterial or para-arterial injection is ushered in by the occurrence of severe burning pain in the hand and forearm, followed by dead-white blanching of the hand and distal portions of the forearm and disappearance of the radial and ulnar pulses. The outcome may be gangrene of the fingers and distal portions of the forearm, necessitating amputation. The underlying pathology is thrombosis of the brachial artery or of one or both of its terminal branches, combined with distal arterial and arteriolar spasm. Explain the immediate maximal arterial constriction noted in these cases. This constriction is due to intense spasm of the smooth muscle of the arterial wall as a result of the irritation and injury to the vessel. Blockage of the vasa vasorum (tiny blood vessels that supply to walls of larger vessels) by the contraction of their muscular walls may contribute to the damage of the intima, enhancing the vascular thrombosis.

Can you name one arterial anomaly that would make intra-arterial injection more likely to occur? A superficial ulnar artery may arise from the brachial artery high in the arm to course down the forearm superficial to the palmar muscles and either superficial or deep to the deep fascia. It occurs in about 3 to 6 percent of all cases and is apt to be mistaken for a vein for purposes of injection or may be injured accidentally when the accompanying basilic vein is injected. As a safeguard against accidental arterial injection, palpation for arterial pulsation of any vessel intended for injection should be made.

Venous embolism

Contrary to expectation, dislodgement of a blood clot (embolism) from a vein that has been thrombosed by frequent injection takes place only exceptionally. Explain this fact. The thrombi in the damaged vein are so firmly anchored by the concomitant inflammation that displacement via the venous bloodstream is very rare.

On the other hand, inadvertent introduction of an air embolus into the venous circulation during i.v. injections and transfusions is a recognized danger of which one must be aware. In taking blood from donors, collection bottles may develop positive air pressure, creating conditions for air embolism with resulting serious cardiac and pulmonary complications. Review the pathway of such an air embolus from the median cubital vein to the pulmonary artery. It would go by way of the median cubital into the basilic, the axillary, the subclavian, the brachiocephalic, the superior vena cava, the right atrium and right ventricle, and into the pulmonary artery. In what veins would the danger of air embolism be greatest? The large veins of the neck and the axillary area are predisposed to air embolism by puncture due to the negative pressure in their lumina and fascial attachments to their walls that prevent them from collapsing when opened.

Other veins used for intravenous injection

Name other superficial veins that are suitable for puncture and injection in case the cubital veins and veins of the forearm are too small or are obliterated after frequent injections. Difficulties in the selection of an adequate vein arise particularly in small infants if large quantities of fluid, plasma, or blood have to be given. The following veins can be used: metacarpal and metatarsal veins and the veins of the dorsal venous arch of the hand and foot, the greater saphenous vein in the ankle, the greater and lesser saphenous veins in the leg, the femoral (strictly speaking, not considered a superficial vein) and greater saphenous veins in the thigh, the veins of the scalp, and the external jugular vein. In rare cases, in the infant, the dural venous sinuses of the skull have been used by puncturing them through the open fontanelles. If the femoral and greater saphenous veins in the thigh and the latter vein in the ankle are used for transfusions, particularly in infants, they are dissected out under local anesthesia in a "cut-down" procedure, and a catheter may be passed into them. What is the relation of the greater saphenous vein to the medial malleolus of the ankle and the medial condyle of the tibia? It runs in front of the medial malleolus, where it can easily be seen and felt but posterior to the medial condyle of the tibia.

43

Tendon Sheath and Thenar Space Infections

Ten days before coming to the hospital, the patient cut his right index finger just above the metacarpophalangeal joint on a tin can. The wound became infected and the patient consulted a physician, who opened the wound and passed a drainage tube through and across the dorsum coming out between index and middle finger on the dorsum of the hand.

EXAMINATION

On examination, the index finger is swollen, as is the entire hand, particularly the dorsum. Several openings appear about the proximal phalanx of the index finger. On probing one of these openings, it is found to communicate with the metacarpophalangeal joint of the index finger. The entire finger and hand are slightly tender, but marked and conspicuous tenderness is elicited over the fibrous flexor tendon sheath of the index finger and sharply circumscribed over it, most acute at its proximal end over the metacarpophalangeal articulation. Flexion of the index finger does not increase the pain, but extension causes marked pain throughout the finger. The pain is most sharply noted by the patient at the proximal end of the tendon sheath. Extension of other fingers causes little increase in pain. There is no particular pain on the dorsum of the index finger where the cuts are found. Axillary lymph nodes on the injured side are markedly swollen. The patient has a temperature of 101° F and acceleration of the pulse.

Although the swelling is most noticeable over the dorsum of the hand, it should be realized as an important principle of all hand infections that the site of greatest swelling does not necessarily indicate the location of pus collection.

DIAGNOSIS

Infected wound of the index finger, synovial tendon sheath the infection of index finger, with involvement of metacarpophalangeal joint, and lymph vessel and lymph node infection are diagnosed.

THERAPY AND FURTHER COURSE

The synovial flexor tendon sheath over the index finger is opened from end to end and pus evacuated. The dorsal openings are also enlarged. Hot dressings are applied. The temperature continues to run between 99° and 101° F. Ten days later there is marked ballooning in the thenar area with tenderness localized in this area. The patient undergoes reoperation, and the thenar space is drained from the dorsum. A drainage tube from the space to the dorsum is inserted. The infection (osteomyelitis) continues and leads to destruction of the metacarpophalangeal joint and the proximal phalanx of the index finger. A month later, after amputation of the index finger, including the head of the second metacarpal, the patient improves rapidly and is discharged from the hospital. He has good function of the thumb and remaining fingers.

DISCUSSION

We are dealing here with a progressive infection of the hand that started from a minor injury but led to a serious infection of the synovial flexor tendon sheath of the index finger with involvement of the bones and the metacarpophalangeal joint of that finger and secondary spread to the thenar space. Another complication was the lymph vessel and lymph node infection that accompanied the local spread. Application of antibiotics may have mitigated the progressive course of this infection, although surgical intervention is usually necessary to stop the spread of the infection.

Infection of synovial flexor tendon sheath

The marked and conspicuous tenderness over the tendon sheath of
the index finger establishes the diagnosis of tendon sheath infection.
What tendons are located in this tendon sheath? The tendons to the
index finger from the flexor digitorum superficialis and flexor
digitorum profundus are within this tendon sheath. Where does this
tendon sheath end proximally and where distally? The sheath ends
proximally at the neck of the second metacarpal and distally at the
base of the distal phalanx (Fig. 43-1). Why is extension of the involved finger so painful compared with flexion? It puts the involved
tendons and their sheath on the stretch.

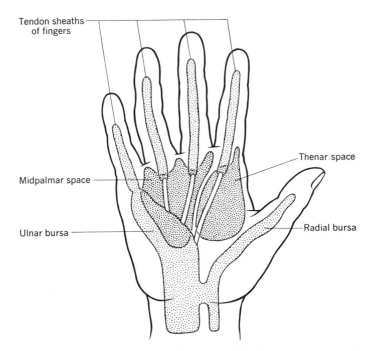

Figure 43-1. Radial and ulnar bursae and the flexor tendon sheaths of the
second, third, and fourth fingers as well as the deep spaces in the palm of
the hand. Notice how infection of the tendon sheath of the index finger
could easily involve the thenar space.

Infection of thenar space

The ballooning of the thenar region with tenderness over it is a typical sign of thenar space infection. Spread of infection from the proximal end of the synovial tendon sheaths of the fingers to the deep spaces in the palm of the hand is quite common because the digital flexor synovial tendon sheaths of the second, third, and fourth fingers begin at the level where the deep spaces end (Fig. 43-1). Where is this level? It is approximately at the level of the distal palmar crease.

Which deep spaces in the palm of the hand frequently harbor and confine infections? The midpalmar space medially and the thenar space laterally are the spaces that lie deep to the flexor tendons in the palm. They are sometimes also called the medial and lateral deep palmar spaces. Infection of which synovial tendon sheath will most commonly lead to involvement of the thenar space, as in this case? Infection of the tendon sheath of the index finger may rupture into the thenar space. Infection of the synovial tendon sheath of the flexor pollicis longus (the radial bursa) may likewise perforate into the thenar space. The reverse may happen with a primary infection of the thenar space breaking into the radial bursa (Fig. 43-1). What are the superficial, deep, lateral, and medial boundaries of the thenar space? The thenar space is bound superficially by the tendons of the index and sometimes also of the middle finger; its deep boundary is the fascia over the adductor pollicis; its lateral boundary is the radial bursa; and medially it is separated from the midpalmar space by a fibrous septum that attaches dorsally to the third metacarpal (Fig. 43-2). What structure would an infection of the thenar space have to penetrate to spread to the midpalmar space? It would have to rupture through the previously mentioned septum between the two deep spaces.

Lymph drainage of the upper extremity

The edema of the dorsum present early in this case is due to infection of the lymphatic vessels. What course do the lymphatic vessels from the fingers and palm take? Lymph vessels from the palmar and dorsal aspects of the digits drain into the plexus on the dorsum of the hand. From here and from a lymph plexus in the palm of the hand,

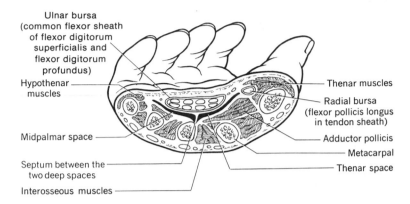

Ulnar bursa
(common flexor sheath
of flexor digitorum
superficialis and
flexor digitorum
profundus)
Hypothenar
muscles

Thenar muscles

Radial bursa
(flexor pollicis longus
in tendon sheath)

Midpalmar space

Adductor pollicis

Metacarpal

Septum between the
two deep spaces

Thenar space

Interosseous muscles

Figure 43-2. Cross section through the palm of the hand showing the deep spaces and the septum between them. Notice the superficial, deep, medial, and lateral boundaries of the thenar space. Also notice how infection from the radial bursa could spread to the thenar space and vice versa.

collecting vessels run superficially on the anterior aspect of the forearm.

What is the anatomical reason that the edema accompanying the infection of the lymphatic vessels is more noticeable on the dorsum than in the palm? Remember, the subcutaneous connective tissue over the dorsum is much looser and not confined by a dense aponeurosis as in the palm. What indication is there of progressive lymph vessel infection? Where are the main lymph nodes draining the hand located? The marked swelling of the axillary lymph nodes indicates spread of the infection via lymphatic vessels to the main collecting station for the lymph of the upper extremity.

Are there any lymph nodes interposed between the hand and the axillary nodes? The cubital (supratrochlear) nodes along the medial side of the biceps brachii three finger breadths above the cubital fossa act as an intermediate drainage station for lymph coming from the medial three fingers and the medial side of the hand and forearm; they drain into the axillary nodes. Of the five groups of axillary nodes, lateral, pectoral, subscapular, central, and apical groups, which is the primary recipient of lymph from the upper extremity? The lateral group located medial and posterior to the axillary vein receives most of the lymph from the upper limb and drains into the central and apical nodes. A few lymph vessels follow the course of the cephalic vein and drain into deltopectoral nodes in the triangle of the same name and from there into the apical nodes.

REFERENCE

Kanavel, A. B. *Infections of the Hand*, 6th ed. Philadelphia: Lea and Febiger, 1933.

44   Carpal Tunnel Syndrome

A 55-year-old seamstress consults her physician, complaining of tingling and burning pain over the palmar aspect of her thumb, index, middle, and lateral side of ring finger of her right hand. The symptoms began gradually over the last two years and lately have become more intense. They are most marked during the night, keeping her awake. She complains that in getting up in the morning her fingers feel puffy and stiff, but her symptoms gradually subside during the morning. If she overworks, particularly if she does heavy ironing, the pain and discomfort increase again. Recently, she has experienced difficulties in holding tableware, resulting in frequent breakage. Also she can hardly keep her grasp on a sewing needle. At the same time, she notices that the movements of her right thumb are not as strong as before. This change is accompanied by some wasting in the outer half of the ball (thenar eminence) of this thumb. For the last few weeks, she also complains of occasional burning in the corresponding area of thumb and fingers of her left hand.

EXAMINATION

On inspection of her right hand, flattening of the outer half of the thenar eminence is noticed. On testing, their is loss of power and limitation of range of motion on abduction and opposition of the thumb. Diminished sensibility (hypesthesia and hypalgesia) over the palmar aspect of the thumb, index, middle, and lateral aspect of the ring finger on the right hand is demonstrated by impaired appreciation of light touch and pin pricks and decreased differentiation between sharp and blunt stimuli. Sensation over the lateral aspect of the palm, including the thenar eminence, is unaffected. Pressure and tapping over the lateral portion of the flexor retinacuum cause tingling and a sensation of "pins and needles" in the involved fingers. On study of the motor functions of the muscles of the right forearm and fingers, no interference with active motion of the elbow, wrist, and fingers (except for the described deficiencies in the motion of the thumb) is noted, but extreme flexion and extension of the wrist reproduce the typical pain in the lateral 3½ digits of her hand.

DIAGNOSIS

Carpal tunnel syndrome is diagnosed.

THERAPY AND FURTHER COURSE

Conservative treatment with immobilization of the wrist during the night by splinting and physical therapy with heat, massage, and mild exercises are tried for several weeks but have no effect. Anti-inflammatory treatment with hydrocortisone injections also does not lead to any improvement. Thus, surgical treatment consisting of division of the flexor retinaculum is agreed on. With the patient under local anesthesia and a tourniquet around the upper arm to obtain a bloodless surgical field, the flexor retinaculum is divided with attention to and avoidance of the superficial palmar vascular arch and the motor or recurrent branch of the median nerve. At operation the synovial sheath of the flexor tendons beneath the flexor retinaculum appears swollen with the median nerve somewhat flattened and compressed in the narrowest part of the carpal tunnel. This decompression operation results in a dramatic disappearance of her pain and other subjective symptoms and gradual cessation of the deficiencies in the next few months. Motor recovery also occurs, although somewhat later. Because the patient is right-handed and can now use her dominant hand without hindrance, the symptoms on the left side also gradually subside.

DISCUSSION

Sensory deficiencies

This patient offers the subjective of symptoms of paresthesias (tingling and numbness) and pain in the lateral 3½ digits of her right hand as well as the objective signs of sensory loss, including loss of pain perception on stimulation over approximately the same cutaneous area. How do you explain the apparently contradictory finding of spontaneous pain and interference with pain perception in approximately the same area? The former is an irritative phenomenon caused by stimulation of certain sensory nerve fibers; the latter is an indication of destruction and loss of function of certain other sensory fibers. This combination is frequent in neurological disorders. In carpal tunnel syndrome, the larger, myelinated fibers that supply voluntary muscle and those that carry tactile discrimination impulses are more affected than the smaller, unmyelinated fibers that transmit pain.

Motor deficits

There is a loss of motor function of the abductor pollicis brevis and opponens pollicis combined with wasting at the site of these two muscles in the lateral part of the ball of the right thumb. What is the function of the abductor pollicis brevis and opponens pollicis, and how are their actions tested? Because it is the function of the abductor pollicis brevis to pull the thumb away from the palm in a plane at right angles to it, ask the patient to point the thumb toward the ceiling against resistance, seeing to it that the forearm is supine and the dorsum of the hand resting on a table. The opponens pollicis pulls the thumb across the hand in an arch, rotating it at the same time so that at the end of the motion the palmar surface of the thumb and little finger are in opposition to each other. Testing is done accordingly by letting the patient execute this motion against the resistance of your outstretched finger.

Location of the site of the lesion

Where, then, is the site of the lesion that causes the combined sensory and motor deficits? We can exclude systemic diseases of the central nervous system, such as multiple sclerosis, which cause more widespread impairments than are present in our case. We can likewise rule out involvement of a spinal nerve before its division into ventral and dorsal rami at the site of the intervertebral foramen, as there is no indication of sensory or motor deficiencies on the posterior aspect of the trunk supplied by dorsal rami. By contrast, it might be tempting in our case to place the lesion in one or more ventral rami in the neck, where they form the roots and trunks of the brachial plexus. Until the late 1940s this was assumed to be the most common site of deficits of this nature. What roots or trunks of the brachial plexus would have to be involved? A dermatome chart would place the sensory deficiencies in the ventral rami of C6 and C7, which form part of the upper and all of the middle trunk of the brachial plexus. On the other hand, the weight of neurological evidence indicates that the muscles affected in our case, the abductor pollicis brevis and opponens pollicis, receive their motor supply from segments C8 and TI by way of the median nerve. It would have to be a widespread lesion involving practically all the roots of the brachial plexus from C6 to TI to accommodate all the deficits in this case. In view of the limited extent of the neurological defect, this seems very unlikely. Consequently, we must assume that the lesion is more peripheral than the brachail plexus.

Is there a peripheral nerve in the upper extremity that supplies the two affected muscles and the skin of the lateral 3½ digits on their palmar aspect? The median nerve innervates the abductor pollicis brevis and opponens pollicis as well as the involved skin.

Level of median nerve involvement

At what level would the median nerve have to be interrupted to cause the defects present in this case? In other words, where can we pinpoint the lesion that causes the described impairments but leaves the other important motor and sensory functions of the median nerve intact?

Does the median nerve supply any mucles in the arm or forearm? Although it does not innervate any muscles in the arm, it supplies the flexors and pronators of the forearm, the flexors of the wrist (with the exception of the carpi ulnaris), and the long flexors of the fingers (with the exception of the medial half of the flexor digitorum profundus). Because the muscles of the forearm supplied by the median nerve display normal function in our patient, the lesion must be located distal to the origin of the branches to these muscles but proximal to the origin of the motor nerve to the opponens pollicis and the abductor pollicis brevis. Where in this branch given off? It is often called the recurrent branch of the medial nerve and leaves the lateral side of the median nerve as the latter emerges distally from beneath the flexor retinaculum (Fig. 44-1). It runs superficial to or through the substance of the flexor pollicis brevis to supply the two muscles of the thumb involved in our case. The same nerve also supplies the superficial portion of the flexor pollicis brevis, but loss of function of the flexor pollicis brevis cannot be demonstrated by ordinary clinical testing. This also holds true for the lateral two lumbrical muscles, which likewise receive their nerve supply from the terminal portion of the median nerve but via the otherwise sensory first two common palmar digital branches.

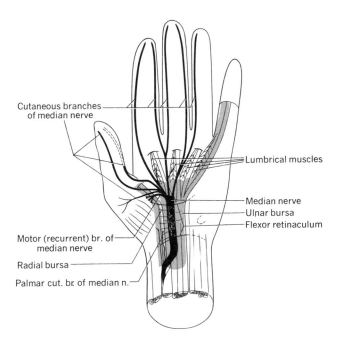

Figure 44-1. Median nerve in carpal tunnel and its distribution in the palm of the hand.

The action of other muscles, such as the interossei, which are supplied by the ulnar nerve, obscures the deficiency of the lumbrical muscles. By contrast, clinical experience proves that the abducting action of the abductor pollicis longus, innervated by the radial nerve, is not usually stong enough to compensate for the paralyzed abductor pollicis brevis.

Can we derive similar localizing indications from the sensory deficiencies in our case history? We notice that sensation over the lateral aspect of the palm and the thenar eminence is unaffected. What cutaneous nerve supplies this area, and where is it given off the median nerve? The palmar cutaneous branch arises from the median nerve just proximal to the upper margin of the flexor retinaculum and supplies the uninvolved skin of palm and thenar eminence (Fig. 44-1). By contrast, the terminal sensory branches of the median nerve supply the skin of the lateral $3\frac{1}{2}$ digits that display the sensory loss. Therefore, we can pinpoint the lesion in that portion of the median nerve located distal to the origin of the unaffected palmar cutaneous branch but above its terminal division into the three common palmar digital branches.

One final question in regard to localization of the level of the lesion within the median nerve must be answered. Why is it that our deficiency cannot be caused by a circumscribed injury to the median nerve more proximally in the arm or forearm? One might assume that such a lesion could affect just component of the nerve that farther distally forms the terminal portion of the nerve involved in our case. This hypothesis presupposes that the fascicles or nerve fibers, which are seen on cross section of the median and other peripheral nerves, correspond to the branches of the main nerve that are given off farther distally and that such fascicles remain intact in their composition within the main nerve trunk throughout its course. This simple "cable" theory has been disproved. It has been shown that within the nerve the identity of a given sensory or motor branch is preserved for only a few centimeters proximal to the origin of the branch from the main stem. Through the intermediation of intraneural plexuses, the various fascicles that make up the main nerve change their composition continuously by divisions and anastomoses; so the aggregations of nerve fibers composing a given branch are distributed over various fascicles a few centimeters proximal to the point where the branch emerges from the main stem. Thus, it is impossible to identify the sensory and motor nerve fibers that supply the lateral 3½ digits and the two muscles of the thumb in a circumscribed cross-sectional area of the median nerve in the arm or proximal forearm. They are dispersed throughout the cross section of the median nerve so that a lesion at any higher level could not imitate a peripheral injury to a branch of this nerve.

In summarizing this discussion on the localization of the defect within the median nerve, we must place it in the nerve where it runs through the carpal tunnel. This common site for median nerve involvement has been known to clinicians since the early 1950s as the carpal tunnel syndrome. What is the carpal tunnel?

Definition and contents of the carpal tunnel

The carpal tunnel is a fibro-osseous canal the trough of which is formed by the palmar concavity of the carpal bones; its roof consists of the flexor retinaculum, a rigid, inelastic ligament. What are the attachments of the flexor retinaculum? The latter extends from the scaphoid and trapezium on the latral side to the pisiform and hook of the hamate on the medial side. How would you relate the retinaculum to the skin creases in the hand? The distal of the two creases on the palmar of the wrist marks the proximal margin of the flexor retinaculum. The retinaculum is 2 to 3 cm long and nearly as wide. A rectangular postage stamp of this size, laid with its narrower edge on the distal crease, would outline the area occupied by the retinacuum.

What are the contents of the carpal tunnel or canal? They are the tendon of the flexor pollicis longus in its synovial sheath (also called the radial bursa), the tendons of the flexor digitorum superficialis and the flexor digitorum profundus in their common synovial sheath (the so-called ulnar bursa), and the median nerve (Figs. 44-1 and 44-2). The latter, with which we are concerned in this case history, lies lateral to the two superficial tendons of the flexor digitorum superficialis against the deep surface of the flexor retinaculum. Does the median nerve supply the muscles listed as contents of the carpal canal with motor fibers within the carpal tunnel? It does not, as the motor nerve supply to a muscle must reach the muscle in its contractile portion, not as its tendon or tendons. The muscle bellies of the indicated muscles are located higher up in the forearm.

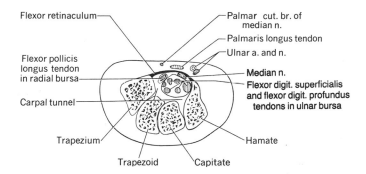

Figure 44-2. Proximal view of the left carpal tunnel showing students in the tunnel and those superficial to the flexor retinaculum.

Reasons for compression of median nerve

The carpel tunnel, being occupied by the structures listed and covered by a rigid ligament, appears crowded as it is. Thus, it is not surprising that any space-occupying alteration within the canal, such as a chronic thickening of the synovial sheath of the common flexor tendons, leads to compression of the median nerve. This would explain the clinical signs and symptoms of irritation and impairment of the median nerve described in our case. The thickening of the synovial sac of the common flexor tendon sheath, a tenosynovitis, is probably caused in this patient by occupational strain and overexertion. It is not surprising that the symptoms are aggravated by motions that increase the pressure within the tunnel, such as hyperflexion and hyperextension. Hormonal disturbances, such as myxedema and acromegaly, that lead to waterlogging and deposition of additional connective tissue in the carpal tunnel, also compress the median nerve. Fluid retention, which often accompanies pregnancy, may have the same effect. Increase in clinical symptoms during the night can be explained on the basis of venous stasis during rest.

Some authors have explained the median nerve deficiency not by direct compression of the nerve itself but rather by interference with its blood supply as a result of pressure on the vasa nervosum. Others ascribe the nerve symptoms to increase in endoneural and

perineural connective tissue within the nerve, such as might occur
in older age groups and also through possible scarring and shrinkage
of the endoneural supporting tissue. Often more than one mechanism is responsible.

Surgically endangered structures superficial to the flexor retinaculum

Identify the structures that run superficial to the flexor retinaculum
and that have to be guarded against injury at surgery (Fig. 44-2). The
superficial palmar arterial arch has been mentioned. What vessels
form it? Its main component is the superficial branch of the ulnar
artery, which is covered by the palmar carpal ligament. This artery
meets the superficial palmar branch of the radial artery or, more
rarely, the radial branch to the index finger or the princeps pollicis
branch. The palmar cutaneous branches of the median and ulnar
nerves accompany the tendon of the palmaris longus as it passes
superficial to the flexor retinaculum. The danger to the recurrent
motor branch of the median, which is given off distal to the flexor
retinaculum, has been mentioned previously.

Other nerve entrapments

In recent years attention has been drawn to other areas where,
because of their anatomical configuration, nerve entrapments take
place. The cause is generally compression of a nerve where it runs
through an inelastic fibrous ring or a rigid fibro-osseous tunnel. The
compression may be due to a local condition, such as callus formation after fracture, bony deformity, rheumatoid arthritis, osteoarthritis, bursitis, or synovitis with swelling. Systemic diseases, such
as hypothyroidism, acromegaly, or collagen disorders, may also
cause nerve compression by waterlogging and deposition of connective tissue in an already crowded space. In addition to the carpal
tunnel, such a condition occurs where the median nerve runs between the two heads of the pronator teres and dips under a fibrous
band that connects the two heads of the flexor digitorum superficialis. The ulnar nerve may be entrapped at the wrist in a trough
where it passes between the pisiform and hook of hamate. The ulnar
nerve may also be compressed in the ulnar groove behind the medial
epicondyle. Other entrapment neuropathies, as these conditions are

called, occur in the posterior interosseous nerve of the radial as it passes through the supinator muscle, in the suprascapular nerve as it passes between the transverse ligament and the scapular notch, in the common and superficial peroneal nerves, and in the tibial nerve beneath the flexor retinaculum in the so-called tarsal tunnel.

VII   LOWER LIMB

45   Intragluteal Injection

A 39-year-old carpenter suffered a respiratory infection with high fever and cough and was given several penicillin injections into his buttocks by a nurse in a physician's office. Immediately after the last injection into his right buttock, he complained of numbness, tingling, and burning in his right leg down to his toes and developed a footdrop the next day, when he was hospitalized.

EXAMINATION

On examination at the hospital, the patient's respiratory infection has almost cleared. His fever and cough have subsided, and the physical findings in his lungs are minimal. Inspection of the right gluteal region shows several injection marks approximately over the course of the right sciatic nerve slightly above the gluteal fold. The sensory loss involves the outer side of the right calf and the dorsum of the right foot. On the motor side there is an inability to dorsiflex the ankle and to evert the foot, with noticeable footdrop. There is also difficulty in extending the toes. When walking, the patient drags the front part and outer margin of his right foot.

DIAGNOSIS

Neural complications of intramuscular injections are diagnosed.

THERAPY AND FURTHER COURSE

The patient is given deep heat followed by electrical stimulation of the involved muscles and reeducation exercises by the department of physical medicine and rehabilitation. After four months he has essentially regained the motor functions of his right leg but still shows some sensory deficits.

DISCUSSION

What is the surface marking of the sciatic nerve at the level of the gluteal fold? It is approximately midway between greater trochanter and ischial tuberosity. Of the two components of the sciatic nerve, the tibial and the common peroneal (fibular), which part seems exclusively involved in this case? The greater susceptibility of the common peroneal nerve in injuries of the sciatic nerve is a characteristic feature that has often been observed. It is explained by the fact that the common peroneal component is placed more superficially. In addition, the more lateral location of this nerve makes it more vulnerable to injuries by intramuscular injection, which should be directed into the upper lateral quadrant of the gluteal region.

How does the sciatic nerve enter the gluteal region? What is its usual relation to the piriformis muscle? It usually enters the gluteal region inferior to this muscle. In 15 percent of cases, however, the common peroneal division of the sciatic nerve passes above or through the piriformis muscle instead of below it, increasing the danger to this division in cases where this variation is present.

Neurological deficiencies

What sensory branch of the common peroneal nerve is responsible for the loss of sensation over the lateral side of the calf? The lateral sural cutaneous nerve, a branch of the common peroneal, and the superficial peroneal nerve, supplies this area with sensory fibers. What accounts for the loss of sensation on the dorsum of the foot? Cutaneous branches of the superficial peroneal nerve (medial and intermediate dorsal) transmit sensory impulses from the dorsum of the foot. What named nerve is responsible for dorsiflexion of the foot and extension of the toes? The deep peroneal nerve innervates the dorsiflexors of the foot and extensors of the toes. Is this the same nerve that mediates sensory impulses from the dorsal aspect of the foot? It is not. What nerve supplies the main evertors of the foot? The peroneus longus and brevis muscles are the main evertors of the foot and are supplied by the superficial peroneal nerve. Would loss of function of only one of the two terminal branches of the common peroneal nerve explain all the neurological deficiencies? The sensory and motor deficits in this case can be explained only on the basis of involvement of the main stem, that is, the common peroneal nerve.

Applied anatomy of intragluteal injections

The gluteal region is a common site for intramuscular injection of drugs. Intramuscular rather than intravenous injections are given when prolonged action is preferred to immediate effect. They are more easily administered and are often better tolerated. In addition, oily preparations cannot be injected directly into the bloodstream but can be given intramuscularly. Irritant drugs are excluded from the otherwise simpler subcutaneous application, where they may cause sloughing or abscess formation. The rich blood supply of the heavy gluteal musculature makes this area a favorable site of parenteral (nongastrointestinal) administration of drugs. Name the main arteries and veins supplying this region. The superior and inferior gluteal vessels are the essential vessels in this area.

How can the inadvertent application of drugs into the subcutaneous tissue or the even more dangerous penetration of the drugs into the gluteal vessels be avoided? Keep in mind that the subcutaneous adipose layer over the gluteal area varies greatly in thickness and may reach a depth of $2^{1}/_{2}$ inches, particularly in women. The injection needle will, of course, have to penetrate beyond this layer if painful indurations and abscesses are to be avoided. Intravenous application into one of the gluteal veins should be guarded against by slightly withdrawing the plunger of the syringe and inspecting the syringe for blood. What would the result be if an oily suspension were injected into one of the thin-walled gluteal veins? Identify all named components of the cardiovascular system such an embolus (plug) would traverse until it reaches the lung, where it might cause dangerous complications. Such an oil embolus would travel via the gluteal veins into the internal and common iliac veins, the inferior vena cava, the right atrium and ventricle, and the pulmonary artery to be arrested in the pulmonary circulation.

If, as stipulated, the injection is made into the upper outer quadrant of the gluteal region, it is given either into the gluteus maximus or the gluteus medius, depending on whether the solution is injected into the lower inner or the upper outer portion of this quadrant (Fig. 45-1). Which direction of the needle should be avoided to prevent injury to the sciatic nerve? It is clear that injection downward and medially would be most apt to reach the sciatic nerve.

Injury to superior and inferior gluteal nerves

Two other motor nerves, the superior and inferior gluteal nerves, are occasionally damaged by intragluteal injection. Where in rela-

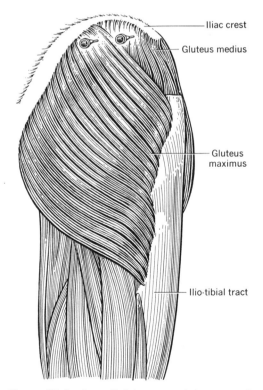

Figure 45-1. Superficial aspect of the musculature of the gluteal region. Two needles for intramuscular injection are in place in the upper outer quadrant of the gluteus maximus and medius.

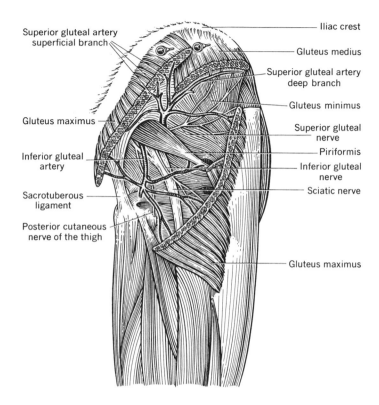

Figure 45-2. Anatomy of the gluteal area, with needles in place, after partial section of the gluteus maximus and medius. Shown are the sciatic nerve and superior and inferior gluteal arteries and nerves. Notice that both gluteal arteries, but only the inferior gluteal nerve, supply the gluteus maximus. The superior gluteal nerve lies on the deep aspect of the gluteus medius, between it and the minimus, and supplies both muscles.

tion to the piriformis muscle does the superior gluteal nerve leave the greater sciatic foramen? Can you explain why it is only rarely injured although it ramifies in the upper outer quadrant? Does it run between gluteus maximus and medius or deep to the medius? It leaves the pelvis above the piriformis and runs between gluteus medius and minimus, both of which it supplies (Fig. 45-2). The deep location and the early branching of this nerve close to its exit from the pelvis seem to explain the rarity of complications originating from injections. Does the same deep location also characterize all branches of the superior gluteal vessels? The superior gluteal vessels have superficial branches that run between the gluteus maximus and medius.

Which is the nerve of supply to the gluteus maximus? This nerve, the inferior gluteal, may likewise be damaged in improperly located injections. Although the inferior gluteal nerve is the only source of supply for this most powerful muscle in the human body, is this also true for the inferior gluteal vessels? The superficial branches of the superior gluteal artery and vein, in addition to the inferior gluteal vessels, participate in the supply of the gluteus maximus muscle and are endangered in subgluteal injections (Fig. 45-2).

Other locations of intramuscular injections

Scrupulous adherence to all rules governing intramuscular injections must be observed to avoid serious and often lasting complications. Other muscle sites that have been recommended are the quadriceps femoris, vastus lateralis, deltoid (here serious neurological mishaps have likewise been reported), and recently the more anterior aspects of the gluteus medius and minimus, inferior and posterior to the anterior superior spine of the ilium.

46   Intracapsular Hip Fracture

A 72-year-old widow who lives with her oldest son is found on the floor of her bedroom, unable to rise. She tells her son she slipped on a scatter rug and fell to the floor. She complains of severe pain in her right hip and is unable to stand. Because no physician is immediately available, an ambulance is called, and she is taken to the hospital on a stretcher. On arrival she is given a small dose of Demerol and is made more comfortable by immobilization of her limb with pillows and sandbags and by gentle longitudinal traction.

EXAMINATION

The patient is a frail, elderly woman in rather poor nutritional state. Her muscles are poorly developed. Mentally she is somewhat confused, which could be ascribed to the shock and the narcotic. Physical examination reveals that her right leg is externally rotated and that she is unable to lift her right heel from the stretcher. The right leg seems shortened, which is confirmed by measuring the distance between the anterior superior iliac spine and the distal tip of the medial malleolus of the tibia with a tape measure and by comparing the results with those obtained in the left leg, which is rotated into the same position as the right. There is shortening of her right leg by 1½ inches. The greater trochanter on the right side appears higher and more prominent than the left. On palpation there is tenderness in the femoral triangle in front of the hip joint.

DIAGNOSIS

A presumptive diagnosis of fracture through the femoral neck is made; and, as with any suspected femoral neck fracture, anteroposterior and lateral radiographs are taken. Close comparison with the contralateral hip x-rays is important. This procedure confirms the daignosis and demonstates the fracture just below the head of the femur (subcapital). The neck of the femur is anteriorly angulated, and the angle between head and neck of the femur is decreased (varus deformity). Neckand shaft are externally rotated, and the fragments overlap with the neck and shaft, having moved superiorly against the head (Fig. 46-1). The pelvic skeleton and femur show marked demineralization (osteoporosis).

THERAPY AND FURTHER COURSE

In our aged patient, who is in poor nutritional state, there is great danger of bed sores, urinary infection, pneumonia, and pulmonary

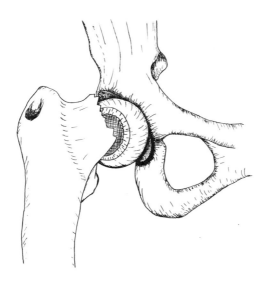

Figure 46-1. Intracapsular subcapital fracture through the neck of the femur. The neck of the femur points forward, and the neck and shaft are externally rotated. Notice the derease in the angle between head and neck (varus deformity).

embolism with possible fatal outcome if the malposition of the fracture is corrected by closed reduction and the patient is confined to bed with the limb immobilized until the fracture has a chance to heal. The head of the femur, when separated from its neck, has a poor blood supply left in the subcapital location of the fracture (10–30% of cases). Consequently, nonunion of the fragments and late necrosis may develop. These complications frequently lead to secondary degenerative osteoarthritis, resulting in a painful and disabled hip.

Thus, in view of the poor prognosis of conservative treatment in our patient, immediate surgery with removal of the femoral head and replacement with a vitallium prosthesis is selected (titanium may also be used). The Austin-Moore prosthesis chosen in this case not only replaces the head but also has a long stem that is inserted into the bone marrow cavity almost halfway down the femoral shaft to anchor the head. The stem of the prosthesis is fenestrated (has windows), and bits of cancellous bone, removed from the upper end of the femur, are placed in these windows as bone grafts. It is expected that these bone chips will become converted into dense new osseous tissue, locking the prosthesis in place and lending strength and stability to the femoral shaft for its weight-bearing function.

With the patient under spinal anesthesia, the hip is approached by an inferolateral skin and fascial incision through the lower part of the buttock. The iliotibial tract is indentified, and the gluteus maximus is split in the direction of its fibers by blunt dissection. A 5-cm-long vertical incision is made to separate the gluteus maximus from its insertion into the iliotibial tract to give better access to the posterior aspect of the hip joint. The upper and lower portions if this muscle are separated and retracted, thus exposing the sciatic nerve and the lateral rotators of the hip. The latter are divided close to their insertion into the greater trochanter. After removal of the overlying fat, the capsule is incised and partly reflected. The head of the femur is dislodged out of the acetabulum and removed, and the ligament of the head is ligated and excised. The neck of the femur is sawed across, and the stem of a properly fitted vitallium prosthesis is inserted into the marrow cavity. Care is taken to preserve the normal forward angle of neck and head. A tight fit of the prosthesis is obtained after moving the artificial head into place.

The operation lasts 45 to 60 min, and the patient is able to sit up in bed and eat on the afternoon of the day of operation. After one day the patient is up and around with the help of a walker and leaves the hospital after 10 days. She is cautioned to use a walker, and only partial weight bearing is permitted for about two months. She is also warned not to expose her leg to too much strain and to avoid heavy weight gain.

On reexamination after a year, the patient reports that she can do her own housework and can walk with no limp or pain. She has practically normal function of her hip.

DISCUSSION

Anatomy of intracapsular and extracapsular fractures of the neck of the femur

We are dealing here with a very common clinical condition of elderly patients, particularly women, in whom neck fracture is 10 times more common than in men. In many cases the fracture is the direct cause of death, as discussed in the case history. Modern advances in the handling of these fractures include insertion of prosthesis, as in this case, or fixation of the fragments with stainless steel screws when the fracture is not displaced, depending on the judgment and preference of the surgeon. These procedures have resulted in avoidance of general complications by allowing early ambulation and quite frequently have given good functional results. As described previously in the case history, the rotational strain in slipping had caused a fracture with complete separation of the fragments. The fracture line is located just below the head of the femur at the highest point of the neck (subcapital) and is therefore completely intracapsular. What are the attachments of the capsule? Are all neck fractures intracapsular? The fibrous capsule, lined by synovial membrane, arises from the margins of the acetabulum of the hip bone and extends sleevelike downward and laterally around the neck of the femur to attach near the intertrochanteric line anteriorly and close to the middle of the neck posteriorly, a finger breadth above the posteriorly located intertrochanteric crest. From the attachments of the capsule, the synovial membrane is reflected onto the neck and up to the margin of the articular cartilage, which, as in all other joints, is not covered by synovial membrane.

From this description we realize that the lateral and distal most portions of the posterior aspect of the neck are outside the capsule; so neck fractures, in contrast to the injury in our case, may be partly intracapsular and partly extracapulsar. Intertrochanteric fractures are always extracapsular.

Anatomy of displacement of the fragments

What is the typical position of the fractured extremity, and how do you explain this position? Typically, the leg is externally rotated by the pull of the lateral rotators and the weight of the leg and foot itself. Which are the lateral rotators? They are the short muscles within the gluteal region: the piriformis, the obturator internus and externus, the superior and inferior gemelli and the quadratus femoris, which are aided by the gluteus maximus. The external rotators are much more powerful than the internal, which explains the position of the leg.

How do you explain the shortening of the extremity in our case? The force of the injury itself may may drive the distal fragment superiorly, but in general it is the muscle pull that leads to this result. Identify the muscles whose pull causes shortening of the leg. The powerful gluteal muscles, the hamstrings, the adductors, the iliopsoas, and some of the flexors of the thigh all arise from the pelvis or lumbar vertebral column above the fracture line and insert into the distal fragment. Their pull results in upward displacement of the lower fragment and shortening of the leg.

Angles of inclination and declination

The muscle pull also leads to a change in the angle of femoral head and neck with the shaft. Normally, this angle is about 125 degrees and is larger in children. This is the so-called "angle of inclination." As so often occurs in hip fractures, the x-ray in our case reveals that the angle is reduced, resulting in what is called a coxa vara (Fig. 46-1). By contrast, an occasional fracture through the neck may take place in abduction of the thigh at the time of injury. If this happens, the neck will be driven in the abducted position into the head, where it remains firmly impacted, increasing the angle of inclination and resulting in the so-called valgus position. Such a fracture has a better prognosis. There is no shortening of the leg and little pain.

Also of importance is the anteriorly open angle between neck and shaft of the femur, the so-called "angle of declination." In contrast to the shoulder, where the head of the humerus faces posteriorly, the head and neck of the femur are directed anteriorly. This angle between the planes laid through neck and shaft is normally about 12 degrees, and care must be taken to preserve it in setting neck fracture or inserting the prosthesis. Any marked alteration in the angles of inclination and declination may seriously interfere with mobility of the hip joint and disable the patient.

Blood supply of the shaft, neck, and head of the femur

A problem that has direct bearing on the course and handling of our fracture is the blood supply to the proximal portion of the femur. Long bones, such as the femur, are well sullpied with blood vessels. These are derived from the following three sources:

1. The nutrient artery, which enters the bone through the nutrient foramen, takes an oblique course through the cortex of the bone until it reaches the marrow cavity, where it divides into ascending and descending branches. The nutrient artery is largely concerned with supply of the bone marrow and the inner two thirds of the cortex. In the femur, there are two nutrient foramina, and the nutrient arteries passing into them are derived from the perforating branches of the deep femoral artery.
2. The periosteal vessels form a communicating network that surrounds the bone. The number of periosteal vessels increases from the middle of the diaphysis toward the metaphyses, which are richly supplied with periosteal blood vessels. Fine branches of the periosteal network enter the outer third of the cortical bone and anastomose with vessels derived from the nutrient artery in the inner portion of the cortex. The two systems of the nutrient and periosteal blood vessels may partially substitute for each other if the circulation in one or the other system is interrupted.
3. The main arteries of supply to the head of the femur come from the medial femoral circumflex, which is most commonly a branch of the deep femoral artery. Injection studies have shown that the posterior branches of the medial femoral circumflex artery, best known as lateral epiphyseal arteries, represent the most important blood supply to the head. These vessels arise from a posterior branch of the medial femoral circumflex, which takes origin

behind the femoral neck. They pierce the fibrous capsule of the hip joint and run upward and medially along the posterior aspects of the neck. There they course beneath the synovial membrane surrounding the neck to enter the head through bony foramina close to the site of the former epiphysis. These vessels have also been called retinacular vessels because they lie within easily movable folds or retinacula of the synovial membrane, which is reflected from the attachment of the fibrous capsule on to the neck.

Other lateral epiphyseal branches enter the head inferomedial to the old epiphyseal line to distribute themselves in the inferomedial portion of the head. The lateral epiphyseal vessels supply two thirds to four fifths of the head (Fig. 46-2) distal to the obliterated epiphysis. Of great interest is the acetabular branch of the obturator artery, which sends a branch to the head: the medial epiphyseal artery, which is carried to the head through the ligament of the head of the femur (ligamentum teres capitis femoris) and is often called the foveolar artery. Its extent and patency are variable, and its contribution to the blood supply of the head is generally not significant unless the lateral epiphyseal arteries do not cross the epiphyseal line, which disappears in adolescence. It is important to note that the medial epiphyseal artery does not anastomose with the lateral epiphyseal branches of the medial femoral circumflex artery in about 20 percent of persons.

Necrosis of the femoral head in subcapital fractures

From the foregoing, it is clear that a subcapital fracture, such as in this case, leads to tearing of the important lateral epiphyseal blood vessels beneath the synovial membrane and therefore to interruption of the main blood supply to the head. On the other hand, trochanteric fractures outside the capsule have a much better chance to allow sufficient nourishment of the bone. The blood supply to the head of the femur via the medial epiphyseal artery may be its only source of blood after fracture of the neck because anastomosis of the lateral epiphyseal vessels across the epiphyseal line does not occur in 20 percent of cases. Therefore, in one fifth of the cases, necrosis of the distal four fifths of the head and the proximal neck is likely to occur. This type of necrosis is due to isolation of the head and neck

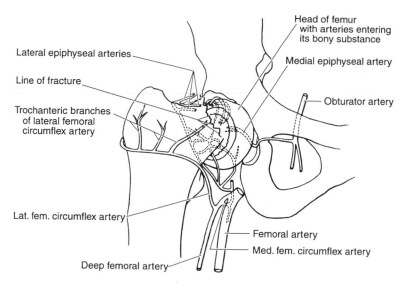

Figure 46-2. Blood supply of the head and neck of the femur. Notice the main artery to the head is the medial femoral circumflex through its lateral epiphyseal arteries. Notice also that the lateral femoral circumflex artery contributes to the blood supply of the neck. Identify the medial epiphyseal artery from the obturator artery that may or may not anastomose with the medial femoral circumflex artery. Notice also that most of the important arteries to the head have been torn by the fracture.

from its blood supply and is aseptic, in contrast to septic necrosis due to bacterial infection.

An interesting radiographic feature of aseptic necrosis of the head is a change in radiodensity in the fracture area, which becomes noticeable several weeks or months after the fracture has been sustained. The surrounding area of the neck and shaft becomes increasingly translucent as a result of bone resorption from disuse and inflammation while the dead head itself, cut off from its blood supply, preserves its normal bone density,

In the past, attempts were frequently made to immobilize the fragments by a plaster cast or by nailing in the hope that the fragments would unite and vessels would grow across the fracture line. This effort often fails, particularly in subcapital fractures in elderly patients, and the previously described necrosis of the head results.

To avoid this complication, in our case the head was excised and replaced by a prosthesis. Other areas where fractures frequently lead to devascularization and necrosis of one fragment are the scaphoid and the talus. Clinically, this commonality is known as retrograde blood supply.

Osteoporosis and its underlying anatomy

The x-ray of the pelvis of our patient called attention to marked osteoporosis, which is common in the elderly, particularly in women. What is the cause of this deficiency in the bony framework that in the femoral head and neck leads to noticeable rarefaction of the spongy bone and thinning of the cortex and so often results in fractures from trivial injuries? The true cause of this type of osteoporosis is not clearly understood but is characterized by a deficiency of the bony matrix. The matrix that is laid down is calcified normally but not enough bony matrix is formed.

Surgical anatomy of the operation

What is the direction of the fibers of the gluteus maximus that are split by blunt dissection? The fibers run from above, laterally and downward. Does the gluteus maximus insert into the greater trochanter? It passes over the lateral surface of this process, a bursa intervening, and inserts into the iliotibial tract and the gluteal tuberosity, which is an upward extension of the lateral lip of the linea aspera. What is the superoinferior sequence of the lateral rotator muscles of the hip joint that are in the operative field? They are the piriformis, the superior gemellus, the tendon of the obturator internus, the inferior gemellus, and the quadratus femoris. These muscles are divided in our surgical procedure with the exception of the lowest muscle, the quadratus femoris, which is cut only if it is necessary to obtain a wide approach to the joint.

Sensory nerve supply of the hip joint and Hilton's law

A short comment on the sensory nerve supply of the hip joint is indicated because it is responsible for the pain suffered by patients with hip fractures and explains the muscle spasms. An old law by John Hilton is quite applicable to the hip joint, that is, that a joint receives its proprioceptive and pain fibers from the same nerves that supply the muscles moving the joint and distribute to the skin over these muscles and their insertions. This law also explains the reflex spasm of the overlying muscles in disease of the joint and the referral of joint pain to the adjacent skin. In the hip joint, the sensory nerve supply is derived from the femoral, obturator, and sciatic nerves in addition to fibers incorporated in muscular branches to the quadratus femoris.

REFERENCE

Hilton, John. *Rest and Pain,* edited by E. W. Walls, E. E. Phillip, and H. J. B. Atkins. Philadelphia: J. B. Lippincott, 1950.

47   "Unhappy Triad" of the Knee Joint

A 20-year-old student, while playing touch football, suffered a severe twisting injury to his right knee. He was running hard and pushed off balance by another player when his foot was planted in the turf. He felt a "pop" and fell to the ground. In excruciating pain, he is taken to the health center on a stretcher.

Examination

The patient is seen later the same day by an orthopedist. His pain is intense and his knee has begun to swell. He prefers to hold it in slight flexion. Abduction of the leg on the femur aggravates the pain. There is tenderness when pressure is applied along the tibial attachment of the tibial collateral ligament but not at its femoral attachment. The clinical evaluation indicates that the ligament is sprained (overstretched). When the knee is flexed to a right angle and an attempt is made to pull the tibia forward, there is a noticeably increased anterior mobility (positive anterior drawer sign) compared with the uninjured knee. There is also marked restriction to passive extension of the knee joint.

A magnetic resonance image (MRI) confirms a clinical diagnosis that the anterior cruciate ligament (ACL) is torn from its femoral attachment and that the medial meniscus is torn (Fig. 47-1).

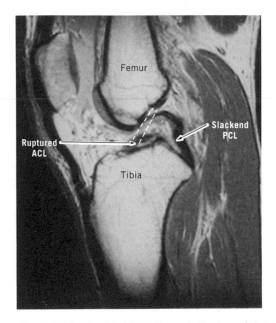

Figure 47-1. Sagittal MRI through the knee joint showing a ruptured ACL. The dashed line marks the location of an uninjured ACL. The PCL is slackened and bent acutely because the tibia has translocated anteriorly.

DIAGNOSIS

A diagnosis is made of an effusion (fluid collection) in the synovial cavity of the knee joint, rupure of the ACL at its femoral attachment, a bucket-handle tear of the medial meniscus, and a sprain of the lower portion of the tibial collateral ligament.

THERAPY AND FURTHER COURSE

Injuries to the knee that disrupt its synovial lining frequently cause the knee to swell. This explains the swelling seen in this patient because the well-vascularized synovial membrane that attaches to the ACL and the outer margins of the medial meniscus was also torn, causing effusion and hemorrhage. Restricted range of motion, also associated with swelling, explains why the patient prefers to hold his knee in slight flexion. In consultation with the patient, arthroscopic surgery for reconstruction of the ACL using a patellar tendon graft is decided on but not until knee motion improves to normal, which may take up to six weeks. Graft replacement was developed because a torn ACL does not heal well, even after surgical repair of the torn ends of the ligament.

The decision to repair the torn medial meniscus will be made only after intra-articular assessment of the exact location and the severity of the injury with the arthroscope. If it is repairable, the arthroscopic surgery will be preformed in two stages; the meniscus will be repaired first, followed by the graft replacement of the ACL. If the medial meniscus cannot be repaired, it will be partially excised by removal of the unstable flaps. The sprain of the tibial collateral ligament will heal without surgical treatment.

In preparation for the arthroscopic surgery, the patient is placed in the supine position. An epidural block for the lumbar and sacral nerves is given and the antibiotic cephalosporin (Cefazolin) is given intravenously. A tourniquet is placed on the proximal thigh to reduce bleeding during surgery. The joint is injected with an anesthetic containing a mixture of xylocaine and marcaine as well as epinephrine that will further reduce bleeding.

After anesthesia is induced, the surgery begins with small skin incisions on each side of the patellar tendon to create anteromedial and anterolateral portals, openings through which arthroscopic instruments are inserted into the joint cavity. The arthroscope, which is equipped with a light source and camera, is inserted into the joint through the anterolateral portal and irrigation is carried out through a cannula inserted into the anteromedial portal.

Diagnostic Arthroscopy

During diagnostic arthroscopy, the ACL and medial and lateral menisci are carefully inspected visually and probed with a nerve hook (curved, round probe) to expose tears. To ensure the best possible visualization of a tear, the surgical assistant maneuvers the injured limb into various positions and degrees of varus, vulgus, or rotational stress.

Inspection shows a large, displaced bucket-handle tear of the medial meniscus in the outer vascular zone of the meniscus, 3 mm from its periphery. The tear is about 2.5 cm long, and it curves from the posteromedial aspect of the meniscus to the posterior horn or root of the meniscus. Because the tear occured in the vascular (or red) zone, it is deemed repairable by suturing the torn edges together. Tears of the thinly tapered inner part (the white zone) are not repairable because this part is avascular. In those cases, the damaged tissue is unstable and is usually excised arthroscopically. The arthroscopy also reveals that the ACL is completely torn (avulsed) from its femoral attachment on the lateral wall of the intercondylar notch.

Repair of the Medial Meniscus

The surgeon chooses the "inside-out" technique of meniscal repair. A 3-cm-long skin incision, extending inward to the fibrous capsule, is made just behind the tibial collateral ligament. The sartorius muscle and saphenous branch of the femoral nerve are retracted by the assistant surgeon posteriorly from harm's way. This incision exposes the posteromedial part of the fibrous capsule, which lies superficial to the torn medial meniscus and provides the site where the assistant surgeon (working outside the joint) will grasp the needles during the intra-articular part of the surgery as they are guided externally through the meniscus and fibrous capsule by the surgeon.

In this inside-out technique of meniscal repair, the surgeon, working inside the joint, guides sutures attached to 8-inch-long flexible needles through the meniscus and pushes them outward through the fibrous capsule of the knee. The assistant surgeon grasps the needles as they come through the capsule and tags the sutures so they be tensioned and tied following the ACL reconstruction. Four inside-out vertical sutures are placed across the tear. Following the procedure, probing the tear confirms proper suture placement and stable fixation of the meniscus.

Reconstruction of the ACL

The ACL is reconstructed in several stages:

1. harvesting and preparing the graft,
2. debridement (removal of nonviable tissue) from the lateral side of the intercondylar notch at the femoral attachment of the ACL,

3. drilling the tibial tunnel,
4. drilling the femoral tunnel,
5. implanting the graft and fixing it into the femoral and tibial tunnels, and
6. closing the incisions and making a postoperative evaluation.

To harvest the patellar tendon graft, a vertical skin incision is made over the patellar tendon, extending from the center of the patella to just inferior to the tibial tuberosity. The graft is harvested by removing a 1-cm-wide central strip of the tendon extending from the tibial tuberosity to the inferior tip of the patella, leaving plugs from both bones attached to the ends of the graft.

Working through the anteromedial portal, the part of the ACL that remained attached to the anterior intercondylar area of the tibia and the site where it was broken from the lateral wall of the intercondylar notch (medial surface of the lateral condyle of the femur) is debrided with a motorized burr (resector). The resector is removed and a small curved osteotome is then inserted through the portal to contour the lateral wall of the intercondylar notch in preparation for drilling the femoral tunnel (Fig. 47-2) to make adequate room for the graft. Debris is removed by irrigation and suction.

The next step is to drill the tibial tunnel. A tibial drill is mounted externally, and its tip is inserted through the anteromedial portal. It is angled so that the tunnel will open into the joint about 7 mm anterior to the tibial attachment of the posterior cruciate ligament (PCL). The angle of the tibial tunnel should align to the slope of the femoral tunnel when the knee is in 70 degrees of flexion, which allows the femoral tunnel to be drilled through the tibial tunnel.

The knee is now ready for graft implantation. An eyelet pin, which was threaded with sutures through the patellar plug of the graft, is passed through the tibial and femoral tunnels and out the anterolateral thigh. This procedure positions the graft within the joint so that the bony plug from the patella lies in the femoral tunnel and the bony plug from the tibia lies in the tibial tunnel. Screws are inserted through the bony plugs into the femur and tibia for fixation. After the graft has been fixed, the knee is brought a full range of motion to test the new graft. The gap in the patellar tendon left after removing the graft is loosely reapproximated with sutures.

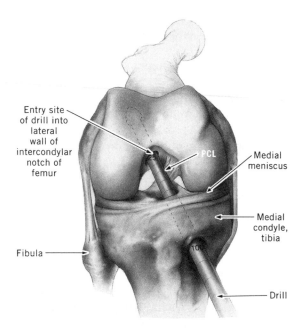

Entry site
of drill into
lateral
wall of
intercondylar
notch of
femur

PCL

Medial
meniscus

Medial
condyle,
tibia

Fibula

Drill

Figure 47-2. A schematic showing the three-dimensional relationships of the drill passing through the right tibia upwards through the joint space and the overlying tibia. (Reproduced with permission, Raven Press.)

Rehabilitation

The patient's knee is immobilized in a brace for about a month except while performing supervised excercises. He begins rehabilitation therapy the day after surgery with two-crutch ambulation. Pedaling a stationary bicycle and doing resistance excercises for the quadriceps, hamstring, and other hip muscles begin during the third or fourth week. Patients who have an uncomplicated postoperative course and who are persistent in doing strengthening exercises are normally able to begin light jogging during the fourth postoperative month. A year after injury, patients usually regain normal knee stability along with a full range of motion and can resume athletic activities.

DISCUSSION

This is a common injury that has been designated the "unhappy traid" of the knee. What are the three important structures involved? The traid consists of injury to the (1) anterior cruciate ligament, (2) medial meniscus, and (3) tibial collateral ligament. The joint swelling in this case reflects damage to the interior of the joint, particularly the synovial lining, and generally accompanies all types of intra-articular knee joint injuries.

There are many causes for ACL injury. A direct blow to the lateral side of the knee (creating valgus stress) as in tackling is not required. The considerable interia of the body rotating its femur medially (excessive lateral rotation may also cause this injury) over a planted foot and stable tibia is a frequent cause of ACL injuries. This injury can occur while a runner is making a quick turn if the heel does not lift off the surface to spin with the runner's body, or in a skier whose ski becomes caught and cannot rotate freely with the skier. Even the quadriceps muscle can exert enough force to break the ACL while arresting knee flexion during landing from a fall by pulling the tibia too far forward on the tibial plateau. This is sometimes called the slingshot effect. In summary, this injury can be caused by a variety of rather common misfortunes all having to do with the knee joint being unable to withstand the rotational, or valgus forces to which it is subjected.

Movements of the knee joint

Is the knee purely a hinge joint allowing only flexion and extension, or do other movements take place? It is commonly considered to be a hinge joint, but its movements are complex and include rolling, gliding, and rotation. In full extension, the matching articular areas of the femur and tibia are most congruent, and the strong stabilizing ligaments, ACL, PCL, tibial collateral, and fibular collateral are taut. The knee is said to be "locked" when fully extended, and it is most stable in this position. The joint occupies this position during quiet standing. Movement from the locked position, as when assuming the sitting position or the beginning of a stride, begins with flexion followed soon by a few degrees of lateral rotation of the femur on the tibia. These movements unlock the knee. The rotational component is allowed by a slackening of the collateral ligaments.

You can readily demonstrate this on yourself while sitting in a chair by keeping your heel on the floor and lifting your forefoot off the surface. While moving your toes from side to side, you can palpate the tibia rotating on the femur by placing your hands on the upper on the upper surfaces of the tibia. If youn repeat this test while standing with your knee in full extension (locked), rotation takes place at the hip joint because the collateral of the knee ligaments are taut.

In summary, the unhappy triad injury seen in this case was caused by excessive medial rotation of the femur on a relatively stable tibia while the joint was partially flexed. It occurred during the moment when the body weight was borne by the stance limb.

The matching surfaces of the tibia and femur contribute little to this mobile joint's stability. Moreover, the contact area between the two bones decreases in flexion, leading to even greater instability. What are the main elements that contribute to the strength and stability of the joint? The joint is crossed by very strong muscles and tendons and is invested by numerous ligaments, (intra-articular, capsular, and extracapsular) that act as stabilizing elements. In addition, the menisci deepen the articular surfaces of the tibial condyles and accommodate the joint to variations in contact between femur and tibia. The fibrous capsule itself contributes greatly to maintaining the integrity of the joint.

Tibial collateral ligament

In this case, the tibial collateral ligament is injured to a lesser extent than the ACL or the medial meniscus. What abnormal and excessive motion stretched the ligament at its attachment to the tibia? Medial rotation and adduction of the femur, with the knee partially flexed, caused this injury; bear in mind the injury occured when the foot was on the ground, thereby making the tibia relatively stable in reference to the femur. This motion, and the consequent separation of the medial tibial and femoral condyles, puts more stress on the ligament than it could withstand. What are the attachments of this ligament? Its superficial fibers attach proximally into the medial epicondyle of the femur and distally onto the medial condyle, about 2 inches below the joint line. Its deep fibers are shorter and thicker and are attached to the capsule, to the outer aspect of the medial meniscus, and to the tibia above the groove for the semimembranosus tendon. Name the three tendons that cross the tibial collateral ligament. They are the sartorius, gracilis, and semitendinosus, on their way to their common insertion on the proximal portion of the tibia, in front of the attachment of the superfical part of the tibial collateral ligament.

Anterior cruciate ligament

The second ligament injured was the ACL. It was torn off its proximal attachment. What is the relation of the cruciate ligaments to the fibrous capsule and synovial membrane? The cruciate ligaments lie inside the fibrous capsule but outside the synovial cavity of the joint; the synovial membrane is reflected around them anteriorly and on their sides. The ACL is attached superiorly to the lateral surface of the intercondylar notch and is directed downward in a medial and anterior direction and inserts on the anterior intercondylar area of the tibia. The posterior cruciate ligament, which crosses the ACL posteriorly, also attaches to the intercondylar area of the tibia, but behind the ACL. The cruciate ligaments cross each other like the limbs of an X, hence their name. This relationship for the right knee can be remembered by crossing your legs by briging your right thigh over the left. In this position, your right lower limb shows the position of the right ACL, and your left limb designates the PCL. You would cross your thighs in the opposite direction to illustrate this relationship for the left side. Although both cruciate ligaments exert a stablizing effect on all motions of the knee joint, they also limit anterior and posterior mobility of the tibia on the femur in flexion. The ACL limits excessive anterior mobility and the PCL limits excessive posterior mobility of the tibia on the femur.

What clinical sign in the examination of this patient made tearing of the ACL likely? The increased anterior mobility (positive anterior drawer sign) of the tibia with the knee in flexion indicates serious injury of this ligament.

Medial meniscus

The final injury was tearing of the medial meniscur. What is the shape of the menisci? Both menisci are wedge-shaped, thicker at their peripheral margins. In contrast to its lateral counterpart, the medial meniscus forms a three-quarter segment of a larger circle, that is, it is more C-shaped than the lateral meniscus, which displays a sharper curve and approximates a more complete, smaller circle. The anterior and posterior horns (ends) of the medial meniscus are attached to the anterior and posterior intercondylar areas of the tibia (the transverse ligament joins the anterior ends of the two menisci). A part of the fibrus capsule termed the coronary ligament attaches the menisci to the underlying tibia. The medial meniscus, in contrast to the lateral meniscus, is firmly anchored on its peripheral margin to the deep portion of the tibial collateral ligament, making it less mobile than its lateral counterpart. The same force that caused the stretching injury to the tibial collateral ligament as well as the rupture of the ACL displaced the medial meniscus more deeply into the joint, where crushing and shearing forces produced the bucket-handle tear. If left unrepaired, the patient is likely to suffer intermittent locking or buckling of the knee.

Are injuries of the medial meniscus more common than those of the lateral meniscus; if so, what is the cause of the difference in frequency? The medial meniscus is injured more commonly than the lateral. The difference is partially explained by the firm anchorage of the medial meniscus to the collateral ligament, which may be considered a thickening of the medial side of the fibrous capsule. The lateral meniscus is not attached to the extracapsular fibular collateral ligament, which gives it increased freedom of movement and presumably allows it greater escape from damage. Another reason sometimes given to explain the less frequent injury of the lateral meniscus is that the popliteus muscle inserts into the lateral meniscus, allowing it to tyug the meniscus away from possible crushing forces while assisting in flexion and lateral rotation of the femur on the fixed tibia. What was the clinical sign in this case that indicated possible meniscus injury? The marked restriction to passive extension of the knee joint.

REFERENCES

Jackson, Douglas W., ed. *Reconstructive Knee Surgery*. New York: Raven Press, 1995.
O'Donoghue, D. H. "Surgical treatment of fresh injuries to the major ligaments of the knee." *J Bone Joint Surg*, 32-A:721–738, 1950.

48   Bipartite Patella and Fabella

A week ago, a 35-year-old skydiver hurt his right knee upon landing. Examination by a physician shows the knee to be swollen and painful on movement. Plain x-rays show distinct fragmentation of the patella in its upper lateral portion, interpreted as a fracture. In addition, anteroposterior (AP) views display a round, pea-sized, bony shadow behind the lateral condyle of the femur, which is also ascribed to the injury and regarded as a small bony fragment from one of the condyles. The patient is admitted to the hospital for diagnosis and treatment.

EXAMINATION

On examination of the knee, the skin is discolored with some swelling of the surrounding soft tissues. There also seems to be a small amount of excess fluid within the synovial cavity of the joint. No particular pain can be elicited on pressure over the patella, including its lateral portion, but some pain occurs with exteme passive motions of flexion and extension. When walking, the patient favors his injured leg. No signs of major internal injuries within the knee joint, such as meniscus damage or tearing of the cruciate ligaments, are seen; the collateral ligaments do not appear to be sprained.

The x-rays demonstrate a bipartite patella on the right side with the upper outer portion of the bone separated from the main part of the patella. In addition, a sesamoid bone, the fabella, is seen on the injured side (Figs. 48-1 and 48-2). Neither finding is related to the trauma. Plain films of the left knee do not show any abnormality.

DIAGNOSIS

The diagnosis is mild traumatic arthritis with small amounts of fluid in the right knee joint but no signs of bone injury. Incidental anomalies not connected with the trauma are a right-sided bipartite patella and a fabella bhind the right knee joint.

THERAPY AND FURTHER COURSE

With physical therapy, followed by strengthening exercises, the patient completely recovers function of the right knee.

DISCUSSION

Sesamoid bones as a source of diagnostic errors

We are dealing here with two bones of more than academic interest: (1) the partition or division of a bone, the patella, and (2) the presence of a small sesamoid bone, the fabella. Sesamoid bones have interested clinical anatomists from the time of Versalius (1514–1564). Knowledge of these bones, which occur mainly in the hands and feet, where they are embedded within tendons or joint capsules, was gained from examination of anatomical specimens. They vary in size and number. Some clearly serve to alter the angle of pull of a tendon; however, others are so small it is difficult to interpret their function.

Radiology has made it possoble to demonstrate these ossicles in living persons, generally as an incidental finding in connection with accidents, as in this case, or in diseases that require radiographic investigation of the part. The temptation, of course, is to establish a causal connection between the presence of these small bones and the accident or disease. In the former case, a sesamoid bone is regarded as a displaced fracture fragment, which it may simulate. In case of chronic joint disease, practicularly in the knee, bones such as the fabella may be misinterpreted as loose bodies or joint "mice" originating from degenerative disease or chronic post-traumatic

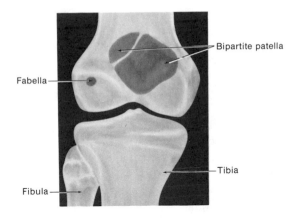

Figure 48-1. Radiographic front view of the right knee joint revealing a bipartite patella with separation in the upper lateral quadrant of the bone. It also shows the hazy outline of the fabella superimposed on the lateral condyle of the femur. The fibula identifies the lateral side.

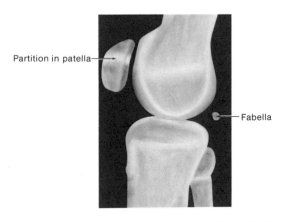

Figure 48-2. Radiographic lateral view of the right knee joint showing the fabella more clearly. It is posterior to the condyles of the femur and above the plane of the menisci. The view also displays, although somewhat hazily, the division of the patella.

changes. Such conditions may lead to secondary ossification of small dislodged cartilaginous fragments. Locking of the joint in a certain position is one of the typical clinical signs of loose bodies.

Many knee joints have been opened under the mistaken diagnosis of a fracture fragment or joint pathology when the surgeon was actually dealing only with an incidental finding of a supermumerary sesamoid bone. The importance of familiarity with these bone anomalies in insurance compensation cases is quite obvious. The praticing physician can leave the decision of whether he or she is dealing with a fracture or a congenital bone anomaly to an expert, usually a radiologist, who is familiar with the numerous osseous variants imitating bone pathology; or the physician can become acquainted with the many details of osteology to interpret these skeletal findings properly. In many cases bony variations are bilateral, but unilateral occurrence, as in this case, does not at first glance rule out the presence of an anomaly. On the other hand, bone reaction with callus formation, which may be detected several weeks after the accident, indicates a traumatic origin of a finding of the skeletal irregularity.

Sesamoid bones

Frequently the term "sesamoid bone" is used for ossicles, such as the fabella. Thus, a clear defination of this designation is indicated. Sesamoid bones are small bones, usually larger than a sesame seed (the term originated with Galen). They are located in tendons, where the latter pass over joints. In some locations they are consistently present. The best known and largest is the patella, which is embedded in the tendon of the quadriceps femoris, where it passes over the knee joint. Others occur in duplicate, such as on either side of the metacarpophalangeal joint of the thumb and metatarsophalangeal joint of the great toe. All sesamoids are preformed in cartilage and develop during early fetal months. They may remain cartilaginous throughout life. If they ossify over a joint, such as the patella over the knee joint, they are included in the joint capsule and are covered on the surface facing the joint by articular cartilage. In this location, the sesamoid bone protects the tendon from wear and tear where it crosses the joint. Its main function, however, is to increase the distance between the tendon and the rotational axis of the joint and thus make muscle action more effective.

Fabella

The fabella ("little bean"), with which we are also dealing here, is a sesamoid bone embedded in the lateral head of the gastrocnemius muscle behind the lateral condyle of the femur. The fabella occurs in about 20 percent of all persons and is bilateral in about half of these cases (some authors give higher figures for bilaterality). Very rarely it occurs in the medial head of the gastrocnemius. As stated, it is preformed in cartilage and cannot be demonstrated radiographically before puberty. In adults most fabellas are seen on properly exposed AP views, and its lateral location is helpful in distinguishing it from a loose body (Fig. 48-1). The lateral view is also useful in showing it clearly behind the femoral condyles, above a line laid through the radiologic joint space that corresponds to the menisici (Fig. 48-2). The fabella varies in size and shape and is often flattened where it faces the lateral femoral condyle. On good films, a bone consisting of a spongy center surrounded by a fine cortex can be seen.

In generalized osteoarthritis, the fabella frequently takes part in the degenerative process and is enlarged and deformed. Its main practical importance, however, lies in the fact that it may be mistaken for a loose body. A loose body in the joint might make surgery necessary. There is one additional differential diagnostic criterion: In flexion of the knee joint, the fabella moves distally with the lateral belly of the gastrocnemius in which it is incorpated; the loose body or "joint mouse" does not.

Bipartite patella

Less well known than the fabella, and therefore more apt to be misinterpreted as traumatic in orgin, is the bipartite patella. Two circumstances in the history and findings confuse the problem even more: (1) there was a definite injury to the knee joint, and (2) the other (uninvolved) knee did not display the abnormality. Bipartition of a bone on a developmental basis is a well-known anomaly; yet the distinction between the former and traumatic partition is often quite difficult, sometimes impossible. Yhe bipartite scaphoid in the wrist has given rise to many investigations with conclusions varying from one extreme (i.e., the always traumatic origin of the bipartition) to definite proof that in a few instances the condition is congenital. The double sesamoid bones of the metacarpophalangeal or metatarsophalangeal joint of the first digit may also be divided.

Most frequently, congenital separation of the patella leads to bipartite bones, such as in our case, but separation into three fragments may also occur. Almost always, the location of the fragmentation is in the upper lateral quadrant of the patella, with one or two segments separated from the main body of the bone. The borders of the fragment and its opposing patellar surface are quite smooth, which makes the assumption of a fracture gap quite unlikely in a recent injury. Soft tissue swelling in the tissues surrounding the fracture is generally present immediately after a fracture. Follow-up in a case of an actual fracture would show a bony reaction or union through callus formation occurring several weeks later.

Causes of partition of the patella

There is extensive discussion of the causes of bipartite and tripartite patellae in the literature, but no definite cause has been identified. One must keep in mind that the patella normally ossifies (at about three to six years of age) from a number of small foci that later fuse. The conclusion seems justified that persistence of multiple anlage of the bone is the primary cause of the separation. The factors responsible for the persistence are as yet not clear. The condition is more common in males.

REFERENCES

Keats, T. E. 1992 *Atlas of Normal and Roentgen Variants that Simulate Disease*, 5th ed. St. Louis: Mosby Year Book.
Koehler, A., and E.A. Zimmer. 1968 *Borderlines of the Normal and Early Pathologic in Skeletal Roentgenology*, 3rd American ed., 11th German ed. New York: Grune and Stratton.

49   Anterior Compartment
        Syndrome

At the beginning of the soccer season, a 20-year-old college man participated in strenuous field practice that extended through the whole afternoon. Later in the evening, he experienced severe pain over the anterolateral aspect of his right leg, radiating down toward the ankle. The next afternoon he went back to the field and continued to play, but the pain in his right leg became so severe that he had to limp off the field. The pain persisted throughout the night and the next morning he consulted a sports medicine physician.

EXAMINATION

On examination there is reddening and swelling over the anterolateral aspect of his right leg. On palpation this area is extremely tender, and it feels hard and warmer than other parts of the leg. The hardening extends from 2 inches below the tibial tuberosity to the junction of the middle and lower thirds of the leg, and it seems to correspond to the anterior compartment of the leg. Dorsiflexion of the foot and extension of the toes are severely limited. The pulses in the anterior tibial and dorsalis pedis arteries are weak. His body temperature is slightly elevated.

THERAPY AND FURTHER COURSE

The patient is hospitalized and his leg is immobilized by splinting; moist packs are applied. Because there is no improvement within the next 24 h, the fascia over the anterolateral aspect of the leg is incised (fasciotomy) with the patient under general anesthesia. The muscles in the anterior compartment of the leg show some grayish brown discoloration and seem rather hard to the touch. Muscle biopsies are taken from the discolored areas for microscopic studies. These show signs of degeneration and necrosis (cell death) in the muscle fibers. The fascia is left wide open, but the skin over it is partially closed.

In the next few days there is discharge of necrotic material from the site of incision, but the pain and fever subside. During the following weeks, exudation from the wound gradually stops and the wound closes. Dorsiflexion of the foot and extension of the toes continue to be restricted, but the patient is able to walk and is discharged.

DIAGNOSIS

We are dealing with a condition that has become known by the name "anterior compartment syndrome."

DISCUSSION

The condition is caused by an acute impairment of the intramuscular circulation in the muscles of the anterior compartment. It is assumed that heavy exercise, particularly in a person who is not well conditioned, causes swelling of the musculature and perhaps also some tearing of muscle fibers and small hemorrhages inside the muscles. This increase in bulk compresses the smaller vessels within the muscle bellies, which in turn leads to degeneration and necrosis of muscle fibers. Identify the muscles in the anterior compartment of the leg. The tibialis anterior is particularly affected, and the extensor hallucis longus is affected to a greater extent and more commonly than the extensor digitorum longus and peroneus tertius. What in the configuration of the anterior compartment of the leg makes this region particularly prone to an increase in intracompartmental pressure? Keep in mind that this compartment is bounded by rigid or semirigid walls formed by the tibia, fibula, interosseous membrane, crural fascia, and anterior intermuscular septum (Fig. 49-1). Remember also that the latter septum separates the anterior compart-

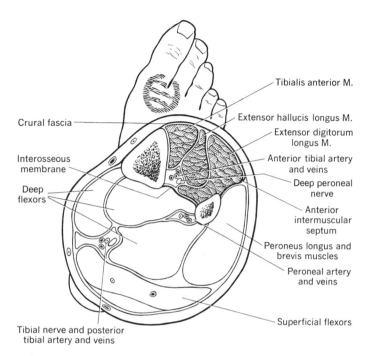

Figure 49-1. Cross section through the right leg at the junction of the intermediate and lower thirds of the leg. Notice the muscles, nerve, and blood vessels in the closed anterior compartment. Also notice the area of sensory loss on the dorsum of the foot resulting from the involvement of the deep peroneal nerve.

ment from the lateral compartment containing the peroneus longus and brevis muscles.

Involvement of the deep peroneal nerve

The major nerve and blood vessels in the anterior compartment may also be affected by the elevation in pressure. Identify them. The deep peroneal nerve and the anterior tibial vessels are important structures in the compartment. How would you test for involvement of the deep peroneal nerve, keeping in mind that dorsiflexion of the foot and extension of the toes may be severely interfered with by

ischemia (inadequate blood flow) to the muscles in the compartment
and that loss of muscle action therefore does not necessarily imply
nerve involvement? What muscle supplied by the deep peroneal
nerve lies outside the compressed compartment, the paralysis of
which could be taken as an indication of direct nerve involvement?
The extensor digitorum brevis and extensor hallucis brevis on the
dorsum of the foot lie outside the anterior compartment and consequently beyond the site of direct attack by pressure but are also
supplied by the deep peroneal nerve. Their paralysis would prove
that the compression involves the deep peroneal nerve within the
compartment. Deficiencies in the sensory supply of the skin would
also demonstrate that the deep peroneal nerve is directly affected.
What area of the skin should be tested for sensory loss? The adjacent
sides of the first and second toes receive their sensory supply from
the deep peroneal nerve (Fig. 49-1).

Arterial involvement

The presence of a pulse in the anterior tibial and dorsalis pedis
arteries, although weak, seems to prove patency of the main stem,
although occasionally a well-established collateral circulation in the
lower part of the leg by means of branches from the arteries in the
posterior compartment may simulate patency in a vessel that is
blocked higher up. What vessels in the posterior compartment
would contribute to such collateral circulation? The posterior tibial
and peroneal artery have important perforating branches that
anastomose with the distal portions of the anterior tibial artery and
with the dorsalis pedis artery.

Where is the pulse of the anterior tibial artery felt? Its pulse is
best taken where it becomes superficial, just above the level of the
ankle joint midway between the malleoli. Where would you palpate
the pulse of the dorsalis pedis artery? Remember, this artery is
directed down the dorsum of the foot to the proximal end of the first
intermetatarsal space. Here it lies on the skeleton of the foot just
lateral to the tendon of the extensor hallucis longus. The pulse of the
posterior tibial artery should be felt halfway between the posterior
margin of the medial malleolus and the medial border of the calcaneus (Achilles) tendon with the foot dorsiflexed and inverted.

Variations in the susceptibility of the three main muscles of the
anterior compartment to impaired circulation can be explained by

differences in the development of the intramuscular arterial anastomoses. Another explanation, frequently offered, is that the tibialis anterior muscle has its sole supply from the anterior tibial artery, the less involved extensor hallucis longus receives additional blood from the perforating branch of the peroneal artery, and the extensor digitorum longus obtains its supply from the three major arteries of the leg, including the posterior tibial by way of perforating branches. This explanation of the preferential involvement of the tibialis anterior muscle presupposes interference with blood flow in the main stem of the anterior tibial artery by elevation of pressure inside the compartment before its branches enter the musculature.

A 33-year-old chef is referred to the orthopedic clinic by his family physician because he complains of pain in his feet when standing or walking that worsens as the day progresses. The pain radiates up his legs and into his back. When he comes home, his feet burn and are swollen. In the last few months, the pain has increased and is most marked on the medial and plantar surfaces of his feet. His wife tells him that he "waddles" with his feet turned out in a kind of duck walk.

EXAMINATION

The patient is an overweight man of medium height who on questioning concedes that in the last few years he has gained about 50 pounds. On examination, the patient is asked to stand on his bare feet with his toes pointing forward and his feet parallel and approximately 4 inches apart. Inspection of his feet from in front and back shows on both sides disappearance of the medial portions of the longitudinal arches (Fig. 50-1). Both feet are everted so that a plumb line dropped from the center of the patella misses the foot entirely, while in the normal condition it strikes the foot between the first and second metatarsal bones (Fig. 50-2).

The patient is then asked to walk, which he does in a clumsy, "Chaplinesque" manner by raising the entire foot at one time instead of rolling it off the ground. On palpation there is tenderness

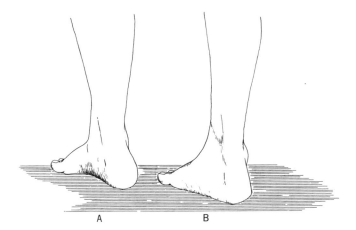

Figure 50-1. A.—Posteromedial view of a normal foot. Notice the longitudinal arch on the medial side of the foot. B.—Posteromedial view of a
flatfoot. Notice the absence of the longitudinal arch.

and prominence on the medial plantar side of the foot over the area
of the navicular and the head of the talus. By having the patient lie
down on a couch, thus removing the body weight from his feet, the
medial longitudinal arch assumes its normal curvature. This arch
also becomes prominent when he stands on his toes because of the
pull of the tibialis posterior muscle. Finally, inspection of the patient's shoes shows the inner border on the soles and heels worn
down to a greater extent than the outer side of the shoes.

DIAGNOSIS

Chronic foot strain is diagnosed.

THERAPY AND FURTHER COURSE

Conservative (nonsurgical) treatment of this condition aims to relieve the ligaments of the foot of tension and stretching, to transfer
the weight of the body to the lateral side of the foot, and to
strengthen the inverters and plantar flexors, which support the longitudinal arch under stress and in motion. An arch support (orthotic)
is prescribed that is sufficiently curved on the medial side to shift the

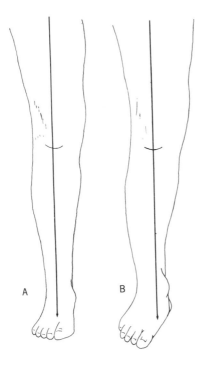

Figure 50-2. A.—A plumb line dropped from the center of the patella strikes the normal foot at a point between the first and second metatarsals. B.—In this flatfoot, the same plumb line misses the foot entirely as a result of the pronation of the foot (eversion or valgus deformity).

weight of the body to the outer side of the foot. The patient is advised to begin with massage and passive exercises after the acute pain has subsided. These should consist of dorsiflexion and plantar flexion and shoulld include the toes. They are done at first with the patient sitting down to relieve the feet from weight bearing. To strengthen his inverters, the patient is instructed to invert his feet against increasing resistance offered by his own hand. He also is advised to walk by rolling his feet off the ground from heel to toes. When he is standing, his feet should be parallel, not turned outward, and should be about 10 inches apart. He is strongly urged to lose 50 pounds, and a weight-loss diet is recommended. The patient is seen at regular intervals. He volunteers the information that his pain has almost subsided and that his feet have become relatively comfortable. He continues with excercise at home. He has lost 30 pounds and is advised to continue his weight loss and exercises. After six months, a slight adjustment is made in his arch support. He has lost another 25 pounds and is now practically asymptomatic.

DISCUSSION

The infirmity that we are dealing with in this case is one of the most common ailments of civilized people. It has been estimated that about 80 percent of the population, at one time or other, have foot trouble of this nature. Another often quoted figure is that among Selective Service subjects, 14 percent had defective arches. A sufficient number will, however, consult their family physician, who should be well versed in the diagnosis and treatment of foot ailments. Familiarity with the pathology, diagnosis, and therapy of this often quite disabling affliction requires a detailed knowledge of the underlying anatomy.

Motions of the tarus: joints, muscles, and nerves concerned

The following terms are used to describe movements of the proximal portion of the foot below the ankle: adduction and abduction, inversion and eversion, and supination and pronation. Try to define these terms. To understand the following discussion of the underlying anatomy, the reader is advised to study an articulated skeleton of the foot or, lacking this, an anatomical atlas. Adduction and abduction refer to movement of the foot around a vertical axis through the leg. In inversion and eversion, rotation of the foot takes place around an oblique axis that passes from the lateral side of the heel forward, upward, and medially through the neck of the talus. Inversion is the movement whereby the medial margin of the foot is elevated and the dorsum of the foot turned laterally. If inversion is done with both feet at the same time, the soles of the feet face each other. The opposite movement is called eversion. Because of the obliquity of the axis, inversion is combined with adduction of the forefoot (metatarsals and toes) and eversion with abduction. The terms inversion and supination are often used interchangeably, as are eversion and pronation. In what joints do these complex movements take place? The main articulation involved is the talocalcaneonavicular joint, which is a synovial joint of the ball and socket variety. The head of the talus is the ball. It is received by the concavity of the posterior surface of the navicular and the anterior and middle anticular facets of the calcaneus, the latter on the superior surface of the susten- taculum tali, a shelf, palpable one inch below the medial malleolus. The socket of this joint is completed by the plantar calcaneonavicular (spring) ligament, which is fibrocartilaginous and extends from the sustentaculum tali to the inferior aspect of the navicular. Two other joints concerned in the motions of the tarsus are the calcaneocuboid articulation between the anterior surface of the calcaneus and the posterior surface of the cuboid and the subtalar joint between a facet on the posteroinferior aspect of the talus and the posterior facet on the upper aspect of the calcaneus. Transverse tarsal joint refers to the talocalcaneonavicular and the calcaneocuboid joints, the latter having a separate synovial cavity. This joint is also the site of a now obsolete surgical disarticulation of the foot, which left only the talus and calcaneus behind and was introduced in the early part of the nineteenth century by the French surgeon Francois Chopart. In orthopedic literature, this compound joint is often referred to as "Chopart's joint." The ability to invert or evert (supinate or pronate) the foot should be appreciated because these motions allow the foot to adjust to sideways sloping surfaces. If inversion or eversion is lost, the patient is severely handicapped in walking over rough ground.

The primary muscles responsible for these motions are the tibialis anterior and the tibialis posterior for inversion and adduction and the peroneus longus and brevis for eversion and abduction. What nerves supply these muscles? The important motor nerves are the deep peroneal for the tibialis anterior, the tibial nerve for the tibialis posterior, and the superficial peroneal nerve for the supply of the peroneus longus and brevis.

Medial and lateral longitudinal arches of the foot

These arches comprise the tarsus and metatarsus. Both share the calcaneus. The medial longitudinal arch is formed, in addition to the calcaneus, by the talus, the navicular, the three cuneiforms, and the medial three metatarsals. The lateral longitudinal arch is com- posed of the calcaneus, the cuboid, and the lateral two metatarsals. The medial arch curves higher than the lateral, which almost rests on the ground. The talus is the keystone of the medial arch and receives the body weight, which is then distributed to the calcaneus posteriorly and navicular, cuneiforms, and the heads of the three medial metatarsals anteriorly. The first metatarsal bears twice the weight borne by the other metatarsals.

It should be realized that the arch is not rigid as it would be if it were made of one solid, curved bone. The weight distribution to individual bones changes as the weight of the body shifts during standing, walking, jumping, and running, requires a supple, resilient construction of the foot for shock absorption. Such a demand is ideally fulfilled by a structure made up of multiple components, the small bones of the foot, which assume a curved configuration. These bones are held together by ligaments, tendons, and muscles that allow continuous alterations in the relationship of the bones to each other.

Supports of the medial longitudinal arch

As stated, the arched shape of the foot is due to the configuration of the bones, with the individual members of the structure supporting each other. Thus, the sustentaculum tali, a medial projection of the calcaneus, buttresses the head of the talus, (L. sustentaculum, prop or support), but the bones alone are not capable of maintaining the stability of the medial arch. Support of the arch in normal quiet standing is maintained by ligamentous structures without assistance from muscles, which show only slight intermittent activity when minor shifts in balance occur. Therefore, physical stress in the standing position is withstood by the ligaments and the bones. Identify the ligaments that maintain the arch in the standing-at-ease posture. The most important is the plantar aponeurosis, which, like a tie beam, extends between the calcaneus and the heads of the metatarsals. Of almost equal importance is the plantar calcaneonavicular (spring) ligament, which directly supports the head of the talus, or the summit of the arch. It is a broad, thick, powerful fibrocartilaginous ligament that blends on its outside with the capsule of the talocalcaneonavicular joint. Other ligaments that help maintain the medial longitudinal arch and resist its flattening are the long and short plantar ligaments in the sole of the foot and the interosseous ligaments between individual tarsal bones, but particularly between talus and calcaneus. They keep the bones together and prevent them from spreading or splaying.

What is the role of the muscles passing through the foot in maintaining the arches as the weight of the body shifts in standing, walking, jumping, and running? The tibialis anterior, tibialis posterior, and peroneus longus and peroneus brevis, as well as the short intrinsic muscles of the foot, play no important role in the normal static support of the longitudinal arch but do show strong activity when the foot is exposed to heavy loads or when standing on tiptoe. They also keep the foot balanced around its oblique anteroposterior axis when, in response to slight changes in posture, the weight on the foot shifts.

Causes of flattened medial longitudinal arch

Heredity, obesity, and prolonged periods of standing can cause a weakening of the ligaments and muscles. The talus, which is the summit of the medial arch, sags under the force of the superimposed weight of the body and rolls off the calcaneus in a downward and medial direction. In this position it exerts undue pressure and stretching on the spring ligament. The result is a medially flattened arch with the talus becoming prominent on the medial aspect of the foot. The foot assumes an everted or valgus position (Fig. 50-1). Which of these causes apply to the patient in this case? He has gained a great deal of weight. His occupation as chef requires long periods of standing with little exercise of the foot muscles. Persons with occupations such as chef, sales clerk, trafic officer, operating room nurse, and surgeon are particularly susceptible to foot strain and flattening of the medial longitudinal arch. As mentioned in our case history, a plumb line dropped from the center of the patella misses the foot entirely because of eversion and abduction of the foot (Fig. 50-2). Also noted was the greater wearing down of the shoes on the inner side of the soles and heels. Contributing to this condition is a weakening and relaxation of the ligaments and atrophy of the supporting muscles due to prolonged bed confinement in chronic illness or extended plaster immobilization of the foot for traumatic or orthopedic disorders. A congenitally shortened Achilles tendon or uncounterbalanced action of the peroneal muscles changes the line of gravity and puts the foot in a position of pronation (pes valgus), increasing the stress on the weight-sustaining ligaments.

There are other causes of painful feet, however; many people whose feet flatten during quiet standing enjoy normal, pain-free function with no clinical symptoms. In those cases, the medial longitudinal arch becomes prominent when patients stand on their toes because of the pull of the tibialis posterior muscle. This rise of the medial arch upon standing on the forefoot indicates a normally functioning foot and usually pain-free foot. Conversely, the painful foot that fails to develop an arch during standing on the toes indicates an abnormal foot wherein the term flatfoot is more properly applied.

The flatfoot in infancy or early childhood, in which longitudinal arch is obscured by a pad of fat that fills the sole of the foot, is frequently the subject of undue concern by parents. Later, as the child grows, much of the fat disappears and the arch becomes demonstrable.

Muscle activity in maintaining the stance

We may ask to what extent the long and short muscles of the foot are called on for support after the ligaments have weakened. Evidence indicates that the tibialis anterior, tibialis posterior, peroneus longus, and certain short muscles in the sole are activated in disorders of the foot that lead to imbalance of the arch. The ligaments of the foot are the first line of defense in maintaining the arch, but extrinsic and intrinsic muscles are needed for additional support.

Pain in chronic foot strain

The primary pain of chronic foot strain is due to stretching of the joint capsules and ligaments, mainly the spring and plantar ligaments, and occasionally the deltoid ligament on the medial side of the ankle joint. When the muscles are charged with the task of maintaining the longitudinal arch, even in relaxed standing, they fatigue and respond to the strain with pain. If the condition remains uncorrected, the anatomy of the foot is altered by the changing relationships of the bones to each other. In that case, other muscles, such as the calf muscles, may become involved and painful. Undue stretching of the ligaments of the knee joint and even of the vertebral column may cause pain in these areas. An aching back is not uncommon in chronic foot strain. Painful calluses may develop over pressure points on bony prominences of the foot that normally do not touch the ground, and finding comfortable shoes may be difficult.

APPENDIX

Peripheral Anatomy of Selected Visceral Reflexes

Visceral reflexes are those that involve structures containing smooth muscle, cardiac muscle, or glandular tissue. The following presentation is a summary of pertinent information taken from texts and reference works.

RESPIRATION

Respiration is the act of bringing air into contact with the alveoli of the lungs for the exchange of oxygen and carbon dioxide. It is controlled by a number of neural mechanisms that are both reflex and central in nature. Inflation is the most basic respiratory reflex (Hering-Breuer). Stretch receptors located within the bronchi and bronchioles are stimulated as the lung inflates during inspiration. The number of afferent impulses traveling to the medulla from these receptors increases as inflation continues. These impulses inhibit the phrenic nerves and other nerves to respiratory muscles. The efferent part of this reflex cause an inhibition of inspiration and limits inflation of the lung. As the number of afferent impulses decreases, the inspiratory muscles are stimulated to contract again.

Chemoreceptors in the carotid and aortic bodies respond to a decrease in arterial oxygen tension, to an increase in arterial carbon dioxide tension, or to an associated decrease in arterial pH. The reflex effects of these receptors include an increase in the frequency and depth of respiration; however, this reflex occurs only in cases of severe hypoxia.

The frequency and depth of respiration are also increased by the stimulation of chemoreceptors located in the medulla. They also respond to an increase in arterial carbon dioxide tension or to a decrease in pH but not to a decrease in arterial oxygen tension.

The acts of breathing in (inspiration) and breathing out (expiration) are accomplished through muscular contraction and tissue elasticity. In quiet inspiration, movements are normally activated by the contraction of the diaphragm assisted by the external intercostal muscles. Movement of the sternum forward and upward and the ribs just a few millimeters forward, upward, and laterally is sufficient to increase the volume of the thoracic cage by 0.5 L, the amount of air that enters and leaves the lungs in quiet breathing. Quiet expiration, on the other hand, is primarily passive in nature. It is initiated as the inspiratory muscles relax. The tissues of the lung and thoracic cage have elastic properties. They recoil or revert to their former size and configuration as air is extruded or forced from the lungs.

Breathing becomes more vigorous with heavy exertion, and as much as 50 to 100 L of air may be exchanged per minute. The sternocleidomastoid, scalene, and extensor muscles of the vertebral column are recruited to assist in increasing thoracic volume. The sternocleidomastoid and scalene muscles fix the superior thoracic aperture so that the external intercostal muscles can pull the ribs upward to expand the thoracic volume. The extensor muscles of the vertebral column act to stabilize the spine. In forced expiration, abdominal muscles contract, pressing the abdominal contents inward, and the relaxed diaphragm upward, diminishing thoracic volume and forcing the gaseous contents from the lungs.

The afferent fibers from the stretch receptors in the lung are carried in the vagus nerve. Receptors located in respiratory muscles (diaphragm, intercostal, and abdominal muscles) are also stimulated, and their afferent impulses are carried in the appropriate cervical, thoracic, and lumbar spinal nerves. The afferent fibers from the chemoreceptors of the carotid body and the aortic body are carried in the glossopharyngeal and vagus nerves, respectively.

The diaphragm receives efferent fibers from the phrenic nerve (C3–C5), the sternocleidomastoid muscles from the cranial XI (spinal part of the accessory nerve), and the scalene muscles from short branches of C3–8. The intercostal and abdominal muscles are supplied with motor fibers from all ventral rami of the thoracic and the first lumbar nerves.

Keeping in mind the mechanisms involved in regulating respiration, a question of considerable interest arises: What induces the newborn to take its first gasp of air? Is it the unplugging of nasal and pharyngeal passages or perhaps the sharp slap on the rear that initiates this response? It has often been said that the cardiovascular-pulmonary events that occur at birth are the most dramatic of a person's lifetime. Many changes take place rapidly. The previously insulated intrauterine fetus, in its first exposure to the outside world, must cope with new stimuli bombarding it from all sides: visual, auditory, thermal, chemical, proprioceptive, and, not least of all, pain. Perhaps a combination of stimuli from all these sources is responsible for the first inspiration, but most important and compelling are the chemical stimuli. After the infant's gaseous exchange with the placenta is cut off, blood oxygen tension rapidly decreases, carbon dioxide tension increases, and the pH of the blood is lowered. Peripheral and central chemoreceptors are soon maximally stimulated. The newborn responds by opening its mouth and gasping for air, thus initiating the first of many, respiratory cycles.

COUGHING

Coughing is a violent expulsion of air caused by forceful contraction of the expiratory muscles after sudden opening of the glottis. It is preceded by deep inspiration and closure of the glottis. Although coughing can be initiated by voluntary action, it is usually a reflex in response to irritation of the mucosa by foreign material or exudates in the pharynx, larynx, trachea, or bronchi. Forced expiration is carried out essentially by the contraction of the muscles of the anterolateral abdominal wall, aided by contraction of the thoracic and pelvic diaphragms.

The mucosa of the oral and laryngeal parts of the pharynx is supplied with afferent fibers by the glossopharyngeal and vagus nerves. The mucosa covering the epiglottis and lining the vestibule of the larynx is particularly sensitive to pain and touch. This mucosal layer of the larynx above the vocal cords is innervated by the internal laryngeal branches of the vagus, and that below the vocal cords is supplied by the recurrent laryngeal nerves. In fact, the larynx is completely supplied by branches of the vagus nerves.

The diaphragm receives motor innervation from the phrenic nerve. The intercostal and anterolateral abdominal muscles receive motor fibers from the intercostal nerves (T1–11), the subcostal nerve (T12) and the iliohypogastric and ilioinguinal nerves (L1). The pelvic diaphragm is supplied with motor fibers, sacral nerves delivered by the perineal branch of the pudendal nerve (S2–4), and through direct branches of S3 and S4.

Opening and closing of the glottis are controlled by the intrinsic muscles of the larynx. To enlarge the airway as much as possible and allow a gasp for breath, there is first a marked abduction of vocal cords brought about by action of the posterior cricoarytenoid muscles. There is prompt closure of the rima glottidis brought about by an approximation of the vocal folds due to the actions of the transverse arytenoid and lateral cricoarytenoid muscles. When this closure is suddenly released in the presence of increased pressure in the thorax, air, mucous, and saliva are expelled at considerable force through the glottis, pharynx, and mouth.

The lateral cricoarytenoid and transverse arytenoid muscles assist in adducting the vocal cords. This act is necessary for complete closure of the rima glottidis or for placing the vocal cords in apposition so they can vibrate as air is forced between them. The oblique arytenoids, thyroepiglottics, and aryepiglottics function as sphincters of the vestibule for swallowing. The involved laryngeal muscles are supplied with motor fibers by the recurrent laryngeal nerves, with the exception of the cricothyroid, which is supplied by the external branch of the superior laryngeal nerve.

SNEEZING

Sneezing is similar to coughing in that it also involves a violent expulsion of air by vigorous contraction of the expiratory muscles. The opening of the pharynx into the mouth is closed by the muscles underlying the palatoglossal muscles and by the descent of the soft palate so that considerable air is expelled through the nose. The last part of the sneeze is when the characteristic "choo" sound is emitted through the mouth after relaxation of the palatoglossal muscles. This reflex is initiated by mechanical or chemical irritation of the sensory nerve endings in the nasal mucosa supplied by nasal branches of the maxillary division of the trigeminal nerve.

The palatoglossus muscles, which underlie the anterior tonsillar pillars, are supplied by pharyngeal branches of the vagus nerve; the tensor veli palatini muscles, which tense the soft palate, are supplied by the mandibular division of trigeminal nerve. The diaphragmatic, intercostal, and anterolateral abdominal musculature contracts, forcing air from the lungs as described in coughing. In a certain percentage of people, strong light, particularly sunlight, may also elicit sneezing, but the exact pathway of this reaction to light is poorly explained.

HICCUP (SINGULTUS)

Hiccups are repeated, involuntary, spasmodic, and short-lasting contraction of the diaphragm accompanied by sudden closure of the glottis. The impact of the air against the rapidly closing glottis causes the characteristic sound.

Hiccups occur as the result of irritation of peripheral afferent nervous pathways or stimulation of the respiratory center in the brain stem. The peripheral afferent nerve endings may be stimulated by swallowing irritating material; by acute or chronic lesions of the esophagus, stomach, or small intestine (ulcers or cancer); by gastric distention; or by obstruction of the small intestine. Such intrathoracic lesions as carcinoma of the lung, aortic aneurysm, or lesions of the diaphragm may also cause stimulation of afferent nerves. Some of these conditions may lead to pressure on the nerve endings in the peritoneum or pleura, causing hiccups.

The sensation leading to hiccups is mediated by sensory branches of several nerves. Sensory impulses are carried by the vagus if the stimulus arises within the thoracoabdominal viscera, by afferent branches of intercostal nerves of the parietal peritoneum or pleura of the peripheral parts of the diaphragm, or by sensory fibers in the phrenic nerve that supply the more central parts of the serous coverings of the diaphragm. The spasms of the diaphragm are mediated by motor fibers of the phrenic nerve. Closure of the glottis is brought about by the stimulation of the inferior laryngeal (recurrent laryngeal) branch of the vagus nerve. The spasms may involve one or both sides of the diaphragm.

Singultus following abdominal operations, brain tumors, multiple sclerosis, or caused by hemorrhage or edema in the medullary respiratory center may be so severe and lasting as to endanger life. Hiccups have been known to last as long as eight years. It is noteworthy that hiccups in the fetus have been detected as early as the fifth to sixth month of intrauterine life.

YAWNING

Yawning consists of a deep inspiratory effort through the widely opened mouth. There are a variety of types of yawns, some respiratory and others entirely nonrespiratory, seeming to be more an expression of boredom or fatigue. Some seem to be a type of stretching, perhaps to increase blood flow to inactive (or stressed) muscles. Respiratory yawning is probably brought about by lowered oxygen tension of the blood as an involuntary expression of air hunger, for example, at high altitude or after a severe hemorrhage.

The mouth is opened widely because of contraction of the lateral pterygoid, mylohyoid, digastric, and infrahyoid muscles. The diaphragm contracts, increasing the volume of the thoracic cage. Stretching movements of the limbs are sometimes added.

The nerves causing these muscular contractions include the mandibular division of the trigeminal nerve (V_3), the ansa cervicalis, the phrenic nerve, and motor nerves from the brachial and lumbar plexuses, which supply the extensors of upper and lower extremities.

Yawning may be induced by suggestion as, for instance, by the sight of another person yawning. In rare cases, it may result in bilateral dislocation of the jaw. As with many of these reflexes, yawning can also be observed in various species of animals.

CONTROL OF BLOOD PRESSURE

Blood pressure is maintained at its average level (120/80 mm Hg) primarily through the mechanism of reflex activity that is influenced by several higher neural centers. In addition, hormonal factors also play an important role in this vital function.

The walls of the carotid sinus, the arch of the aorta, the great veins, and the right atrium contain stretch receptors that are stimulated by an increase in pressure (baroreceptors). Afferent fibers to receptors in the carotid sinus are branches of the glossopharyngeal nerve, and those to receptors in the other mentioned areas are branches of the vagus nerve. Impulses in these nerves travel to the medulla and stimulate groups of nerve cells there, the cardiac center and the vasomotor center.

The cardiac center can further be divided into an inhibitory part and an accelerator part. Fibers from the inhibitory part project to efferent neurons of the vagus in the medulla that send impulses to the heart, inhibiting it and slowing its rate of contraction (bradycardia). Fibers from the accelerator part project to efferent neurons in the spinal cord at levels T1–5, which in turn send preganglionic sympathetic fibers to the cervical and upper five thoracic sympathetic chain ganglia. These ganglia supply fibers to the heart that cause it to beat more strongly and faster (tachycardia). Fibers from nerve cells in the vasomotor center descend within the spinal cord to levels T1 to L2 to stimulate neurons of preganglionic sympathetic fibers that will ultimately supply peripheral arterioles and cause vasoconstriction or vasodilation.

As blood pressure increases above its average level, the baroreceptors in the walls of the carotid sinus and in other localities are stimulated. The number of impulses traveling to the medulla in the glossopharyngeal (IX) and vagus (X) nerves increases. These impulses act on the cardiac center to decrease the heart rate and its strength of contraction. They also act on the vasomotor center to depress the action of the sympathetics to cause vasodilatation of peripheral arterioles. This combination of events results in lowering blood pressure, with which the peripheral baroreceptors in the carotid sinus, arch of the aorta, and so on are not stimulated as much as before. Fewer impulses pass to the medulla and to the cardiac and vasomotor centers. As a result, the heart beats faster, peripheral arterioles constrict, and blood pressure rises. Under normal conditions, there is a continuous rise and fall of blood pressure as it is maintained at approximately the average level.

SWALLOWING (DEGLUTITION)

Swallowing is a complex neuromuscular mechanism subject to volition only in its first stage. After food is ground by the teeth and mixed with the help of saliva, it is formed into a bolus. By action of the tongue, particularly its styloglossus muscles, the bolus is then directed upward to the back of the mouth and forced through the isthmus of fauces (narrows of the throat) into the pharynx. This is the end of the voluntary phase of the swallowing mechanism.

The reflex stage consists of a well-coordinated propulsion of the bolus into the oral pharynx, through the piriform recesses, and into the esophagus. In its passage through the pharynx, the food must be prevented from entering the wrong channels, that is, the nasal cavity, larynx, and trachea. The nasal part of the pharynx is shut off from the oral pharynx by raising the soft palate. This action is mainly brought about through the combined actions of levator veli palatini and tensor veli palatini on both sides. Entrance into the larynx and trachea is prevented by sphincteric reduction of the laryngeal aditus and closure of the rima glottidis. In addition, the contraction of the longitudinal muscles of the pharynx raises the hyoid and upper part of the larynx and causes the epiglottis to be pushed backward against the pharyngeal wall.

The bolus of food passes downward directly around the posteriorly tipped epiglottis and is diverted laterally by the aryepiglottic folds so that it bypasses the closed entrance of the larynx, flowing into the piriform recesses of the pharynx. This passage through the piriform recesses is the course also taken by fluids. The bolus is propelled along the length of the pharynx by the well-coordinated successive contraction of the middle and inferior constrictor muscles. Finally, the lowest fibers of the inferior constrictors relax and the food enters the esophagus.

In the upright position, the force of gravity, in combination with peristaltic waves of the esophagus, helps the downward passage of food; but swallowing and propulsion of the bolus are also possible in the upside-down position of the body. The sensory part of the swallowing reflex is mediated mainly by the glossopharyngeal nerve, the pharyngeal branches of which are incorporated in the pharyngeal plexus. The muscles of the tongue that assist in forming the food into a bolus and pushing it backward toward the pharynx are supplied by the hypoglossal nerve. Motor fibers to muscles of the palate and pharynx are also part of the pharyngeal plexus and are from the vagus nerve. The vagus contains accessory nerve fibers from the medulla (cranial root of XI) that supply motor fibers to the involved muscles of the larynx. The glossopharyngeal nerve, via its branch to the stylopharyngeus, and the trigeminal nerve, through its innervation of the tensor veli palatini, also participate in the efferent portion of the reflex arc.

Dysphagia denotes difficulty in swallowing or an inability to swallow. It is a fairly common and important clinical symptom and may be caused by lesions in the central nervous system or in the periphery. Investigators report that paralysis of the last four cranial nerves results in great difficulty in swallowing.

VOMITING (EMESIS)

Vomiting is the forceful ejection of gastric contents through the mouth and is often accompanied or preceded by nausea. This visceral reflex can be initiated in many parts of the body and is transmitted through sensory fibers to the vomiting center in the medulla. One of the more common causes is irritation of the mucous membranes of the stomach or duodenum by food or drugs. Irritation or distention of numerous viscera, such as the heart, uterus, small intestine, gallbladder, gonads, and appendix, and also the parietal peritoneum can likewise initiate the reflex.

Afferent nerve fibers from the organs and tissues mentioned above belong primarily to the vagus nerve (X). Nauseating sights (II), taste (VII, IX and X), odor (I), and psychological upsets can also bring about vomiting. Stimulation of the vestibular apparatus (VIII), as in motion sickness, may also induce the reflex as can a number of diseases associated with the central nervous system, such as meningitis, encephalitis, and brain tumors.

Vomiting is brought about by vigorous contraction of the stomach musculature, the abdominal wall and thoracic, and the pelvic diaphragms with simultaneous relaxation of the cardiac sphincter of the stomach and the esophagus. This coordinated action leads to an increase in intragastric pressure, which results in reflux of the gastric contents through the relaxed esophagus and open mouth, often in a projectile manner. As a protective action, the glottis tightly closes and the soft palate is elevated in an attempt to prevent entrance of the vomitus into the larynx or nasopharynx.

Efferent fibers course in the phrenic and thoracoabdominal nerves to the skeletal muscles of the diaphragm and the abdominal wall. The vagus, through its parasympathetic innervation of the stomach and esophagus, is also involved.

The cause of vomiting in early pregnancy is unclear but has been ascribed to either hormonal or metabolic influences. It is well known that gagging and, ultimately, vomiting can be brought about intentionally by physically stimulating the soft palate.

DEFECATION

As in many visceral reflexes, the mechanism of *defecation* is, in part, under voluntary control. Personal habits and emotional states influence the time and frequency of the act. Normally, the distal part of the descending colon and the sigmoid colon store the fecal masses while the rectum is generally empty. When the pressure in the rectum rises and its distention increases, because of the presence of feces, certain skeletal and smooth muscles contract and others relax to bring about the evacuation of contents of the rectum through the anus. This action occurs when no antagonistic muscles, subject to voluntary control, are activated. The intentional act of defecation starts with the voluntary contraction of the thoracic and pelvic diaphragms, closure of the glottis, and contraction of the musculature of the abdominal wall, combined with the peristaltic contraction of the circular musculature of the distal colon and rectum and relaxation of the longitudinal musculature of the same structures. As these processes elevate the rectum and anus over the descending fecal column, the contents of the descending and sigmoid colon simultaneously empty into the evacuating rectum. An important part of the act consists in relaxation of the puborectal sling of the levator ani (to enable straightening or elimination of the perineal flexure of the anorectal junction) and relaxation of the internal and external anal sphincters.

The afferent part of the reflex arc of defecation starts with sensitive nerve endings, particularly the stretch receptors, in the wall of the rectum. Indeed, perception is so acute that the receptors can distinguish (as it were) between air and water. These receptors are the terminations of nerve fibers that are derived from the middle and inferior rectal plexuses, which connect with the sacral spinal cord via the pelvic splanchnic nerves (S2–S4), which also convey parasympathetic fibers. The sensory branches of the inferior rectal nerves, which supply the lowest part of the rectum and anus, are branches of the pudendal nerves (S2–4).

On the efferent side of the reflex are peripheral nerve fibers, which activate the skeletal muscles of the abdominal wall (T6–L1), the thoracic (phrenic nerve) and pelvic diaphragms (S2–S4), and the sphincters of the glottis (inferior laryngeal nerve). The circular smooth musculature of the rectum is activated by impulses conducted by preganglionic parasympathetic fibers that synapse with ganglion cells in the wall of the intestine. The external anal sphincter, which voluntarily relaxes in defecation, is innervated by the inferior rectal branches of the pudendal nerve. This muscle and the puborectalis, by their voluntary contractions, prevent unwanted evacuation of the rectum. They are not strong enough, however, to maintain contractions for any length of time against increasing rectal pressure but are, in fact, inhibited by distension of the rectum. The external anal sphincter is located in the lower 2 cm of the rectum. When surgical removal of the rectum is necessary, this muscle is preserved whenever possible.

URINATION (MICTURITION)

Urination is rather complex, and its anatomy and physiology are still subjects of dispute. It is most easily understood in the infant, where it is a pure reflex, not subject to conscious voluntary control. Here the reflex occurs whenever the bladder has become sufficiently distended. As the organ fills with urine from the ureters, its wall is stretched by relaxation of its muscle fibers. The stretch receptors in the wall are stimulated, and impulses travel to the spinal cord. This action triggers contraction of the tunica muscularis of the bladder wall, called the detrusor muscle. It also reflexly inhibits the striated external sphincter (sphincter urethrae) muscle. As the urine enters the urethra, the voiding reflex is potentiated by the opening of the urethra caused by relaxation of the external sphincter muscle.

Paralleling the development of the brain during the second or third year of life, the child acquires voluntary control of the emptying reflex. In the adult, a feeling of fullness and a desire to void is perceived when 300 to 500 ml of urine is accumulated in the bladder. If voluntary emptying is inopportune at that moment, voiding can be deferred by contraction of the external sphincter and inhibition of further bladder contraction. If the amount of urine in the bladder reaches 700 ml, pain ensues, and if it reaches 800 ml or more, the ability to defer urination becomes uncontrollable.

We have stated before that emptying fair amounts of urine can be suppressed by volition. On the other hand, voiding can also be initiated voluntarily even if the bladder contains only small amounts of urine by straining through contraction of diaphragmatic and abdominal musculature and voluntary relaxation of the controlling sphincters. Once urine has entered the urethra, reflex action will

bring about contraction of the detrusor muscle and its longitudinal
fibers along the bladder neck. The external striated sphincter can,
by its contraction, voluntarily interrupt the flow of urine during
voiding.

Involuntary micturition may occur during emotional upsets
(fear, nervousness, excitement), when centrally originating impulses
will increase the tonus and state of contraction of the bladder. In
females, weakening of the pelvic floor, as in cases where the pelvic
and urogenital diaphragms have been damaged by complicated
childbirth, may result in incontinence, especially during coughing
or laughing, which causes an increase in abdominal pressure.

Afferent pathways of the reflex arc mediating micturition start
in proprioceptive stretch and bare nerve endings of sensory nerve
fibers transmitting the sensation of fullness and, in cases of overfill-
ing, pain and urgency. Most of these afferent fibers course with the
parasympathetic nerve fibers in the pelvic splanchnic nerves to the
spinal cord through sacral nerves 2–4. Some pain fibers travel with
the sympathetic fibers through the inferior hypogastric plexus to the
lower thoracic and upper lumbar spinal cord segments. The efferent
or effector part of the reflex is completely under parasympathetic
control. The nerve impulses leading to contraction of the detrusor
muscle of the bladder wall and longitudinal fibers in the bladder
neck are conducted by preganglionic fibers that are components of
the pelvic splanchnic nerves. The fibers synapse with ganglion cells
in the bladder wall that then activate the smooth musculature of the
bladder by their postganglionic fibers.

Since the nerves on their way to the bladder pass on both sides
of the rectum, they may be injured during resection of the rectum,
as, for instance, in cancer operations, leading to difficulties in urination. The external voluntary sphincter (the sphincter urethrae) is
controlled by the pudendal nerve.

ERECTION

Erection of the penis or clitoris from a normal flaccid state may occur
in response to sexual stimuli or to nonsexual physical stimuli. These
stimuli lead to engorgement of the corpora cavernosa penis and the
corpus spongiosum penis or the corpora cavernosa of the clitoris and
bulbs of the vestibule by dilation of the terminal branches of the
deep and dorsal branches of the internal pudendal arteries. These

arteries empty via coiled or helicine arteries into an endothelial-lined network of cavernous spaces. Expansion of erectile tissue leads to compression of the veins located between this distended tissue and its external covering of tough inelastic tunica albuginea, resulting in interference with the venous return. Contraction of the bulbospongiosus and ischiocavernosus muscles also compresses the veins and helps maintain erection. Thus the penis, increased in length and transverse diameter, remains in the erect position and the clitoris becomes turgid and more prominent.

Secretion of a viscous fluid from the urethral glands in males lubricates the glans penis; in females lubrication is produced by the paraurethral and greater vestibular glands in the prospect of copulation. Once orgasm has occurred, in both sexes, or the erotic stimuli leading to erection have stopped, the arteries again become constricted, the arterioles coiled, and the blood is permitted to return by way of the expanding veins. The organs then return to their former flaccid state.

Afferent impulses producing erection travel in part by way of sensory fibers that are derived from the pudendal nerve (S2–S4). The impulses may be initiated by mechanical stimulation of the skin of the genitals, particularly the glans of the penis or clitoris, but this is not the only means of causing erection. Stimulation of other parts of the body, as well as visual, auditory, and olfactory excitation, may also bring about arousal and erection. Finally, erotic thoughts may have the same effect. It should be recalled that olfactory perception as an act of sexual stimulation is of greater importance in the lower animal kingdom, but we are also aware that humans use artificial scents, as in perfumes, for the same purpose.

The efferent nerve impulses that lead to erection through arteriolar dilatation travel by way of the parasympathetic fibers contained in the pelvic splanchnic nerves from sacral nerves 2, 3, and 4 (older literature, nervi erigentes). The efferent fibers supplying the paired skeletal bulbospongiosus and ischiocavernosus muscles of the penis or clitoris, the contraction of which causes impedance of venous return and maintenance of erection, belong to the pudendal nerve. Constriction of the arteries of the erectile tissues leading to cessation of erection and flaccidity is caused by sympathetic fibers derived from the 12th thoracic and the upper lumbar segments of the cord.

As mentioned, erection in both females and males is essentially the same in terms of mechanism and nerve supply. The erectile tissue of the female is contained in the clitoris (corpora cavernosa and glans clitoridis) and the vestibular bulbs that lie adjacent to the ostium of the vagina. In females, sexual stimulation causes the secretion of a viscous fluid from the greater vestibular glands and the production of a serous exudate by the vagina. These fluids facilitate the introduction and movement of the erect penis during sexual intercourse. The efferent part of the reflex arc is also under parasympathetic and voluntary motor control.

EJACULATION

Ejaculation is the expulsion of seminal fluid (the mixture of sperm and glandular fluids) from the external opening of the urethra at orgasm in males. The process begins when spermatozoa are propelled from the ducts of the epididymis into the ductus deferens. They are forced by rhythmic contractions of the strong muscular wall of the ductus deferens into the ampulae of the ductus deferens and then into the prostatic urethra through the ejaculatory ducts. Simultaneously, the stimulation of glands associated with the ductus deferens, the seminal vesicles, the prostate, and the bulbourethral glands expel a nutritive alkaline secretion that suspends the spermatozoa. This part of the ejaculatory process, called emission, is followed by ejaculation proper, which is created by the spasmodic contractions of the bulbospongiosus and ischiocavernosus muscles.

Most of the seminal fluid is produced by the prostate glands. The ejaculate, amounting on average to about 3 to 4 ml, contains about a quarter billion spermatozoa or less, allowing for downward variations depending on the age of the man and the frequency of ejaculation.

Ejaculation is preceded or accompanied by a mass discharge of nervous impulses, resulting in an acme of emotional sensations and motor reactions that represent orgasm. The range of reactions is exemplified by wide changes in pulse rate, blood pressure, and respiration.

As to the nervous elements responsible for the ejaculation reflex, the afferent pathways use fibers that reach the spinal cord via the pudendal nerves. Impulses leading to ejaculation may arise elsewhere in the body with complete absence of tactile stimuli of the penis. The reflex is under control of centers of the brain that can prevent or retard ejaculation. On the effector side, the somatic motor and sympathetic and parasympathetic systems participate. The first part of the reflex (i.e., the movement of the semen from the deferent ducts, seminal vesicles, and prostatic urethra) is under sympathetic control. It is believed that impulses are carried in preganglionic fibers from cord segments Ll and L2. They synapse in ganglia located in the inferior hypogastric plexus; from there, postganglionic fibers go to the smooth muscle of the ducts and glands. Ejaculation proper is assisted by forceful contraction of the perineal muscles, which is mediated by branches of the pudendal nerve that stimulate the ischiocavernosus and bulbospongiosus in clonic contractions.

In females, the combination of events analogous to ejaculation and orgasm in males is called the orgasm or climax. There are wide changes in blood pressure, pulse, and respiratory rates. Increased secretions are produced. Rhythmic uterine and vaginal contractions and clonic contractions of the trunk, hip, pelvic, and perineal musculature all occur, followed by a sudden a release of pleasurable sensations and relaxation.